Anaerobic Bacteria

Selected Topics

Anaerobic Bacteria
Selected Topics

Edited by

Dwight W. Lambe, Jr.

East Tennessee State University
Johnson City, Tennessee

Robert J. Genco

State University of New York
New York, New York

and

K. J. Mayberry-Carson

East Tennessee State University
Johnson City, Tennessee

PLENUM PRESS · NEW YORK AND LONDON

Library of Congress Cataloging in Publication Data

International Symposium on Anaerobic Bacteria.
Anaerobic bacteria.

Includes bibliographical references and index.
1. Bacterial diseases–Congresses. 2. Bacteria, Anaerobic–Congresses. I. Lambe, Dwight W. II. Genco, Robert J. III. Mayberry-Carson, K. J. IV. Title. [DNLM: 1. Bacterial infections–Congresses. 2. Gram-negative anaerobic bacteria–Congresses. WC200 I613a 1979]
RC115.I55 1979 616'.014 80-18505

ISBN-13: 978-1-4613-3161-2 e-ISBN-13: 978-1-4613-3159-9
DOI: 10.1007/978-1-4613-3159-9

Proceedings of the International Symposium on Anaerobic Bacteria:
Laboratory Aspects, Pathogenicity, Human Immune Response to Infection, and Serology, held at East Tennessee State University, Johnson City, Tennessee, April 2–4, 1979.

Softcover reprint of the hardcover 1st edition 1980

A Division of Plenum Publishing Corporation
227 West 17th Street, New York, N.Y. 10011

PREFACE

A symposium seems an appropriate vehicle to review recent, as well as new, data on important topics. It is therefore our goal to present a symposium on selected topics of importance every three years. Some topics will be updated and new topics will be presented.

A vast amount of information has been accumulated over the past ten years on the significance of anaerobic bacteria in infectious diseases. This symposium was organized to discuss laboratory aspects, normal flora, pathogenicity, serology, and the patients' immune response to anaerobic infection. Important imformation on the patients' immune response and serology of anaerobes which has accumulated over the last few years made these topics an important part of the symposium. Development of serological diagnostic tests undoubtedly will provide quicker and less expensive identification of certain anaerobic species in the future. Utilization of the patients' immune response to anaerobic septicemia has the potential of providing a diagnosis of the causative agent within 24 hours after onset of symptoms. The development of such diagnostic methods and the use of these methods in the clinical laboratory in the future would provide rapid diagnostic information to the clinician on these life-threatening infections.

Campylobacter was included in the symposium to emphasize the important role of this organism in human acute gastroenteritis. The pathogenesis of Campylobacter in gastroenteritis has been recognized in certain European countries since 1972, although we have recognized the importance of Campylobacter gastroenteritis in the United States only within the past two years.

The papers on periodontal disease emphasize the important role of certain anaerobes in periodontal disease.

The subject matter presented in this book is of practical interest in clinical and research laboratories, and we hope that some of the information presented will stimulate new ideas and provoke new research. The topics should be of major interest to medical and clinical microbiologists, physicians, dentists, and medical technologists.

This book represents the papers presented at the International Symposium on Anaerobic Bacteria, which was held in April, 1979 at East Tennessee State University in Johnson City, Tennessee. The Symposium was sponsored by the Department of Microbiology, College of Medicine,

East Tennessee State University. Co-sponsors of the Symposium included: Beecham Laboratories, Bellco Glass, Inc., Carr-Scarborough Microbiologicals, Inc., Johnston Laboratories, Inc., Marion Scientific Corporation, Roerig Division of Pfizer, Inc., Schering Corporation, and Shimadzu Scientific Instruments, Inc.

We express our sincere appreciation and gratitude to Mrs. Paula Williams for her skill and dedication in typing the final chapters as they were photographed, and to Mrs. Brenda Bowman who assisted. We are indebted to Mr. Jerry Keplinger and Mrs. Kaethe Ferguson for their expert proofing of the manuscripts.

Dwight W. Lambe, Jr.
Robert J. Genco
K.J. Mayberry-Carson

CONTENTS

PART I
INTRODUCTION. SELECTED CLINICAL LABORATORY TOPICS AND IDENTIFICATION

Moderators: D.W. Lambe, Jr. and V. DelBene

PART II
PATHOGENICITY OF ANAEROBES

Moderator: L.V. Holdeman

LIST OF SPEAKERS

Symposium on Anaerobic Bacteria: Selected Topics
April 2-4, 1979

E.C.S. Chan, Ph.D.
Associate Professor
McGill University
Montreal, Quebec
Canada 3A2B4

Cecil S. Cummins, Sc.D.
Professor
Anaerobe Laboratory,
VPI and SU
Division of Basic Sciences
Blacksburg, Virginia

Dan Danielsson, M.D., Ph.D.
Assistant Director
Department of Clinical Bacteriology
and Immunology
Central County Hospital
Orebro, Sweden

Victor DelBene, M.D.
Associate Professor of Medicine
Department of Medicine
Division of Infectious Diseases
Medical University of South Carolina
Charleston, South Carolina

Robert J. Genco, D.D.S., Ph.D.
Professor and Chairman
Department of Oral Biology
State University of New York at Buffalo
Buffalo, New York

Gale B. Hill, Ph.D.
Associate Professor
Department of Obstetrics/Gynecology
Assistant Professor
Department of Microbiology/Immunology
Duke University Medical Center
Durham, North Carolina

Lillian V. Holdeman, Ph.D.
University Distinguished
Professor
Anaerobe Laboratory,
VPI and SU
Division of Basic Sciences
Blacksburg, Virginia

Dennis L. Kasper, M.D.
Associate Professor of
Medicine
Department of Medicine
Harvard Medical School
Harvard University
Boston, Massachusetts

George E. Kenny, Ph.D.
Professor and Chairman
Department of Pathobiology
School of Public Health and
Community Medicine
University of Washington
Seattle, Washington

Dwight W. Lambe, Jr., Ph.D.
Professor and Chairman
Department of Microbiology
College of Medicine
East Tennessee State
University
Johnson City, Tennessee

W. Wayne Laslie, M.S.
Pfizer Pharmaceuticals
New York, New York

Sabine Lauwers, M.D.
Department of Microbiology
St. Pierre Hospital
Brussels, Belgium

W.E.C. Moore, Ph.D.
Professor
Anaerobe Laboratory
VPI and SU
Division of Basic Sciences
Blacksburg, Virginia

Ronald L. Nichols, M.D.
Henderson Professor of Surgery
Department of Surgery
University of Tulane
New Orleans, Louisiana

Andrew B. Onderdonk, Ph.D.
Supervisor, Infectious Diseases
Research Laboratory
Veterans Administration Hospital

K.P. Phillips, B.Sc.
Public Health Laboratory
Luton and Dunstable Hospital
Luton, England

J. Peter Rissing, M.D.
Chief, Division of Infectious
Diseases
Veterans Administration Hospital
Assistant Professor of Medicine
School of Medicine
Medical College of Georgia
Augusta, Georgia

Charles V. Sanders, Jr., M.D.
Associate Professor of
Medicine and Microbiology
School of Medicine
Department of Medicine
Louisiana State University
New Orleans, Louisiana

Anna Schwan, M.D.
University of Uppsala
Institute of Clinical Bacteriology
Uppsala, Sweden

Joseph Silva, M.D.
Associate Professor of Medicine
Division of Infectious Diseases
University of Michigan
Medical Center
Ann Arbor, Michigan

Jorgen Slots, D.D.S., Ph.D.
Associate Professor
Department of Oral Biology
State University of New
York at Buffalo
Buffalo, New York

Betsy L. Williams, Ph.D.
Research Assistant
Professor
Department of Periodontics
School of Dentistry
University of Washington
Seattle, Washington

INTRODUCTION: CULTURE OF CLINICAL SPECIMENS FOR ANAEROBIC BACTERIA

Dwight W. Lambe, Jr.

Department of Microbiology, College of Medicine
East Tennessee State University
Johnson City, Tennessee

The literature has numerous articles on culture of anaerobes from clinical specimens and will not be reviewed. Instead, I will discuss certain topics which we feel are important in the isolattion and evaluation of anaerobes from clinical specimens.

The clinical bacteriologist is responsible for reporting to the clinician the aerobic and anaerobic growth from clinical specimens as well as the antibiotic susceptibility of each pathogen. Our goal in the clinical laboratory should be to report this information to the clinician as soon as possible.

Normal Flora

Body sites may contain large or small numbers of normal anaerobic flora; these normal flora should be avoided in specimen collection. For example, the feces normally contain large numbers of more than 200 species of anaerobes. Propionibacterium acnes is a normal inhabitant of human skin. The mouth and throat may contain anaerobic cocci, Fusobacterium, Eubacterium lentum, Actinomyces and other anaerobes. The male and female genitalia may contain anaerobic cocci, Fusobacterium, Bacteroides, Bifidobacterium, as well as other anaerobes.

Isolation of Anaerobes from Clinical Specimens

Successful isolation of anaerobes from a clinical specimen depends upon several factors: culture of an appropriate specimen, appropriate collection and sampling of the infected material, rapid transport of the specimen in an anaerobic atmosphere to the clinical laboratory, culture on freshly made media that will support the growth of fastidious anaerobes, and anaerobic incubation of the inoculated media at the appropriate temperature for at least seven days to permit growth of slow-growing anaerobes. These steps should be followed by accurate identification of the anaerobic organisms isolated from infected material.

The number of a particular organism reported from a specimen may be important. Terms such as predominant, moderate, or rare can be helpful, or misleading if not accurate. In a mixed culture, the number of each colony type is described in most laboratories at 48 h when the anaerobe plate is first examined. But how many laboratories report the relative number of each colony type after seven to 10 days incubation? This latter evaluation is important with mixtures of rapid- and slow-growing anaerobes. For example, with a mixture of B. fragilis, E. lentum, and Peptococcus magnus, a large number of B. fragilis colonies may be present after 48 h incubation whereas only a small number of E. lentum and P. magnus colonies may be present. However, after incubation for seven days, colonies of E. lentum or P. magnus may have increased and may now even exceed the number of B. fragilis colonies. We have seen many specimens that showed no growth of a pure culture of P. magnus until the fourth to seventh day after incubation. We have also noted this problem of delayed growth from cases of mixed septicemia; at 48 h only B. fragilis grew on subculture from blood broth to solid medium, but at four to seven days, many colonies of E. lentum were present.

Specimens to Culture for Anaerobes

Over the past 10 years, we and others, have found that the following specimens should be cultured for anaerobes:

- Blood
- Wounds
- Fluids (pleural fluid especially with a diagnosis of empyema, lung abscess, or aspiration; spinal fluid especially in a diagnosis of brain abscess or hypophysectomy; peritoneal fluid; bile; synovial fluid; pericardial fluid)
- Bone marrow
- Female genital specimens (abscesses, operative specimens and samples obtained by culdocentesis to exclude contamination with vaginal flora)
- Surgical specimens such as intra-abdominal, intra-thoracic, etc.
- Urines in special instances and by subra-pubic bladder puncture

Specimens That Should Not Be Cultured

Specimens which should not be cultured for anaerobes routinely include:

Stomach or jejunal fluid

Routine vaginal or cervical swabs
Nasopharyngeal, mouth or throat specimens
Sputum or bronchoscopic specimens
Feces and rectal swabs
Routine urine
Bartholin and pilonidal cysts
Drainage from colostomy and jejunostomy wounds

There are exceptions to the above. For example, it may be useful to culture jejunal fluid from a case of blind loop syndrome since anaerobes have been implicated in this disease. Feces from infants should be cultured for Clostridium botulinum in suspected cases of infant botulism. There are now over 60 cases of infant botulism reported in the United States. The laboratory diagnosis of this disease has been made by identification of C. botulinum as well as by typing botulinal toxin from infant feces.

GUIDELINES FOR SPECIMEN COLLECTION

Some general guidelines for specimen collection which will aid the recovery of anaerobes from specimens include: cleanse the normal flora away from the wound surface; collect the specimen from deep in the wound; collect several ml of pus or fluid if possible; if several ml of pus are not available, collect the pus on two swabs if possible; place the swab in an anaerobe transport tube; transport the specimen directly to the laboratory; culture the specimen within 20 min after collection; and culture the specimen on freshly prepared media that will support the growth of fastidious anaerobes. Several ml of pus can be collected in a syringe. The air is expelled from the syringe, the needle is corked with a sterile cork, and the specimen is transported to the laboratory and cultured without delay.

ANAEROBE TRANSPORT CONTAINERS

Several anaerobe transport containers are now available commercially. The Anaerobic Culturette (Marion Scientific Corp., Kansas City, Mo.) provides a swab on which to collect the specimen; the swab is then placed in an anaerobic atmosphere and kept moist. The Anaerobic Culture Set (Marion Scientific Corp.) provides a swab for specimen collection; the swab can then be inoculated onto a freshly prepared medium which is placed in a plastic bag where an anaerobic atmosphere is generated.

Several anaerobe transport kits are marketed by Carr-Scarborough Microbiologicals, Inc., Stone Mountain, Ga. These kits include: the Anaerobic Transport Tube for a liquid specimen; the AnaTrans in sterile surgical pack; the Anaerobic Transport Medium for swab which employs modified Cary-Blair medium; and the AnaT swab in sterile surgical pack. An anaerobic specimen collector (Beckton-Dickinson, Rutherford, N.J.) employs one swab which is used for specimen collection; the swab is then placed in a tube where an anaerobic gas is generated. No liquid is employed in this system to keep the swab moist.

Although the above systems keep the swab under anaerobic conditions, with or without added moisture, the swab should be transported to the laboratory and cultured without delay since ambient temperature is not ideal for the growth of anaerobes.

GRAM STAIN

Once the specimen arrives in the laboratory a Gram stain should be made if sufficient material is available. The Gram stain should be reported to the clinician or put on the chart without delay. Too many times, Gram stains are delayed until the technologist has "time" to perform and read these stains, and the results may not reach the chart until the following day. Culture results should be compared to Gram stain results and every effort should be made to isolate all cell morphotypes observed in the Gram stain. Precautions which should be observed in interpreting Gram stain results are: certain species of clostridia stain Gram-negatively; some Gram-positive anaerobic cocci are easily decolorized; tiny bacterial cells such as Veillonella parvula or Bacteroides melaninogenicus may be mistaken as debris; E. lentum tends to decolorize; and Bacteroides bivius and Bacteroides disiens tend to retain the crystal violet and have coccal shape rather than a bacillus shape.

ISOLATION MEDIA FOR ANAEROBE CULTURE

Blood specimens should always be cultured in suitable aerobe broth as well as in Pre-reduced Anaerobically Sterilized (PRAS) broth for growth of anaerobes. The PRAS medium that we have had the most experience with and which provides suitable anaerobic culture conditions is the Bac-Tec PRAS medium (Johnston Laboratories, Cockeysville, Md.); this medium should be tested on the Bac-Tec machine.

Solid media used for the isolation of anaerobes may include: freshly prepared media, a PRAS roll-streak tube, selective media, or a commercial tube of PRAS agar which has been melted and cooled, blood added, and the blood medium poured into plates. The hardened blood medium is then inoculated with the specimen and incubated anaerobically.

The formula which we have prepared and used successfully in our laboratory for the past 10 years for the culture of fastidious anaerobes and the directions for preparation of that medium follow:

Anaerobic Blood Agar Medium
Plus Supplements (NBAPS)

1.	Brain Heart Infusion Agar (Difco)	52 g
	Yeast Extract	5 g
	Distilled water	1,000 ml

2. Heat to dissolve. Sterilize at 121 C for 15 min.

3. Add 50 ml sheep blood.

4. Add Vitamin K_1-Hemin (VPI Anaerobe Laboratory Manual, 4th ed.) to above medium.

5. Pour 20 ml agar into 15 x 90 mm plastic Petri dishes.

This NBAPS plated medium is used within three h after preparation. Alternately, it may be stored at room temperature in an anaerobe atmosphere immediately after preparation of plates, and used within two days after preparation. Media made as described above and stored anaerobically is called reduced media.

We have compared growth of anaerobes on our freshly prepared media (NBAPS) with growth on commercial 5% Sheep Blood Columbia Agar Base (CBA) and commercial 5% Sheep Blood Trypticase Soy Agar Base (TSBA). Organisms were inoculated on these three media, incubated anaerobically for five days, and observed for growth. The organisms in the inoculum were not quantitated, therefore the growth was recorded qualitatively as: no growth; few colonies; or light, moderate, or heavy growth.

Organisms which grew on NBAPS but failed to grow on CBA and TSBA included: Bacteroides asaccharolyticus; Bacteroides melaninogenicus subsp. levii; and Bacteroides melaninogenicus subsp. intermedius, strain 275. The organisms which produced heavy growth on NBAPS but only a few colonies on CBA and TSBA were: Bacteroides melaninogenicus subsp. melaninogenicus; B. melaninogenicus subsp. intermedius, strain 532; and Eubacterium limosum. Anaerobes which produced heavy growth on NBAPS but light growth on CBA and TSBA were: P. magnus, V. parvula, B. disiens, B. bivius, and E. lentum. Species which grew heavily on NBAPS but only moderately well on CBA and TSBA included: Bacteroides oralis, Fusobacterium nucleatum, Fusobacterium varium, and Actinomyces meyeri. Thus, freshly prepared NBAPS medium was superior to commercially prepared CBA and TSBA for supporting growth of most anaerobes tested. The age of the commercial CBA and TSBA is unknown when the media are received by the clinical laboratory from the commercial source.

A SIMPLIFIED TECHNIQUE FOR THE ROUTINE CULTIVATION OF ANAEROBIC BACTERIA

E.C.S. Chan

Department of Microbiology and Immunology
McGill University
Montreal, Quebec, Canada

INTRODUCTION

Anaerobic bacteria are as common and widespread in nature as aerobic bacteria. In some natural habitats, they outnumber the aerobes by several orders of magnitude. But studies on the anaerobes have always lagged behind those on aerobic organisms mainly because of technical difficulties and inconveniences.

Recently there has been an increasing number of studies on anaerobic bacteria and a greater appreciation of their role in the disease process. For example, there is a current awareness that anaerobes are involved in infections of humans much more frequently than had generally been supposed (6). These advances are mainly due to the introduction and development of techniques in anaerobiosis (1,2,3).

The ideal anaerobic culture method should meet the following criteria: a. no exposure to oxygen of the culture medium during preparation to keep oxidized materials in as low a concentration as possible and to prevent the formation of toxic oxidation products; b. exclusion or displacement of oxygen from the medium during inoculation and incubation; and c. maintenance of a sufficiently low oxidation-reduction potential in the culture environment.

At the present time, three major techniques have been developed for the cultivation of anaerobic bacteria particularly on solid culture media: (i) the simplest and least complex system is the anaerobic jar such as the BBL GasPak jar. These jars are freed of oxygen by use of disposable carbon dioxide hydrogen generator packets. The disadvantages of the system are that the jar must be opened and the contents exposed to air when the cultures are examined. It takes at least one to six hours for good anaerobiosis to occur. The use of petri plates in the system makes it particularly attractive. (ii) The anaerobic glove box technique (1) uses a large chamber filled with oxygen-free gases and is of sufficient size to house all necessary items and to provide space for carrying out microbiological manipulations. The main advantages are that any microbiologist employing conventional techniques can use it; media can be prepared in the usual manner and any specimen can be examined as often as necessary through the transparent chamber without compromising anaerobiosis. Such chambers are now available commercially from several sources. The disadvantages are that they require manipulation through rubber gloves and occupy valuable laboratory space. (iii) The established standard for rigorous anaerobic bacteriology is the roll-tube method. It was used initially in Germany but was introduced in North America by Hungate (4,5). It has been effectively modified by Moore (7) and specific details can be found in the Anaerobe Laboratory Manual (3). Essentially, the method features the use of pre-reduced, anaerobically sterilized (PRAS) media, that is, media freed of oxygen by boiling and then autoclaved under an inert gas such as nitrogen or carbon dioxide. All subsequent manipulations are carried out under a stream of oxygen-free gas delivered into round tubes through a metal cannula. To carry out isolation procedures, molten PRAS agar medium is spun in a horizontal position to form the roll tube consisting of a thin film of solidified agar medium on the inner wall of the tube. The advantages are that the technique requires little laboratory bench space and each tube is its own independent anaerobic system so that it can be examined as often as necessary without losing anaerobiosis. However, the present technique as practiced (3,5) requires special equipment and skill to perform. It also does not facilitate the study of colonial morphology.

This paper describes a simpler and more economical technique than those described for the cultivation of anaerobic bacteria. It incorporates the criteria enunciated above for the ideal anaerobic culture method.

METHODS

Pre-reduced media were prepared as described by Holdeman and Moore (3). Required amounts of basal medium ingredients are dissolved in a volume of distilled water in a glass vacuum flask. Agar, if required, was added later. An oxidation-reduction indicator, such as resazurin (0.6 ml per 100 ml medium of a solution containing 11 mg resazurin dissolved in 44 ml distilled water) was added. The side arm of the flask with a cotton-wool filter was clamped off. A removable chimney which was an inverted plastic bottle with a hole in the bottom was placed on the flask (Fig. 1).

The medium was boiled on a magnetic stirrer heater, with refluxing through the chimney, until the resazurin turned from pink to colorless. The flask was removed from the heat and oxygen-free carbon dioxide was immediately introduced through the side arm, now unclamped. The gas was freed of oxygen by use of a heated copper column, also called a furnace tube (furnace tube, cat. no. S-36518; furnace, cat. no. S-36517; from Sargent-Welch Scientific Co., 7300 North Linder Avenue, Skokie, Illinois 60076 or 3300 Cavendish Blvd., Montreal, Quebec H4B 2M8) sitting in a furnace (Fig. 2). The chimney was replaced by a rubber stopper with a single glass tubing.

The fluid medium was cooled to room temperature in an ice bath with continued carbon dioxide flow. It was removed from the ice bath and cysteine hydrochloride (0.05 g/100 ml) was added. The flask was shaken gently to dissolve all the cysteine. The pH was adjusted to the desired value with HCl or NaOH by immersing a small combination electrode into the medium under the rubber stopper. The

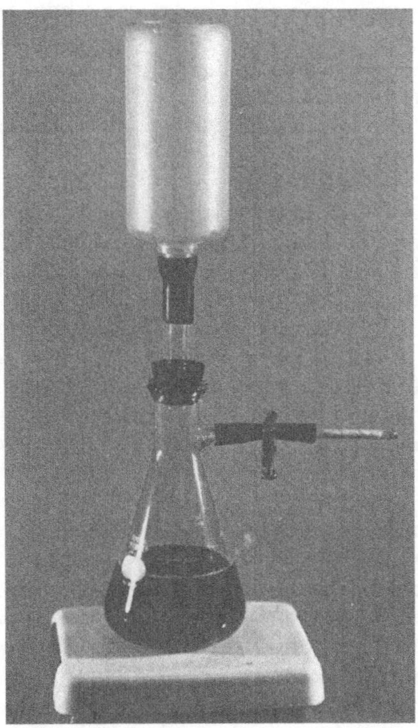

Fig. 1. Vacuum flask with side-arm clamp and cotton filter. Chimney sits on top.

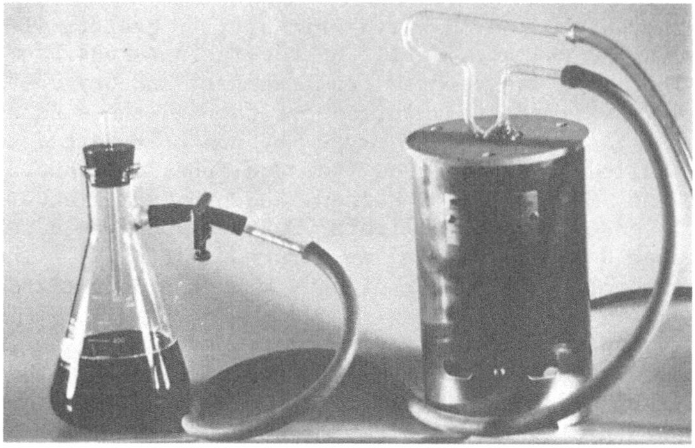

Fig. 2. Vacuum flask with a single glass tubing-rubber stopper shown with oxygen-free gas supply from a furnace (right).

rubber stopper with single glass tubing was then removed and replaced with the chimney. At this time, agar was added if required. The carbon dioxide flow was stopped and the gas delivery tube removed; the side arm was again clamped. The medium was boiled as before until it lost all pinkness due to any oxidized resazurin.

Prior to sterilization the chimney was replaced with a stainless steel check valve that had a nominal cracking pressure of one lb/in (cat. no. SS-4CP2-1 Nupro check-valve from Nupro Co., 4800 E. 345th Street, Willoughby, Ohio 44094; in Canada, Laurentian Valve and Fittings Limited, 96 Leacock Road, Pointe Claire, Quebec H9R 1H1). The valve was mounted on a rubber stopper (Fig. 3). The check valve permitted a blanket of nitrogen of one lb/in above the medium. The gas was disconnected from the side arm, and after clamping, the flask assembly was autoclaved for the necessary time in the conventional manner.

A further innovation involved the dispensing of sterile and reduced media after autoclaving using a Salvarsan tube. The check valve on the flask was replaced by a sterile, single glass tubing through a rubber stopper under continuous gas flow. For ease of handling, the gas used from here on was a mixture of 90% argon, 5% hydrogen, and 5% carbon dioxide. Argon is heavier than nitrogen and air and is inert. Sterile blood was added if required. The glass tubing was then connected by sterilized rubber tubing to the Salvarsan dispenser (Fig. 4). In this manner gas flushed freely through the Salvarsan tube.

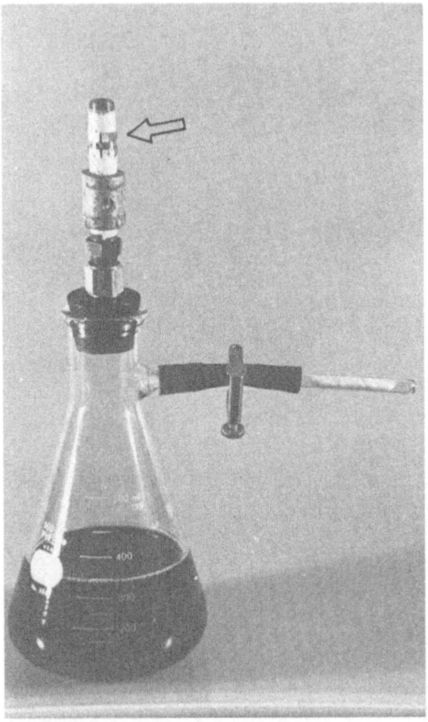

Fig. 3. Vacuum flask with a mounted check valve (arrow).

With the delivery end clamped, the medium was transferred to the Salvarsan tube by tilting the flask. Gas continued to flush through the system. Gas was also directed to the sleeve assembly of the delivery tube (Fig. 5).

The culture bottles were 40 ml (2 oz) rubber-lined screw-capped prescription bottles (cat. no. 16164-481; John's Scientific, 219 Broadview Avenue, Toronto, Ontario, Canada M4M 2G4). Ten ml were dispensed after flushing. This amount provided a flat layer of agar medium which could be used for inoculation under a stream of oxygen-free gas.

When quantitative measurements of fluid were necessary, the Salvarsan tube was replaced by a Kelly infusion bottle (Corning) (Fig. 6). The exact volume of liquid medium was measured by means of the graduated pipette side arm and delivered as before (Fig. 5). Oxygen-free gas flushed freely through the apparatus at all times.

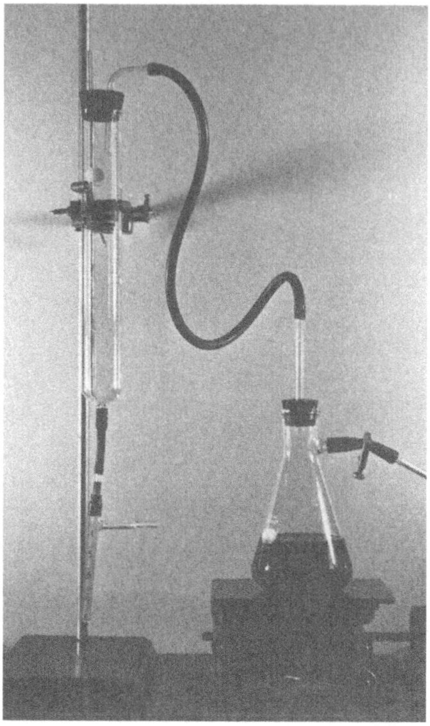

Fig. 4. Salvarsan tube with rubber stopper containing two glass tubings. The bent one extends below the stopper and is connected to the vacuum flask. The other open tubing serves as a vent.

RESULTS AND DISCUSSION

The innovations described above were made in the course of studies with specimens of dental plaque collected from patients with periodontal disease. These were diluted in a reduced fluid medium and aliquots were spread on the surface of blood agar medium enriched with hemin and vitamin K in the prescription bottles as described. Incubation of the prescription bottles was in a conventional incubator. The culture bottle (Fig. 7) shows some of the varieties of discrete colonies of anaerobic bacteria from a dilution of plaque sample; such colonies are easily visualized and enumerated. Furthermore, pure cultures of anaerobic bacteria have been successfully cultivated. These include Bacteroides asaccharolyticus, Bacteroides melaninogenicus, Bacteroides fragilis, Clostridium histolyticum, Clostridium novyi, Clostridium septicum, Clostridium sporogenes, and Clostridium tetani.

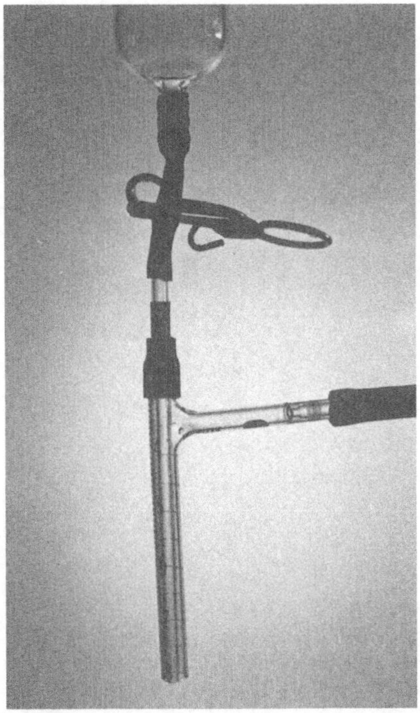

Fig. 5. Delivery tube from Salvarsan tube (or Kelly infusion bottle) with a sleeve or jacket for gas influx from side arm.

There are several improvements in the preparation of PRAS media by the technique described. The most important of these is the use of a check valve. It retains a constant atmosphere of nitrogen, or any other oxygen-free gas, over the medium before autoclaving. When the steam is turned off, the difference in vapor pressure within the flask and the autoclave chamber is relieved by the check valve eliminating any danger of explosion. In addition, media may be made in bulk because all the ingredients, such as agar, heme, and menadione or vitamin K may be added at one time. The dispensing of PRAS media is facilitated by the use of the Salvarsan tube or Kelly infusion bottle under a gas stream which completely excludes oxidation by air. The gas mixture, 90% argon, 5% hydrogen, and 5% carbon dioxide, is a non-explosive mixture. The hydrogen helps in maintaining a reduced atmosphere as well as keeping the copper column in a reduced state; the carbon dioxide meets the requirement of some anaerobes and its low concentration does not affect the pH of the medium.

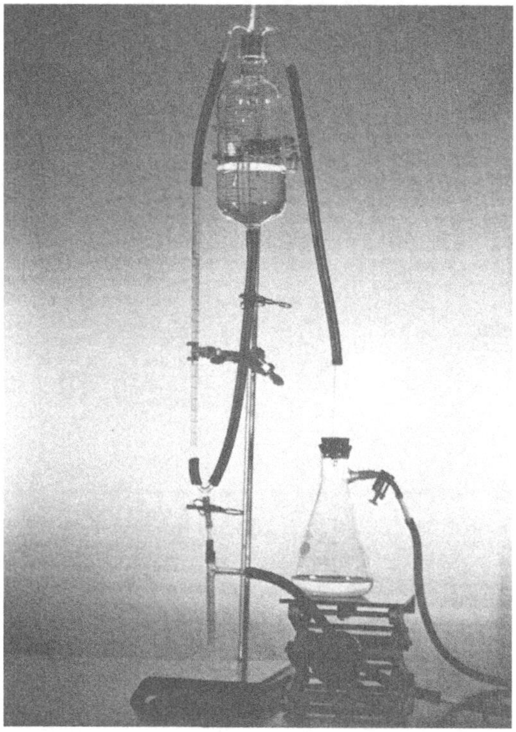

Fig. 6. Kelly infusion bottle with a graduated pipette side arm. Its rubber stopper has three short glass tubings: one is connected to the vacuum flask; one is connected to the graduated pipette; one is open to the air and serves as a vent for oxygen-free gas. The pipette tip is connected to the delivery mouth of the infusion bottle by means of a Y-joint and butyl rubber tubing.

Argon, being heavier than air, facilitates the flushing of air from the glass vessels and culture bottles. Pure carbon dioxide, even though it is heavier than air and nitrogen, was not used because it would lower the pH of the medium. The use of ordinary flat prescription glass bottles with rubber-lined screw caps was efficient and practical. The rubber liner maintained the medium in the reduced state. Such media can be stored until use.

The simplified procedures described in this paper for the preparation and use of PRAS media could lead to greater interest in anaerobiosis in the routine diagnostic laboratory as well as in research.

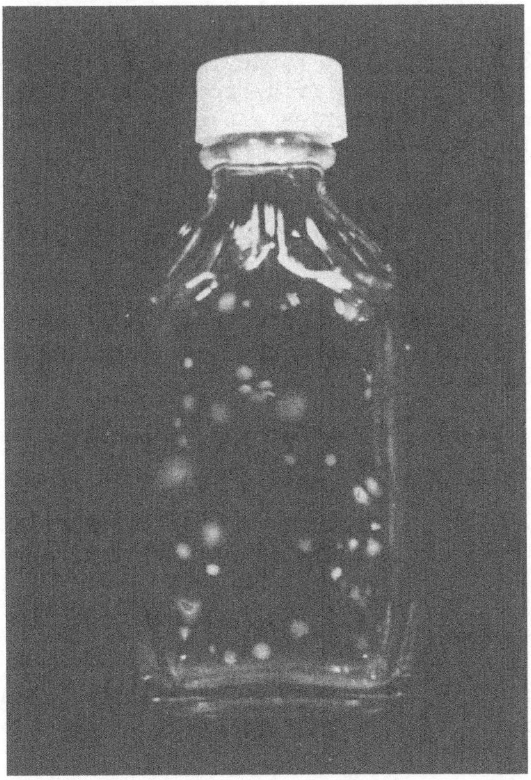

Fig. 7. Surface colonies of anaerobic bacteria from dental plaque growing in prescription bottle.

SUMMARY

A simplified technique for the routine cultivation of anaerobic bacteria is described. Its main features include the use of a check valve for the production of pre-reduced anaerobically sterilized media, a Salvarsan tube for the dispensing of such media, and screw-capped prescription glass bottles for the cultivation of the anaerobes.

ACKNOWLEDGMENTS

This research was supported by the Medical Research Council of Canada, grant no. MA-6176.

The expert technical assistance of Miss Carolina Alfieri and Mr. Turho Salo is gratefully acknowledged.

LITERATURE CITED

1. Aranki, A., S.A. Syed, E.B. Kenney, and R. Freter. 1969. Isolation of anaerobic bacteria from human gingiva and mouse cecum by means of a simplified glove box procedure. Appl. Microbiol. 17: 568-576.

2. Gosden, P.E., and G.C. Ware. 1977. A method for the production of pre-reduced anaerobically sterilized culture media. J. Appl. Bacteriol. 42: 77-79.

3. Holdeman, L.V., and W.E.C. Moore (ed.) 1972. Anaerobe Laboratory Manual, Virginia Polytechnic Institute and State University, Blacksburg.

4. Hungate, R.E. 1950. The anaerobic mesophilic cellulolytic bacteria. Bacteriol. Rev. 14: 1-63.

5. Hungate, R.E. 1969. A roll tube method for cultivation of strict anaerobes. In Methods in Microbiology 3B: 117-132.

6. Miraglia, G.J. 1974. Pathogenic anaerobic bacteria. CRC Crit. Rev. Microbiol. 3: 161-181.

7. Moore, W.E.C. 1966. Techniques for routine culture of fastidious anaerobes. Int. J. Syst. Bacteriol. 16: 173-190.

GAS CHROMATOGRAPHY OF PUS AS AN INDICATION OF ANAEROBIC INFECTION

K.D. Phillips

Public Health Laboratory
Luton and Dunstable Hospital
Lewsey Road, Luton LU4 ODZ
Bedfordshire, England

INTRODUCTION

Gas liquid chromatographic analyses of fermentation end products are of immense value to the study of the obligately anaerobic bacteria. The most intensively investigated end products in this context are the volatile fatty acids of the series formic to heptanoic, certain other short chain carboxylic acids (notably lactic and succinic) and the low molecular weight alcohols. These end products are generated by anaerobes as a result of fermentation of carbohydrates and amino acids, and are excreted in low concentrations in their growth environment. Gas chromatography has the potential to analyse minute quantities of closely related chemical substances and is eminently suited to the rapid separation, sensitive detection and accurate quantification of these anaerobic bacterial metabolites. The application of this technique with respect to anaerobes was initiated and extensively explored by workers at the Anaerobe Laboratory, Virginia Polytechnic Institute (4,5,6).

Their studies of a wide range of anaerobic bacteria showed that qualitative and quantitative differences in end products of metabolism were associated with different genera and species, and that these characteristics were stable, and, therefore, of taxonomic value. The fundamental importance of this concept had great impact on the development of a more rational classification of anaerobic bacteria, particularly the non-sporing anaerobes. Gas chromatographic techniques subsequently became readily accepted as a practical tool by laboratories concerned with definitive identification of their anaerobic isolates. Many anaerobic bacteria isolated from clinical material in the past were unidentifiable on the basis of conventional criteria; in conjunction with key biochemical tests, most genera and species are now readily distinguishable by their chromatographic profiles. Moreover, the availability of simple reliable gas chromatographic instrumentation renders analysis of acid and alcohol end products a procedure, not limited to reference or research laboratories, but within the capabilities of many routine diagnostic microbiology laboratories and does not of necessity require personnel with extensive training in gas chromatographic techniques.

Non-sporing anaerobes form a large part of the normal flora of the gastrointestinal tract, the female genital tract and the oropharynx. Under appropriate conditions these anaerobes may cause endogenous infection by invasion of adjacent tissues. Notable examples of infective processes in which non-sporing anaerobes, particularly Bacteroides, Fusobacterium and Gram-positive anaerobic cocci, have been implicated in intraabdominal and pelvic infections. Anaerobic sepsis of this type is characterized by the formation of deep seated abscesses; culture of the exudate by conventional direct plating methods yields mixtures of non-sporing anaerobes, frequently in association with commensal facultatively anaerobic species. By virtue of their fermentative metabolism, anaerobic bacteria generate end products not only in vitro but also in vivo, and this was first demonstrated by gas liquid chromatography of purulent material from anaerobic sepsis (2). This observation was confirmed and extended by a number of workers (1,3,7,8,9). Selected examples of chromatographic analyses of ether extracts of exudates obtained from anaerobic and aerobic infections are depicted in Fig. 1 and Fig. 2 respectively. In addition, gas chromatography of macroscopically positive blood cultures (Fig. 3) is of value for differentiation of anaerobic from aerobic bacteremia (8,10).

DISCUSSION

The importance of non-sporing anaerobic bacteria in the etiology of pyogenic infections occurring in virtually any tissue or organ of the body is now widely recognized. Laboratory diagnosis of sepsis due to non-sporing anaerobes is conventionally established by cultural methods employing direct plating of pathological exudate on suitable selective and non-selective solidified media. By cultural methods there is a delay of at least 24 - 48 h before the nature of the infection can be ascertained. In some instances, prolonged incubation is necessary for the isolation of slow growing organisms. Should cultural conditions be inappropriate, or the apparatus employed fail to achieve or maintain the necessary degree of anaerobiosis, isolation of fastidious pathogens may not be realized. On non-selective media, the growth of obligately anaerobic species may be largely obscured by the growth of associated commensal facultatively anaerobic organisms; selective media, which are never perfect, frequently suppress to some degree the growth of organisms whose selection is required, and may on occasion be completely inhibitory to

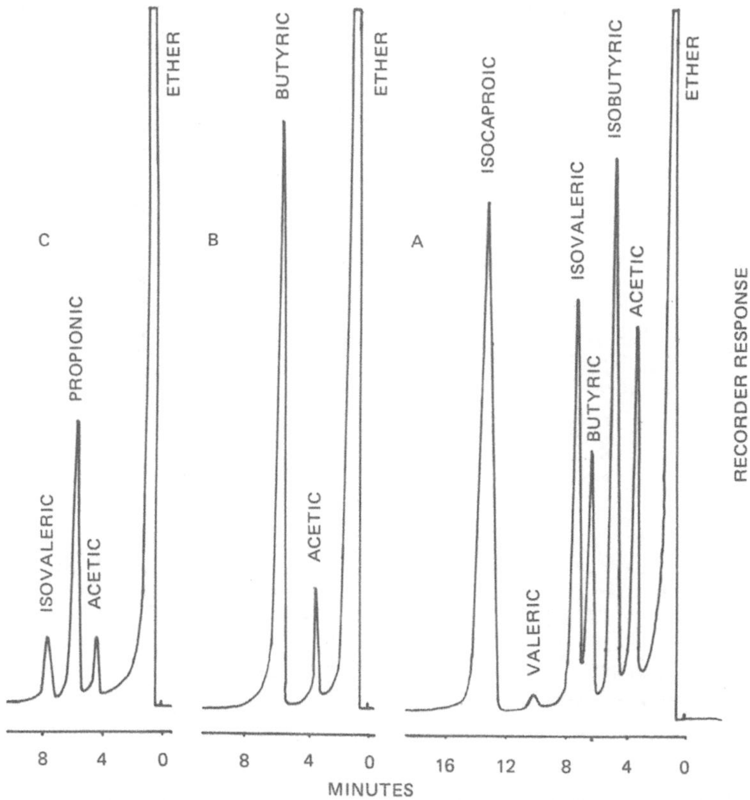

Fig. 1. Selected examples of chromatograms obtained by analysis of exudates from anaerobic sepsis.

(A) Appendectomy wound pus. Bacteroides fragilis and Bacteroides melaninogenicus isolated in association with coliforms and enterococci.
(B) Pilonidal sinus pus. B. fragilis isolated in pure culture.
(C) Joint fluid from septic arthritis. Fusobacterium necrophorum isolated.

some anaerobes. Thus, with cultural methods alone, there is always a possibility that anaerobic sepsis may be overlooked; even with conditions optimal for isolation there is an inherent delay before qualitative and quantitative assessment of the infecting flora can be made. However, gas chromatographic detection of multiple volatile fatty acids including butyric acid, in a specimen of pus can be useful in many instances for providing an indication of anaerobic sepsis within minutes of receipt of the specimen in the laboratory. Such rapidly generated, non-cultural information about the probable nature

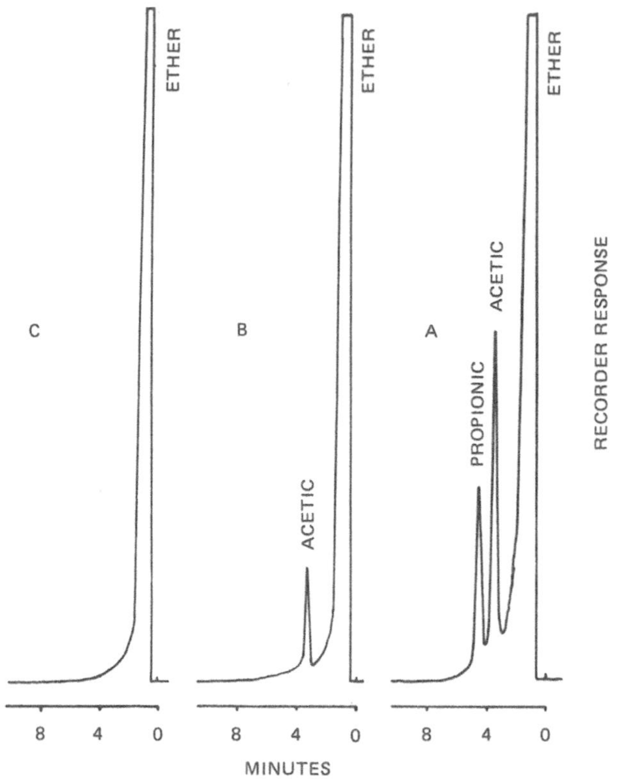

Fig. 2. Selected examples of chromatograms obtained by analysis of exudates from aerobic sepsis.

(A) Subphrenic abscess. Klebsiella spp. isolated.
(B) Axillary abscess. Staphylococcus aureus isolated.
(C) Abdominal wound. Escherichia coli isolated.

of the infection is of value, both to the clinician for effective management of the patient's condition, and to the microbiologist whose attention is positively directed to the elucidation of the anaerobic bacterial constituents of the specimen.

Usually it is not possible to reliably identify individual components of the infective flora on the basis of the chromatogram alone. Although monomicrobial infections due to anaerobes occasionally occur, much more frequently mixtures of anaerobes are present in lesions. Within the narrow spectrum of the volatile fatty acids, the chromatographic profiles of individual species may be superimposed. In addition, there is evidence from monomicrobial infections that the chromatographic profiles generated in vivo are not necessarily identical with those produced by pure cultures of the

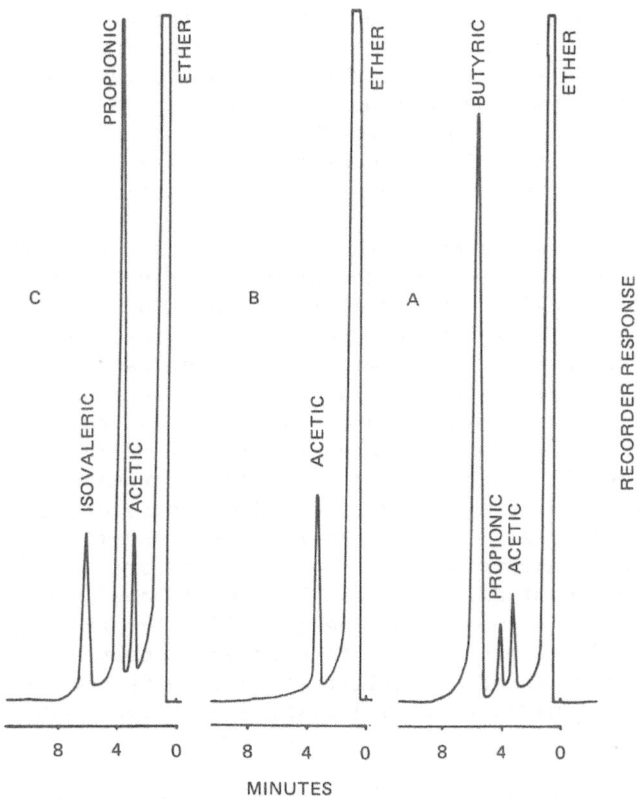

Fig. 3. Chromatograms obtained by analysis of macroscopically positive blood cultures.

(A) Fusobacterium spp. from blood of patient with acute otitis media. Subsequently identified as F. necrophorum.
(B) A facultatively anaerobic organism from the blood of a patient with urinary tract infection. Subsequently identified as E. coli.
(C) Propionibacterium spp. (P. acnes) isolated in a single blood culture bottle, derived from skin flora at venipuncture.

same organisms when grown in artificial culture media. Nevertheless, detection of multiple volatile acids in a specimen of pus is of value for the rapid presumptive diagnosis of anaerobic sepsis per se. The correlation obtained between chromatographic analyses of unselected specimens of pathological exudate and the results of culture for both anaerobic and aerobic sepsis is in excess of 90%. False negative results on specimens (chromatographically negative, anaerobes isolated) do occur, usually as a result of culture of exudate obtained early in the course of infection, prior to the accumulation of detectable levels. False positive results do not occur. Detection of relevant volatile fatty acids in the absence of anaerobic isolation is encountered from time to time during the course of successful antimicrobial treatment of an established anaerobic infection. Indeed, the diminution of residual acids in drainage from a lesion may be utilized to monitor the efficacy of antimicrobial therapy.

Blood cultures are among the most important specimens received in a diagnostic bacteriology laboratory. Early diagnosis of bacteremia may be critical to the patient's chances of recovery. Growth in blood culture media is commonly detected by microscopy, visual inspection or subculture. Determination of the isolate as aerobic, facultatively anaerobic or obligately anaerobic requires subculture of the organism under appropriate conditions and this may further delay a diagnosis. However, detection in the medium of volatile acids of anaerobic metabolism by gas liquid chromatography indicates the presence of an anaerobe isolate and may provide an identification at generic or species level. Unfortunately, usually it is not possible to detect end products in the medium before growth has been noted. Because many different facultatively anaerobic organisms generate detectable amounts of acetic acid only, gas liquid chromatography is not discriminatory in this group. However, detection of anaerobic bacteremia at an earlier stage than is possible by cultural methods is of clinical value and enables a rational choice of chemotherapy.

The applications of gas chromatography developed sequentially in three related fields of investigation. Following the profound implications which the discovery of stable qualitative and quantitative differences in metabolic profiles had for the taxonomy of these organisms, practical methods of gas chromatography evolved for purposes of identification and were readily adopted as a routine procedure. From analyses of end products generated by anaerobes during growth in vitro, interest extended to encompass the detection of metabolites resulting from in vivo growth and the potential of gas chromatography for early diagnosis of anaerobic sepsis became apparent.

SUMMARY

Gas chromatographic analysis of pathological exudate is of clinical value for the rapid presumptive diagnosis of anaerobic sepsis per se, but does not, in most instances, reliably identify components of the infecting flora. Results are available within minutes compared with day(s) required to establish diagnosis by cultural methods. In addition, gas chromatographic analysis of macroscopically visible blood cultures may differentiate between aerobic and anaerobic bacteremia earlier than is possible by subculture. Anaerobic isolates may be identifiable at generic or species level at this stage.

ACKNOWLEDGEMENTS

I thank Dr. A.T. Willis for his support in this work, Maria Jarzembski for preparation of the manuscript and John Harrison, medical photographer, Luton & Dunstable Hospital, for the illustrations.

LITERATURE CITED

1. Eykyn, S.J., and I. Phillips. 1976. Metronidazole and anaerobic sepsis. Br. Med. J. 2: 1418-1421.

2. Gorbach, S.L., J.W. Mayhew, J.G. Bartlett, H. Thadepalli, and A.B. Onderdonk. 1974. Rapid diagnosis of Bacteroides fragilis infections by direct gas-liquid chromatography of clinical specimens. Clin. Res. 22: 442A.

3. Gorbach, S.L., J.W. Mayhew, J.G. Bartlett, H. Thadepalli, and A.B. Onderdonk. 1976. Rapid diagnosis of anaerobic infections by direct gas-liquid chromatography of clinical specimens. J. Clin. Invest. 57: 478-484.

4. Holdeman, L.V., E.P. Cato, and W.E.C. Moore (ed.). 1977. Anaerobe laboratory manual, 4th ed., Virginia Polytechnic Institute and State University, Blacksburg.

5. Moore, W.E.C. 1970. Relationships of metabolic products to taxonomy of anaerobic bacteria. Int. J. Syst. Bacteriol. 20: 535-538.

6. Moore, W.E.C., E.P. Cato, and L.V. Holdeman. 1966. Fermentation patterns of some Clostridium species. Int. J. Syst. Bacteriol. 16: 383-415.

7. Nord, C.-E. 1977. Diagnosis of anaerobic infections by gas-liquid chromatography. Acta Pathol. Microbiol. Scand. Sect. B, Suppl. 259: 55-59.

8. Phillips, K.D., P.V. Tearle, and A.T. Willis. 1976. Rapid diagnosis of anaerobic infections by gas-liquid chromatography of clinical material. J. Clin. Pathol. 29: 428-432.

9. Taylor, A.J. 1978. The application of head-space analysis gas-liquid chromatography to the diagnosis of anaerobic infection. J. Med. Microbiol. 11: ix.

10. Wüst, J. 1977. Presumptive diagnosis of anaerobic bacteremia by gas-liquid chromatography of blood cultures. J. Clin. Microbiol. 6: 586-590.

RECENT CHANGES IN IDENTIFICATION AND CLASSIFICATION OF SOME ANAEROBES

Lillian V. Holdeman, Elizabeth P. Cato, and W.E.C. Moore

Anaerobe Laboratory
Virginia Polytechnic Institute and State University
Blacksburg, Virginia 24061

INTRODUCTION

Contrary to the belief of many, Bergey's Manual of Determinative Bacteriology has no official taxonomic status but does affect taxonomy in that taxonomic status can become established on the basis of common usage. Bergey's Manual is one of the manuals commonly used when persons are trying to identify organisms or attempting to establish changes in nomenclature. Therefore, it seems appropriate to review changes in nomenclature of known taxa that have occurred since the eighth edition of Bergey's Manual was published and to discuss the reasons for some of these changes. A few of the new species that have been described recently, particularly those isolated from clinical infections or species that are similar to clinically important species, also will be discussed.

CAPNOCYTOPHAGA

The taxa given in Table 1 illustrate how progress in characterization and concepts of taxonomic groupings leads to nomenclatural changes. As late as 1950, various groups of anaerobes were differentiated principally by cellular morphology. The thin, tapered-ended Gram-negative bacilli (fusiforms) were placed in Fusobacterium (Fusiformis), the pleomorphic rods in Sphaerophorus, and the rods of regular morphology in Bacteroides (Ristella, Capsularis). Therefore, it was quite reasonable that Prévot and colleagues placed a relatively long, Gram-negative rod with tapered ends in the genus Fusiformis. Because cells of strains of this species looked very similar to F. nucleatum and because colonies were yellowish, the new taxon was called F. nucleatus var. ochraceus (27).

Table 1. Taxa of Capnocytophaga

Fusiformis nucleatus var. ochraceus Prévot, Tardieux, Joubert, and de Cadore 1956

↓ G + C = 42%

Ristella ochracea (Prévot et al.) Sebald 1962

synonymous with

Bacteroides oralis var. elongatus Loesche, Socransky, and Gibbons 1964

↓

Bacteroides ochraceus (Prévot et al.) Holdeman and Moore 1972

↓

Capnocytophaga ochracea (Prévot et al.) Leadbetter, Holt, and Socransky 1979

In 1962 Sebald published her classic work concerning the guanine plus cytosine (G + C) content of various anaerobic Gram-negative rods (29). She reported that strains of F. nucleatus var. ochraceus had a G + C content of 42 moles percent, which was similar to that of species of Ristella and unlike that of other species in the genus Fusiformis (Fusobacterium). She therefore suggested that F. nucleatus var. ochraceus be reclassified as Ristella ochracea.

In 1964 Loesche and colleagues proposed a new species, Bacteroides oralis, with two varieties (var. oralis and var. elongatus) for saccharolytic Gram-negative rods they had isolated from human mouths (23). When we were preparing the descriptions for Bergey's Manual (8th ed.) we compared strains of R. ochracea from the Institut Pasteur (Paris) and of B. oralis var. elongatus from the American Type Culture Collection. Our studies of these strains indicated that they were the same species. Since "ochraceus" was the first name that had been used for this taxon, we proposed the new combination of Bacteroides ochraceus, which is found in Bergey's Manual (8th ed.) (12). At this time (1974) we realized that strains of B. ochraceus would grow on the surface of blood agar plates incubated in 5 to 10% CO_2, which is not typical for members of the genus Bacteroides. However, we felt that this was a valid species and that its description should occur in Bergey's Manual so that when strains were isolated they could be recognized. We were not surprised, therefore, when a new genus, Capnocytophaga, was proposed to include this species. Two other species, Capnocytophaga sputigena and Capnocytophaga gingivalis, also are included in this new genus (22,32). Subsequent studies have shown that CDC Group DF-1 strains also are capnocytophagae (26, 40).

BACTEROIDES UREOLYTICUS

In 1958 Eiken described Bacteroides corrodens as a group of nonfermentative Gram-negative rods that were either obligately anaerobic or facultatively anaerobic (5). They were given the specific epithet of "corrodens" because they corroded, or pitted, the agar around the colony. In subsequent years, Drs. Jackson and Goodman and colleagues found that DNA of the obligately anaerobic strains had a G + C content of 28 to 30 moles percent, whereas the DNA of the facultative strains had a much higher G + C content (16). A new genus, Eikenella, was proposed for the facultative strains (14), and the CDC Group HB-1 was Eikenella corrodens (28). The obligately anaerobic strains were then referred to as B. corrodens for several years. This, however, was confusing, because B. corrodens once also had included the facultative strains. Further, the type strain of B. corrodens Eiken (anaerobes and facultatives) had become the type strain of E. corrodens. Therefore, in 1978 Jackson and Goodman proposed a new taxon, Bacteroides ureolyticus, for the obligately anaerobic strains (15). B. ureolyticus, Vibrio succinogenes, and Campylobacter sputorum subsp. sputorum, have a rather specialized metabolic pathway for gaining energy and growing. This pathway was first described by Wolin et al. (41) for the organism that they named V. succinogenes (because it was "vibrio" in shape and produced succinic acid). These three species use either hydrogen or formate as an electron donor and fumarate or nitrate as an electron acceptor (31,36). They grow reasonably well (but never as well as B. fragilis) in a medium that contains either formate in the medium or a high concentration of hydrogen in the gaseous atmosphere and fumarate (or some substrate that can be metabolized to fumarate) or nitrate in the medium. Of these three taxa, only B. ureolyticus produces urease and is not motile. V. succinogenes and C. sputorum subsp. sputorum are both motile with polar flagella but differ markedly in the G + C content of their DNA. C. sputorum subsp. sputorum requires fumarate or nitrate for anaerobic growth but can grow in 5 to 10% oxygen without these particular electron acceptors (30). V. succinogenes is an obligate anaerobe.

BACTEROIDES THAT PRODUCE BLACK-PIGMENTING COLONIES ON BLOOD

Historically, Bacteroides melaninogenicus has included anaerobic Gram-negative bacilli that form black pigment when grown on blood-containing agar. Although these strains will grow on peptone media supplemented with vitamin K and hemin, they will not form the characteristic pigment unless blood is present. In Bergey's Manual

(8th ed.) three subspecies of Bacteroides melaninogenicus are listed: subsp. melaninogenicus, subsp. intermedius, and subsp. asaccharolyticus. In the VPI Anaerobe Laboratory Manual (4th ed.) (8) subsp. levii also is listed. Included in subsp. levii are those strains that are like the rumen strain studied in detail by Lev. They produce a mixture of volatile fatty acids, similar to those produced by the asaccharolytic strains, but also ferment glucose and lactose.

As one would presume, strains of B. melaninogenicus subsp. asaccharolyticus did not ferment any carbohydrates, which made them quite different from strains of subsp. intermedius and subsp. melaninogenicus. Also, strains of subsp. asaccharolyticus had a much higher G + C content than did strains of the other subspecies. It was the consensus of the members of the International Taxonomic Subcommittee for Anaerobic Gram-negative Rods that subsp. asaccharolyticus should be elevated to species status. Accordingly, the new taxon of B. asaccharolyticus was proposed in 1977 (6). It will not be surprising if the remaining subspecies of B. melaninogenicus also are reclassified as separate species in the future.

Reclassification of this type causes difficulty in identification for microbiologists who previously were not determining the subspecies to which the black-pigmenting colony belonged. Identification now is more difficult because one has to test additional characteristics before properly identifying an organism as B. melaninogenicus. This does not make identification easier, but it does make species more meaningful. If these are distinctly different organisms, and subsequent work is showing that they are, then they have distinctly different properties. If we need to recognize these species at all, then we need to recognize them for what they really are. Only when we differentiate truly distinct entities can we (or anyone else) assess the significance of these organisms in different infections or situations.

CLOSTRIDIUM CLOSTRIDIIFORME

According to the present definition in Bergey's Manual (8th ed.), all anaerobic bacilli that form spores are placed in Clostridium, except for the sulfate reducers, which are classified in Desulfotomaculum. Accordingly, when strains thought to be Bacteroides clostridiiformis were found to have spores, they were reclassified as Clostridium clostridiiforme (4,21). These organisms are Gram-negative rods that tend to have tapered ends. The two subspecies of B. clostridiiformis, subsp. clostridiiformis and subsp. girans, formerly differentiated on the basis of motility, were not thought to be sufficiently different to be maintained as two subspecies. In this instance, therefore, we see a simplification of nomenclature.

SACCHAROLYTIC BACTEROIDES

Perhaps one of the most extensive nomenclatural changes has occurred with the species recognized in Bergey's Manual (8th ed.) as Bacteroides fragilis. Five subspecies (fragilis, vulgatus, distasonis, thetaiotaomicron, and ovatus) were recognized. All shared common characteristics: fermenting glucose, lactose, maltose, and sucrose; growing in 20% bile; producing succinic acid, often with acetic, isobutyric, and isovaleric acids as well. DNA/DNA homology studies of members of this group showed that they did not have sufficient DNA homology to remain together as subspecies of B. fragilis (17). Therefore, the former subspecies have been restored to species rank (3) as B. fragilis, B. distasonis, B. vulgatus, B. thetaiotaomicron, and B. ovatus. Comparison of phenotypic results with the DNA homology groups (18) showed that the criteria that were given in Bergey's Manual (8th ed.) were not always the best criteria to use for differentiation of some of these species. For example, fermentation of salicin, rather than fermentation of mannitol, was a better phenotypic test for differentiating between B. thetaiotaomicron and B. ovatus (8). Even so, some strains of B. thetaiotaomicron do ferment salicin, so correlation is not 100 percent. The homology studies of the indole-positive members of this group also showed that two distinct entities have been confused as B. thetaiotaomicron. The second was determined as Bacteroides uniformis, originally described by Eggerth in 1933 and an entity that was still recognized by some European investigators. Strains of B. uniformis usually do not ferment trehalose; those of B. thetaiotaomicron do ferment trehalose (8). B. uniformis is part of the normal fecal flora of many individuals and is relatively frequently isolated from clinical specimens. Many of the strains referred to as B. thetaiotaomicron in our previous publications of human fecal flora (10,25) are B. uniformis.

Three new species of saccharolytic Bacteroides have been described within the last five years: B. eggerthii, B. splanchnicus, and B. multiacidus.

B. eggerthii Holdeman and Moore 1974

This species produces indole and does not ferment sucrose. It has been isolated from human feces and, occasionally, from clinical specimens (13).

B. splanchnicus Werner, Rintelen, and Kunstek-Santos 1975

Key characteristics of this species are production of acetic, propionic, isobutyric, butyric, isovaleric, and succinic acid; no fermentation of maltose and sucrose (37). Strains have been isolated from human feces and, occasionally, from clinical specimens. Like members of the former "B. fragilis group", strains of this species are resistant to kanamycin (1 mg disc) and grow in 20% bile.

B. multiacidus Mitsuoka, Terada, Watanabe, and Uchida 1974

Strains of this species ferment many carbohydrates to a low pH, forming lactic, succinic, and acetic acid. Human feces appear to be the natural habitat (24).

Strains of nonpigmenting saccharolytic Bacteroides that do not grow well in 20% bile are part of the normal flora of the mouth and of the vagina and are rather frequently isolated from clinical specimens. When strains with these characteristics are isolated one is inclined to think immediately of three possibilites: Bacteroides oralis, Bacteroides ruminicola, or strains of B. melaninogenicus that have not yet pigmented. Especially troublesome are those saccharolytic strains that appear to be B. melaninogenicus subsp. intermedius except they do not form pigment. We had quite a few of these strains, almost all isolated from clinical specimens, many referred to us by Lambe. Some fermented lactose and some did not, an acceptable variation within B. melaninogenicus. We were most hesitant to call them "nonpigmenting strains of B. melaninogenicus," and equally hesitant to say that they were not. Would this one observable phenotypic difference be a sufficient basis for establishing a new species? In this case it was. Johnson determined that representatives of these two phenotypic groups showed no significant DNA/DNA homology with B. melaninogenicus. Therefore, two new species have been proposed: Bacteroides disiens and B. bivius (11). B. disiens is fairly common in infections of the female reproductive tract. Although the first isolates of B. bivius that we examined also were from the female reproductive tract, we now have isolates of this species from many different areas of the body. One would suspect that the source of both of these species probably is the vagina.

B. ruminicola was first described by Bryant et al. (2), who differentiated two subspecies (subsp. ruminicola and subsp. brevis) and 11 biotypes. These strains were from rumen contents. Similar strains, particularly with phenotypic characteristics corresponding to B. ruminicola subsp. brevis biotype 3, are isolated from human specimens from various sources. Strains with these characteristics are listed as B. ruminicola subsp. brevis biotype 3 in the 4th edition of the VPI Anaerobe Laboratory Manual, even though we have some reservation about their synonymy with the bovine strains.

B. oralis (B. oralis subsp. oralis) includes saccharolytic strains that do not ferment the pentoses. According to the original description of this species, cellobiose is fermented by all strains. It appears, however, that many persons identify a strain as B. oralis without ever testing for cellobiose fermentation. It seems that so many different entities have been mistakenly identified as B. oralis that the existence of the species itself is somewhat in jeopardy. At the 1979 meeting of the International Taxonomic Subcommittee on Anaerobic Gram-negative Rods in Munich, no agreement could be reached among the committee members concerning a neotype strain for B. oralis. Because there are probably several distinct entities in this group of saccharolytic Bacteroides that do not grow well in bile, it appears that bacteriologists should be more conservative than they have in the past and should avoid "lumping" together as B. oralis the saccharolytic Bacteroides that do not grow well in 20% bile. The key characteristics that we use for differentiating among these organisms are given in Table 2. These are only key characteristics; other phenotypic traits need to be determined to confirm the identification.

ANAEROBIC COCCI

A new genus, Coprococcus Holdeman and Moore 1974 (13), has been proposed for the anaerobic Gram-positive cocci that require a fermentable carbohydrate for growth and that produce butyric acid (acetic acid, sometimes with propionic, also is produced). The

Table 2. Key Characteristics of Some Species of Saccharolytic, Bile-negative, Nonpigmenting Bacteroides[a]

Characteristic	Suggested Species
Arabinose and/or xylose acid	B. ruminicola Bryant, Small, Bouma, and Chu 1958
Arabinose and xylose negative	
Cellobiose acid	B. oralis Loesche, Socransky, and Gibbons 1964
Cellobiose negative	
Lactose acid	B. bivius Holdeman and Johnson 1977
Lactose negative	B. disiens Holdeman and Johnson 1977

[a]Succinic = major fermentation acid, indole not produced, nitrate not reduced.

coprococci are members of the fecal flora of man (and probably other animals) but have not been reported from clinical specimens. Many anaerobic Gram-positive cocci produce butyric acid and are members of Peptococcus. The peptococci do not require a fermentable carbohydrate for growth. That is, the peptococci grow in a medium containing peptone and yeast extract without any carbohydrate added, the coprococci (and ruminococci) do not grow in this medium unless a carbohydrate that they can ferment also is present.

In Bergey's Manual (8th ed.), some described species of peptococci and peptostreptococci fermented carbohydrates and produced lactic acid, as do strains of streptococci. The G + C content of these was similar to that reported for streptococci. Additionally, most strains of these species could grow in atmospheres of increased carbon dioxide or reduced oxygen, even though they might appear to be obligate anaerobes upon initial isolation. The description of Streptococcus was emended to include obligately anaerobic strains and three of these species were reclassified in Streptococcus: S. intermedius, S. constellatus, and S. morbillorum (13).

Both Peptococcus anaerobius and Peptostreptococcus anaerobius are included in Bergey's Manual (8th ed.). Having two species with the same specific epithet in two different genera that started with "P." was confusing. For example, "P. anaerobius" could be either. The original description of Peptococcus anaerobius was rather vague and could have referred to any of number of different species. The Judicial Commission has approved the request (38) to reject the name "Peptococcus anaerobius" (19).

No strains of the type species of Peptococcus, P. niger, were extant in 1974. This species, originally isolated by Ivan C. Hall, was described as producing black colonies - thus the name "niger". Strains of this species have now been isolated (39). Its natural habitat is the navel of some individuals, and it occurs rarely in clinical specimens. The black pigment may not be produced in subcultures, but on initial isolation plates the colonies are jet black, just like some strains of B. melaninogenicus. The pigmentation apparently results from accumulation of hydrogen sulfide in the colony. Chopped meat agar is a good medium for demonstrating black colonies of this species.

Peptococcus indolicus is new to most of us, and of interest because it is the only anaerobic coccus known to produce coagulase (33,35). P. indolicus has been associated with mastitis in cattle, but also has been isolated from the skin lesion of a sheep herder (1).

CLOSTRIDIUM

Two new species of Clostridium (C. spiroforme and C. cocleatum) with characteristics similar to Clostridium ramosum have been described by Kaneuchi et al. (20). All strains of C. cocleatum studied were from non-human sources. Strains of C. spiroforme were from human feces and from chickens.

EUBACTERIUM

In our studies of the microbial flora of periodontitis, we have isolated numerous strains of three groups of eubacteria with characteristics unlike those of previously described species: Eubacterium timidum, Eubacterium brachy, and Eubacterium nodatum (9). All are obligately anaerobic and nonfermentative.

Cells of E. timidum are like "small diphtheroids" and may decolorize easily. Chromatograms of cultures grown in peptone-yeast extract (with or without carbohydrate) may show trace amounts of acetate, formate, succinate, or lactate. No hydrogen is detected. They do not reduce nitrate or show evidence of an arginine dihydrolase pathway, as do strains of Eubacterium lentum (34). They do not ferment sugars, as do strains of Actinomyces.

Gram's stains of E. brachy show very short rods in chains. Volatile acids detected are similar to those produced by P. anaerobius, but neither glucose nor maltose is fermented. E. brachy also differs from P. anaerobius in that growth is not inhibited by sodium polyanethol sulfonate (7) and tyrosine is not degraded (Babcock, J.B., Abst. Int. Cong. Microbiol. 12th. Munich, abst. no. I60, p. 90, 1978). E. brachy has been isolated and identified from a lung abscess specimen collected by needle aspiration (L. Stringer, personal communication).

Cells of E. nodatum resemble Actinomyces, but the species differs from any of the Actinomyces by not fermenting any sugars and by producing butyric acid. Surface colonies are heaped and colonies in agar deep cultures have the shape of small raspberries.

It may seem that classification and taxonomy of bacteria change more rapidly than do the bacteria, even with the rapid mutation rate that they may have. Classification and taxonomy do change, but with reason. As analytical methods improve we are better able to determine and differentiate distinct entities. As the microbial population of more environments is analyzed, new species will be isolated. A species name, properly applied, represents all of the information available about that species. If the proper name is not applied to the entity being identified, then erroneous characteristics will be associated with the organism. Improved characterization with improved taxonomy and identification facilitate our understanding of each entity and its importance in its environment. After all, this is what taxonomy, characterization, and identification are all about.

LITERATURE CITED

1. Bourgault, A.M., and J.E. Rosenblatt. 1979. First isolation of Peptococcus indolicus from a human clinical specimen. J. Clin. Microbiol. 9: 549-550.

2. Bryant, M.P., N. Small, C. Bouma, and H. Chu. 1958. Bacteroides ruminicola n. sp. and the new genus and species Succinimonas amylolytica. Species of succinic acid-producing anaerobic bacteria of the bovine rumen. J. Bacteriol. 76: 15-23.

3. Cato, E.P., and J.L. Johnson. 1976. Reinstatement of species rank for Bacteroides fragilis, B. ovatus, B. distasonis, B. thetaiotaomicron, and B. vulgatus: designation of neotype strains for Bacteroides fragilis (Veillon and Zuber) Castellani and Chalmers and Bacteroides thetaiotaomicron (Distaso) Castellani and Chalmers. Int. J. Syst. Bacteriol. 26: 230-237.

4. Cato, E.P., and C.W. Salmon. 1976. Transfer of Bacteroides clostridiiformis subsp. clostridiiformis (Burri and Ankersmit) Holdeman and Moore and Bacteroides clostridiiformis subsp. girans (Prévot) Holdeman and Moore, to the genus Clostridium as Clostridium clostridiiforme (Burri and Ankersmit) comb. nov.: emendation of description and designation of neotype strain. Int. J. Syst. Bacteriol. 26: 205-211.

5. Eiken, M. 1958. Studies on an anaerobic, rod-shaped Gram-negative microorganism: Bacteroides corrodens n. sp. Acta Pathol. Microbiol. Scand. 43: 404-416.

6. Finegold, S.M., and E.M. Barnes. 1977. Report of the ICSB Taxonomic Subcommittee on Gram-negative Anaerobic Rods. Proposal that the saccharolytic and asaccharolytic strains at present classified in the species Bacteroides melaninogenicus (Oliver and Wherry) be reclassified in two species as Bacteroides melaninogenicus and Bacteroides asaccharolyticus. Int. J. Syst. Bacteriol. 27: 388-391.

7. Graves, M.H., J.A. Morello, and F.E. Kocha. 1974. Sodium polyanethol sulfonate sensitivity of anaerobic cocci. Appl. Microbiol. 27: 1131-1133.

8. Holdeman, L.V., E.P.Cato, and W.E.C. Moore (ed.). 1977. Anaerobe laboratory manual, 4th ed. Anaerobe Laboratory, Virginia Polytechnic Institute and State University, Blacksburg.

9. Holdeman, L.V., E.P. Cato, J.A. Burmeister, and W.E.C. Moore. 1980. Descriptions of Eubacterium timidum sp. nov., Eubacterium brachy sp. nov., and Eubacterium nodatum sp. nov. isolated from human periodontitis. Int. J. Syst. Bacteriol. 30: (January, in press).

10. Holdeman, L.V., I.J. Good, and W.E.C. Moore. 1976. Human fecal flora: variation in bacterial composition within individuals and a possible effect of emotional stress. Appl. Env. Microbiol. 31: 359-375.

11. Holdeman, L.V., and J.L. Johnson. 1977. Bacterioides disiens sp. nov. and Bacteroides bivius sp. nov. from human clinical infections. Int. J. Syst. Bacteriol. 27: 337-345.

12. Holdeman, L.V., and W.E.C. Moore. 1974. Genus I. Bacteroides Castellani and Chalmers 1919, 959. p. 385-404. In R.E. Buchanan and N.E. Gibbons (ed.). Bergey's manual of determinative bacteriology, eighth ed. Williams and Wilkins, Baltimore.

13. Holdeman, L.V., and W.E.C. Moore. 1974. New genus, Coprococcus, twelve new species, and emended descriptions of four previously described species of bacteria from human feces. Int. J. Syst. Bacteriol. 24: 260-277.

14. Jackson, F.L., and Y.E. Goodman. 1972. Transfer of the facultatively anaerobic organism Bacteroides corrodens Eiken to a new genus, Eikenella. Int. J. Syst. Bacteriol. 22: 73-77.

15. Jackson, F.L., and Y.E. Goodman. 1978. Bacteroides ureolyticus, a new species to accommodate strains previously identified as "Bacteroides corrodens, anaerobic". Int. J. Syst. Bacteriol. 28: 197-200.

16. Jackson, F.L., Y.E. Goodman, F.R. Bel, P.C. Wong, and R.L.S. Whitehouse. 1971. Taxonomic status of facultative and strictly anaerobic "corroding bacilli" that have been classified as Bacteroides corrodens. J. Med. Microbiol. 4: 171-184.

17. Johnson, J.L. 1978. Taxonomy of the Bacteroides. I. Deoxyribonucleic acid homologies among Bacteroides fragilis and other saccharolytic Bacteroides species. Int. J. Syst. Bacteriol. 28: 245-256.

18. Johnson, J.L., and D.A. Ault. 1978. Taxonomy of the Bacteroides. II. Correlation of phenotypic characteristics with deoxyribonucleic acid homology groupings for Bacteroides fragilis and other saccharolytic Bacteroides species. Int. J. Syst. Bacteriol. 28: 257-268.

19. Judicial Commission, International Committee on Systematic Bacteriology. 1979. Minutes of the meeting, 3 September 1978. Int. J. Syst. Bacteriol. 29: 267-269.

20. Kaneuchi, C., T. Miyazato, T. Shinjo, and T. Mitsuoka. 1979. Taxonomic study of helically coiled, sporeforming anaerobes isolated from the intestines of humans and other animals: Clostridium cocleatum sp. nov. and Clostridium spiroforme sp. nov. Int. J. Syst. Bacteriol. 29: 1-12.

21. Kaneuchi, C., K. Watanabe, A. Terada, Y. Benno, and T. Mitsuoka. 1976. Taxonomic study of Bacteroides clostridiiformis subsp. clostridiiformis (Burri and Ankersmit) Holdeman and Moore and of related organisms: proposal of Clostridium clostridiiforme (Burri and Ankersmit) comb. nov. and Clostridium symbiosum (Stevens) comb. nov. Int. J. Syst. Bacteriol. 26: 195-204, 341.

22. Leadbetter, E.R., S.C. Holt, and S. S. Socransky. 1979. Capnocytophaga: new genus of gram-negative gliding bacteria. I. General characteristics, taxonomic considerations and significance. Arch. Microbiol. 122: 9-16.

23. Loesche, W.J., S.S. Socransky, and R.J. Gibbons. 1964. Bacteroides oralis, proposed new species isolated from the oral cavity of man. J. Bacteriol. 88: 1329-1337.

24. Mitsuoka, T., A. Terada, K. Watanabe, and K. Uchida. 1974. Bacteroides multiacidus a new species from the feces of humans and pigs. Int. J. Syst. Bacteriol. 24: 35-41.

25. Moore, W.E.C., and L.V. Holdeman. 1974. Human fecal flora: the normal flora of 20 Japanese-Hawaiians. Appl. Microbiol. 27: 961-979.

26. Newman, M.G., V.L. Sutter, M.J. Pickett, U. Blachman, J.R. Greenwood, V. Grinenko, and D. Citron. 1979. Detection, identification, and comparison of Capnocytophaga, Bacteroides ochraceus, and DF-1. J. Clin. Microbiol. 10: 557-562.

27. Prévot, A.R., P. Tardieux, L. Joubert, and F. de Cadore. 1956. Recherches sur Fusiformis nucleatus (Knorr) et son pouvoir pathogène pour l'homme et les animaux. Ann. Inst. Pasteur (Paris) 91: 788-798.

28. Reiley, P.S., H.W. Tatum, and R.E. Weaver. 1973. Identity of HB-1 of King and Eikenella corrodens (Eiken) Jackson and Goodman. Int. J. Syst. Bacteriol. 23: 75-76.

29. Sebald, M. 1962. Étude sur les bactéries anaérobies gram-négatives asporulées. Thèses de l'Université Paris. Imprimerie Barnéoud S.A. Laval, France.

30. Smibert, R.M. 1978. The genus Campylobacter. Ann. Rev. Microbiol. 32: 673-709.

31. Smibert, R.M., and L.V. Holdeman. 1976. Clinical isolates of anaerobic Gram-negative rods with a formate-fumarate energy metabolism. Bacteroides corrodens, Vibrio succinogenes, and unidentified strains. J. Clin. Microbiol. 3: 432-437.

32. Socransky, S.S., S.C. Holt, E.R. Leadbetter, A.C.R. Tanner, E. Savitt, and B.F. Hammond. 1979. Capnocytophaga: a new genus of gram-negative gliding bacteria. III. Physiological characterization. Arch. Microbiol. 122: 29-34.

33. Sørensen, G.H., 1973. Micrococcus indolicus. Some biochemical properties and the demonstration of six antigenically different types. Acta Veg. Scand. 14: 301-326.

34. Sperry, J.F., and T.D. Wilkins. 1976. Arginine, a growth-limiting factor for Eubacterium lentum. J. Bacteriol. 127: 780-784.

35. Świtalski, L.M., O. Schwan, C.J. Smyth, and T. Wadström. 1978. Peptocoagulase: clotting factor produced by bovine strains of Peptococcus indolicus. J. Clin. Microbiol. 7: 361-367.

36. van Palenstein-Helderman, W.H., and I. Rosman. 1976. Hydrogen-dependent organisms from the human gingival crevice resembling Vibrio succinogenes. Antonie van Leeuwenhoek J. Microbiol. Serol. 42: 107-118.

37. Werner, H., G. Rintelen, and H. Kunstek-Santos. 1975. A new butyric acid-producing Bacteroides species: B. splanchnicus n. sp. Zbl. Bakt. Hyg. I. Abt. Orig. A 231: 133-144.

38. West, S.E.H., and L.V. Holdeman. 1973. Placement of the name Peptococcus anaerobius (Hamm) Douglas on the list of nomina rejicienda. Int. J. Syst. Bacteriol. 23: 283-289.

39. Wilkins, T.D., W.E.C. Moore, S.E.H. West, and L.V. Holdeman. 1975. Peptococcus niger (Hall) Kluyver and van Niel 1936: emendation of description and designation of neotype strain. Int. J. Syst. Bacteriol. 25: 47-49.

40. Williams, B.L., D. Hollis, and L.V. Holdeman. 1979. Synonymy of strains of Center for Disease Control group DF-1 with species of Capnocytophaga. J. Clin. Microbiol. 10: 550-556.

41. Wolin, M.J., E.A. Wolin, and N.J. Jacobs. 1961. Cytochrome-producing anaerobic vibrio, Vibrio succinogenes, sp. n. J. Bacteriol. 81: 911-917.

ANAEROBIC FLORA OF THE FEMALE GENITAL TRACT

Gale B. Hill

Department of Obstetrics/Gynecology
Department of Microbiology/Immunology
Duke University Medical Center
Durham, North Carolina

INTRODUCTION

Early investigators realized that knowledge of the endogenous flora of the lower genital tract was basic to an understanding of obstetric and gynecologic infectious diseases. They surmised that alterations of the normal flora state might produce local infections such as vaginitis, and later it became apparent that certain organisms in the flora could produce ascending infections involving the upper genital tract. Today the importance of the endogenous flora as a source of genital tract infections is widely recognized.

Concepts of the endogenous vaginal flora have undergone considerable change. Prior to 1900 it was proposed that Döderlein's bacillus (lactobacilli) constituted the normal flora throughout women's menstrual life and during pregnancy and that the presence of other organisms was pathologic or abnormal. This concept was considered too restrictive and was later modified to include yeast and Staphylococcus epidermidis which also might be present with lactobacilli in the normal vagina.

Present data indicate that it is unrealistic to conclude that one particular flora (lactobacilli) is normal and that other patterns of flora are abnormal. A vaginal flora consisting primarily of lactobacilli has been observed in a minority of women although it, in fact, may be the most effective in maintaining a healthy vagina and minimizing infections of the upper genital tract. The pattern of endogenous flora depends on the population studied with regard to age, hormonal status, and socioeconomic group. The relationships of other factors such as sexual practices, nutrition, immunologic status, local or systemic drugs or chemicals, and hygiene are inadequately studied but probably are important in determining the flora and may account for many of the differences among various socioeconomic groups or individuals of the same age and hormonal status.

The endogenous flora of an individual is dynamic rather than static. Changes in flora which occur with age from the neonatal period to the post climacteric state are believed to be primarily dependent on hormonal status. Under the influence of estrogen glycogen increases in the vaginal mucosa and appears to encourage the growth of lactobacilli. Lactobacilli supposedly metabolize the glycogen to form acid which, in turn, tends to restrict the flora to these more acidotolerant species. Indeed, there is a rough parallel between the estrogen level during life and the incidence of lactobacilli; a higher incidence of lactobacilli are observed during menstrual life and particularly in pregnant women as opposed to premenarchal and post climacteric women. This concept, however, does not explain the multiplicity of other aerobes and anaerobes which may occur in the presence (or absence) of lactobacilli. Changes in the endogenous flora also occur coincidental with different phases of the menstrual cycle (1) and throughout pregnancy (9).

Recent studies have demonstrated that anaerobic bacteria are important constituents of the endogenous flora and are numerically predominant (1,16) in certain, and probably most, populations. In earlier investigations culture of anaerobic bacteria was either not attempted or the methods were most often inadequate. Interest in culture of anaerobic bacteria from the vagina followed the observations in the late 1920's of investigators (13,19) who demonstrated that anaerobic cocci were important agents in puerperal fever and were probably endogenous in origin (13). Because of this association with puerperal morbidity and mortality the anaerobic Gram-positive cocci were emphasized and frequently were isolated from infectious material (6,13,19) and from vaginal secretions in both obstetric (3,13) and gynecologic patients (3). Anaerobic Gram-negative bacilli were rarely mentioned in these earlier studies (3, 4), but recent investigations have demonstrated their common occurrence in the endogenous flora (1,9,10,12,16,17,22) and importance in genital tract infections (4,5,7,8,11,18,20,21,23). The media and anaerobic culture techniques available earlier probably did not support growth or facilitate the isolation of these organisms in most cases, but the actual incidence of anaerobic Gram-negative rods in the endogenous flora and in infection possibly may have increased.

VAGINAL FLORA OF PREMENOPAUSAL WOMEN

A study of the vaginal flora of premenopausal women which emphasized the recovery of anaerobic organisms in addition to aerobic and facultative bacteria was performed at Duke University Medical Center with the collaboration of Stanley Gall, M.D., Alfreda Kohan, M.T.

(ASCP), and Ouida Ayers, M.T. (ASCP). Sixty-five public and private patients who were entering the hospital for vaginal hysterectomy mainly for benign conditions were cultured from the posterior fornix of the vagina. Swab specimens were collected in a B-D Anaerobic Specimen Collector (Becton Dickinson & Co., Rutherford, N.J.) and immediately transported to the Anaerobic Microbiology Laboratory. In the laboratory a direct smear for Gram stain was prepared, and the specimen was placed in an anaerobic glove box (Coy Laboratory Products, Inc., Ann Arbor, MI) for inoculation of media. Anaerobic media included anaerobically stored brucella blood agar supplemented with 0.5 ug/ml menadione, 5 ug/ml hemin, and 5% defibrinated sheep blood, phenylethyl alcohol agar with 0.5% yeast extract in addition to supplements mentioned above, and kanamycin-vancomycin blood agar in which 75 ug/ml of kanamycin and 7.5 ug/ml of vancomycin were present with the above supplements in lysed blood agar. Anaerobic chopped meat carbohydrate broth (Carr-Scarborough Microbiologicals, Atlanta, Ga.) was inoculated as a backup broth. Media for aerobic and facultative organisms (subsequently termed aerobes) included sheep blood agar, colistin-nalidixic acid blood agar, MacConkey agar, and chocolate agar. Media for aerobes were placed in a CO_2 incubator at 35 C for a total of four days, and organisms were identified using standard laboratory procedures. Anaerobic media was incubated in the anaerobic glove box at 35 C for a total of seven and 14 days for plate media and broth, respectively. The anaerobic bacteria were identified by Gram stain morphology, gas liquid chromatography and biochemical tests using the API 20A (Analytab Products, Chamblee, Ga.) in addition to media and techniques as described in the Virginia Polytechnic Institute Anaerobe Laboratory Manual (14). Strains belonging to anaerobic genera were listed as microaerophilic if they demonstrated more luxuriant growth under anaerobic conditions but would grow in a CO_2 incubator either initially or after several transfers. The concentration of each organism in the flora was estimated semiquantitatively (1+ to 4+) by observing the growth in sequentially streaked zones on primary plating media. The nomenclature used for the anaerobic isolates is taken from the Virginia Polytechnic Institute Anaerobe Laboratory Manual (14).

Of the 65 women cultured 91% had obligately anaerobic bacteria, and 97% had aerobic bacteria present in the vagina. All women were positive for some aerotolerance type - aerobic, anaerobic, or microaerophilic; and a mixture of aerotolerance types was found in 94% of these women. On the average 9.1 different species, consisting of 3.9 aerobic, 0.5 microaerophilic, and 4.7 anaerobic, were isolated per patient. Up to 16 different species were isolated in a single patient. Thus, anaerobes were isolated from almost all of the patients, and a greater number of obligate anaerobes (305 strains) were isolated than were aerobes (251 strains) or microaerophiles (35 strains).

Anaerobic Gram-positive cocci, Gram-positive bacilli, and Gram-negative bacilli each were harbored by over one-half of these 65 women (Table 1). When patients were positive for either Gram-positive cocci or Gram-negative bacilli, generally two to three different species belonging to the group were simultaneously present (Table 1). On the average slightly less than two species of Gram-positive bacilli were simultaneously present, but Gram-negative cocci tended to occur singly. The anaerobic Gram-negative cocci consisted primarily of Veillonella parvula (20% of patients), and there was only one isolation of Acidaminococcus fermentans.

Peptococci were the most common anaerobic Gram-positive cocci isolated (in 58% of patients), whereas peptostreptococci were isolated less frequently overall (in 31%). The most common species of Peptococcus were Peptococcus asaccharolyticus, Peptococcus prevotii, and Peptococcus magnus, whereas Peptostreptococcus anaerobius was the major representative of the genus Peptostreptococcus (Table 2). This accounts for the higher percentage of peptococci observed although P. anaerobius was isolated from a similar percentage of patients as was each of the predominant species of Peptococcus (Table 2). Gaffkya anaerobia also was isolated frequently. A substantial number of cocci could not be speciated satisfactorily (Table 2). Obligately anaerobic Gram-positive cocci accounted for 37% of the total anaerobic isolates.

Lactobacillus was the most commonly isolated anaerobic Gram-positive bacillus (Table 3). Most isolates were obligately anaerobic

Table 1. Frequency of Anaerobic Bacteria by Group from the Vaginal Flora of 65 Premenopausal Women

Group	Total Isolates/ Positive Patients	Percent[a] of Patients
Gram-positive cocci[b]	121/52	80
Gram-positive bacilli[b]	85/47	72
Gram-negative bacilli	105/41	63
Gram-negative cocci	16/15	23

[a] Patients positive for one or more species.

[b] Includes microaerophilic strains.

Table 2. Anaerobic[a] Gram-positive Cocci from the Vaginal Flora of 65 Premenopausal Women

Species	Number of Isolates	Percent of Patients
Peptococcus		
P. asaccharolyticus	21	32
P. prevotii	18	28
P. magnus	16	25
Peptostreptococcus		
P. anaerobius	19	29
P. micros	2	3
Gaffkya anaerobia	18	28
Streptococcus		
S. intermedius	5	8
S. constellatus	1	2
S. morbillorum	1	2
Species, unidentifiable	20	29

[a] Includes microaerophilic strains of Streptococcus.

(from 38% of patients), but if microaerophilic strains (Table 4) are included 55% of patients had one or more species of anaerobic and/or microaerophilic lactobacilli. The many different species of lactobacilli isolated demonstrates the diversity of this group representing Döderlein's bacillus, and many isolates could not be reliably speciated (Tables 3 and 4). Obligately anaerobic isolates of Corynebacterium vaginale (Haemophilus vaginalis) were observed in seven patients. A variety of clostridia, including four isolations of Clostridium perfringens, and other Gram-positive bacilli were isolated from fewer patients (Tables 3 and 4).

Two newly described species (15), Bacteroides bivius and Bacteroides disiens, were the most frequently isolated anaerobic Gram-negative bacilli (Table 5). Bacteroides melaninogenicus has been described previously from the vaginal flora, and in the present study Bacteroides melaninogenicus subsp. intermedius was most common. Bacteroides asaccharolyticus which formerly was classified as a subspecies of B. melaninogenicus was present somewhat less frequently. Only 5% of patients harbored Bacteroides fragilis, and altogether

Table 3. Anaerobic Gram-positive Bacilli from the Vaginal Flora of 65 Premenopausal Women

Species	Number of Isolates	Percent of Patients
Lactobacillus		
L. minutus	4	6
L. delbrueckii	3	5
L. acidophilus	2	3
L. fermentum	2	3
L. leichmannii	1	2
L. casei subsp. casei	1	2
species, unidentifiable	16	25
Corynebacterium		
C. vaginale	7	11
species, unidentifiable	2	3
Clostridium		
C. perfringens	4	6
C. innocuum	2	3
C. indolis	1	2
C. ramosum	1	2
C. mangenoti	1	2
Bifidobacterium		
B. adolescentis	1	2
species, unidentifiable	2	3
Propionibacterium acnes	2	3
Eubacterium lentum	1	2
Species, unidentifiable	5	8

the former subspecies of B. fragilis were present in 11% of these patients (two subspecies were isolated from each of two patients). However, a large percentage of the Bacteroides isolated could not be speciated. Fusobacterium naviforme and Fusobacterium nucleatum were the most common fusobacteria (Table 5); the fusobacteria were observed less frequently than the Bacteroides. Anaerobic Gram-negative bacilli accounted for 34% of all anaerobic isolates.

Aerobic Gram-positive cocci and Gram-positive bacilli were also

Table 4. Microaerophilic Gram-positive Bacilli from the Vaginal Flora of 65 Premenopausal Women

Species	Number of Isolates	Percent of Patients
Lactobacillus		
L. leichmannii	6	9
L. fermentum	4	6
L. acidophilus	3	5
L. casei subsp. casei	1	2
L. casei subsp. rhamnosus	1	2
L. jensenii	1	2
species, unidentifiable	6	9
Bifidobacterium		
B. longum	1	2
species, unidentifiable	2	3
Corynebacterium vaginale	1	2
Species, unidentifiable	1	2

commonly isolated and were present in 82% and 78% of patients, respectively. Aerobic Gram-negative bacilli were isolated from 38% of these patients. The most frequent isolates of aerobic Gram-positive cocci were alpha- and nonhemolytic-streptococci, S. epidermidis, and in somewhat fewer patients, enterococci. The most frequent aerobic Gram-positive bacilli were diphtheroids and C. vaginale; aerobic strains of lactobacilli were less common than the anaerobic or microaerophilic strains of lactobacilli. Escherichia coli was the most common aerobic Gram-negative bacillus; a variety of other species were isolated infrequently.

DISCUSSION

Investigations during the 1970's of the endogenous genital tract flora emphasized premenopausal or pregnant women (1,9,10,16,17,22); fewer studies utilizing modern anaerobic techniques were published on preadolescent (12) and post-climacteric (22) populations. Most often the upper vagina has been sampled. The frequencies and species of anaerobes are similar in the cervix and vagina. However, recent data (2) have demonstrated that within an individual the species in the endocervix may be quite different from those in the vagina, suggesting that specific ecologic niches are present. There has been greater agreement among different studies regarding the frequency and

Table 5. Anaerobic Gram-negative Bacilli from the Vaginal Flora of 65 Premenopausal Women

Species	Number of Isolates	Percent of Patients
Bacteroides		
B. bivius	22	34
B. disiens	12	18
B. melaninogenicus[a]	8	12
B. asaccharolyticus	4	6
B. ruminicola subsp. brevis	4	6
B. coagulans	3	5
B. capillosus	3	5
B. fragilis	3	5
B. vulgatus	3	5
B. ovatus	2	3
B. oralis	2	3
B. thetaiotaomicron	1	2
species, unidentifiable	24	37
Fusobacterium		
F. naviforme	5	8
F. nucleatum	4	6
F. gonidiaformans	2	3
F. russii	2	3
species, unidentifiable	1	2

[a] Includes subsp. intermedius 7 isolates, 11% of patients; subsp. melaninogenicus 1 isolate, 2% of patients.

types of aerobic bacteria isolated than for the anaerobic bacteria. Greater discrepancies in frequency and types of anaerobic species isolated, as compared to aerobes, may be the result of (i) differences in patient population, but more important, (ii) differences in anaerobic methods such as specimen collection, transport to laboratory, primary isolation media, anaerobic culture environment, and identification methods. For example, if only non-selective isolation media are used only the most predominant species would be isolated normally, whereas the use of selective and non-selective media will produce a greater number of different species. The influences of all these variables on past and present (1,10,16,17,22) study results for the premenopausal population are demonstrated by differences in the frequency of isolation of anaerobes (range 70% of patients to approximately 94%), the average number of species of aerobic and anaerobic bacteria per sample (range four to nine), the frequency of isolation of each group of anaerobic bacteria (by Gram stain morphology, e.g., Gram-positive cocci), and the species representing each group.

The particular species of anaerobic Gram-positive cocci isolated have been similar among the recent flora studies when speciation has been performed. Importantly, these same species (from the present study - P. anaerobius, P. asaccharolyticus, P. magnus, P. prevotii, and G. anaerobia) are also the most commonly isolated anaerobic Gram-positive cocci from obstetric and gynecologic infections. Among the anaerobic Gram-negative bacilli there has been less agreement. Previous reports have not demonstrated B. bivius and B. disiens as prominant members of the vaginal flora. These organisms were described and named in 1977 (15), but they probably were represented in earlier reports as unidentifiable Bacteroides species or mistakenly identified as Bacteroides oralis or B. melaninogenicus subsp. intermedius which they resemble in certain cultural and morphological characteristics. In some instances they may not have been isolated since they are more difficult to culture than many other Bacteroides. The primary clinical source of both of these organisms apparently is from obstetric and gynecologic infections. At our hospital B. bivius is more common from these infections than is B. fragilis, whereas B. disiens is less frequently isolated. B. melaninogenicus and B. asaccharolyticus which were the next most frequently isolated species from the endogenous flora are also common in infection. With few exceptions (9,10) among this and other recent studies (1,16,17,22) B. fragilis has been infrequently isolated from the endogenous flora (generally less than 10% of the study population), even when all former subspecies (B. fragilis, Bacteroides vulgatus, Bacteroides ovatus, Bacteroides thetaiotaomicron, and Bacteroides distasonis) were included.

Whereas the frequency of isolation of most anaerobic Gram-positive cocci and Gram-negative bacilli from the vaginal flora generally reflects their incidence in genital tract infection, the situation is different for the anaerobic Gram-positive bacilli and Gram-negative cocci. Gram-positive anaerobic bacilli were commonly found in the vaginal flora in the present study but are much less common and significant in clinical infection. The reported incidence of anaerobic lactobacilli, clostridia, propionibacteria, and bifidobacteria in the endogenous flora has varied considerably among recent studies. This is also true for anaerobic Gram-negative cocci (range from 1% to 27% in the study populations).

A common generalization is that B. fragilis is resistant to ordinary doses of the penicillin class of antibiotics, although other anaerobic Gram-negative bacilli are susceptible. Yet, in the endogenous flora broader resistance to these antibiotics is apparent. In the present study approximately one-third of all Bacteroides isolated were resistant to ampicillin (at 4 ug/ml). Resistance to penicillin among B. bivius and B. disiens strains has been described (15); approximately one-fourth of our isolates of B. bivius and one-fifth of the B. disiens isolates were resistant to ampicillin. Increasing resistance has also been noted with B. melaninogenicus strains. Thus, it can be anticipated that anaerobic Gram-negative bacilli involved in genital tract infections will frequently be resistant to penicillin-type antibiotics.

Because certain members of the endogenous flora are opportunistic pathogens in lower and upper genital tract infection it is important to understand the factors, probably external and host-related, which control the microbiologic composition of this flora. There is evidence, mainly indirect, that the composition of the endogenous flora is an important determinant of the infection rate among various populations. Yet, the basis for the potential pathogenicity of certain members of the flora is understood poorly. The incidence and relative concentration of certain anaerobic bacteria from the vaginal flora reflect their incidence in genital tract infection, but for other organisms this correlation does not exist. This situation parallels data on the endogenous flora of the gastrointestinal tract and infections deriving from that source. Another aspect of the composition of the flora which is incompletely studied, but probably quite important, is bacterial synergism or antagonism. Synergism is an important factor in production of anaerobic or polymicrobic infection. It can be anticipated that improved understanding of the cervical and vaginal bacterial ecology will further the progress in prevention and treatment of genital tract infection.

LITERATURE CITED

1. Bartlett, J.G., A.B. Onderdonk, E. Drude, C. Goldstein, M. Anderka, S. Alpert, and W.M. McCormack. 1977. Quantitative bacteriology of the vaginal flora. J. Infect. Dis. 136: 271-277.

2. Bartlett, J.G., N.E. Moon, P.R. Goldstein, B. Goren, A.B. Onderdonk, and B.F. Polk. 1978. Cervical and vaginal bacterial flora: Ecologic niches in the female lower genital tract. Am. J. Obstet. Gynecol. 130: 658-661.

3. Carter, B., and C.P. Jones. 1937. A study of the vaginal flora in the normal female. South. Med. J. 30: 298-304.

4. Carter, B., C.P. Jones, R.L. Alter, R.N. Creadick, and W.L. Thomas. 1953. Bacteroides infections in obstetrics and gynecology. Obstet. & Gynecol. 1: 491-510.

5. Chow, A.W., J.R. Marshall, and L.B. Guze. 1975. Anaerobic infections of the female genital tract: Prospects and perspectives. Obstet. Gynecol. Surv. 30: 477-494.

6. Colebrook, L. 1930. Infection by anaerobic streptococci in puerperal fever. Br. Med. J. 2: 134-137.

7. Eschenbach, D.A., T.M. Buchanan, H.M. Pollock, P.S. Forsyth, E.R. Alexander, J.S. Lin, S.P. Wang, B.B. Wentworth, W.M. McCormack, and K.K. Holmes. 1975. Polymicrobial etiology of acute pelvic inflammatory disease. N. Eng. J. Med. 293: 166-171.

8. Finegold, S.M., J.G. Bartlett, A.W. Chow, D.J. Flora, S.L. Gorbach, E.J. Harder, and F.P. Tally. 1975. Management of anaerobic infections. Ann. Intern. Med. 83: 375-389.

9. Goplerud, C.P., M.J. Ohm, and R.P. Galask. 1976. Aerobic and anaerobic flora of the cervix during pregnancy and the puerperium. Am. J. Obstet. Gynecol. 126: 858-868.

10. Gorbach, S.L., K.B. Menda, H. Thadepalli, and L. Keith. 1973. Anaerobic microflora of the cervix in healthy women. Am. J. Obstet. Gynecol. 117: 1053-1055.

11. Hall, W.L., A.I. Sobel, C.P. Jones, and R.T. Parker. 1967. Anaerobic postoperative pelvic infections. Obstet. Gynecol. 30: 1-7.

12. Hammerschlag, M.R., S. Alpert, A.B. Onderdonk, P. Thurston, E. Drude, W.M. McCormack, and J.G. Bartlett. 1978. Anaerobic microflora of the vagina in children. Am. J. Obstet. Gynecol. 131: 853-856.

13. Harris, J.W., and J.H. Brown. 1929. Clinical and bacteriological study of 113 cases of streptococcic puerperal infection. Bull. Johns Hopkins Hosp. 44: 1-31.

14. Holdeman, L.V., E.P. Cato, and W.E.C. Moore (ed.). 1977. Anaerobe Laboratory Manual, 4th ed. Virginia Polytechnic Institute and State University, Blacksburg.

15. Holdeman, L.V, and J.L. Johnson. 1977. Bacteroides disiens sp. nov. and Bacteroides bivius sp. nov. from human clinical infections. Int. J. Syst. Bacteriol. 27: 337-345.

16. Levison, M.E., L.C. Corman, E.R. Carrington, and D. Kaye. 1977. Quantitative microflora of the vagina. Am. J. Obstet. Gynecol. 127: 80-85.

17. Ohm, M.J., and R.P. Galask. 1975. Bacterial flora of the cervix from 100 prehysterectomy patients. Am. J. Obstet. Gynecol. 122: 683-687.

18. Parker, R.T., and C.P. Jones. 1966. Anaerobic pelvic infections and developments in hyperbaric oxygen therapy. Am. J. Obstet. Gynecol. 96: 645-659.

19. Schwarz, O., and W.J. Dieckmann. 1926. Anaerobic streptococci: Their role in puerperal infection. South. Med. J. 19: 470-479.

20. Sweet, R.L. 1975. Anaerobic infections of the female genital tract. Am. J. Obstet. Gynecol. 122: 891-901.

21. Swenson, R.M., T.C. Michaelson, M.J. Daly, and E.H. Spaulding. 1973. Anaerobic bacterial infections of the female genital tract. Obstet. Gynecol. 42: 538-541.

22. Tashjian, J.H., C.B. Coulam, and J.A. Washington. 1976. Vaginal flora in asymptomatic women. Mayo Clin. Proc. 51: 557-561.

23. Thadepalli, H., S.L. Gorbach, and L. Keith. 1973. Anaerobic infections of the female genital tract: Bacteriologic and therapeutic aspects. Am. J. Obstet. Gynecol. 117: 1034-1040.

A STANDARDIZED DISK METHOD FOR ANTIBIOTIC SUSCEPTIBILITY TESTING FOR ANAEROBES; FOUR YEARS OF ANTIBIOTIC DATA

Dwight W. Lambe, Jr., Professor and Chairman
W. Wayne Laslie*

Department of Microbiology, College of Medicine
East Tennessee State University
Johnson City, Tennessee 37601
*Pfizer Diagnostic Products, International
New York, New York 10017

INTRODUCTION

In vitro antibiotic susceptibility testing of aerobes and facultative bacteria has been a service provided by the clinical laboratory since the 1940's. However, little effort was made to standardize susceptibility tests until 1966 when investigators at the University of Washington in Seattle developed a technique which became known as the Kirby-Bauer technique. The standardized technique employed Mueller-Hinton agar as the test medium and a single high-content disk with a standard concentration of antimicrobic; adjusting the density of the inoculum before inoculating the plate, and the development of interpretive standards based on growth inhibition zone diameters around the disk. These interpretive standards were developed by determining the relationship between zone diameters and the minimal inhibitory concentrations (MIC) and relating this information to the achievable serum levels of the antibiotic after the usual dose was administered to the patient. The Kirby-Bauer technique has been the generally accepted technique throughout the United States for testing rapidly growing aerobes and facultative bacteria.

With advances in techniques, microbiologists are isolating and identifying more anaerobic bacteria from clinical specimens. These organisms are now recognized as causative agents of a significant number and variety of human infections. An awareness of the role of anaerobes in infections has stimulated an interest in the susceptibility of these anaerobic organisms to antimicrobial agents.

Susceptibility testing of anaerobes has been limited to studies done in a few laboratories throughout the country. Some investigators have determined the MIC of antibiotics for anaerobes by broth or agar dilution, while others have developed and used standardized disk techniques. Variables in the disk methods of different investigators have been: growth medium, age of the inoculum, size of the inoculum, anaerobic atmosphere and length of anaerobic incubation. Interpretative values of susceptible, indeterminant, and resistant differ with the method employed.

In the past, clinicians have relied on general guidelines based on predictable patterns of susceptibility of anaerobes to antimicrobial agents. Susceptibility testing has been recommended only in cases involving serious infections, infections failing to respond to therapy and in patients who relapse after antibiotic therapy. The need for day to day susceptibility testing of anaerobes has not been recommended by some workers.

We feel that there is a need for a rapid and reliable method for routine antimicrobial susceptibility testing of anaerobic bacteria for several reasons. First, the use of general guidelines for treatment of anaerobic infections requires knowledge about the identity of the infective organism because there are definite differences in susceptibility depending upon species; data to support this will be presented later. Identification of certain anaerobic species requires longer than in vitro susceptibility testing. Secondly, the information that routine antibiotic testing provides may enable the use of a less toxic antibiotic such as penicillin or erythromycin as opposed to a more toxic antibiotic such as clindamycin or chloramphenicol. Thirdly, data on a large number of strains of different species is needed to determine the general antibiotic patterns of each species as well as to monitor the emergence of strains resistant to certain antibiotics. The classic example of changing resistance is the emergence of tetracycline resistant strains of Bacteroides fragilis. In the late 1960's and early 1970's, tetracycline was the antibiotic of choice to treat B. fragilis infections. Since 1972, however, about 60% of B. fragilis strains are resistant to tetracycline. We, and others, have reported clindamycin resistance in B. fragilis, and we have observed penicillin resistance among various subspecies of Bacteroides melaninogenicus and Bacteroides asaccharolyticus. Recently, other investigators have reported chloramphenicol resistance in B. fragilis.

There are several advantages of the disk test as compared to a tube or plate MIC test. First, the disk test is more reproducible than the MIC test. We (3) have shown statistically that the standardized disk test is ten to 15 times more reproducible than the MIC test. Other investigators have shown similar reproducibility of the disk test for meningococci and sulfonamides (1) and for B. fragilis to tetracycline (4). One source of error with MIC determinations is the accurate weighing of the antibiotic powder, and a second source can be in preparation of dilutions. Secondly, the results of the disk test are interpreted for the clinician so that he knows if the organism is susceptible, indeterminant, or resistant to a particular antibiotic. These interpretations are derived by relating the diameter of the zone of inhibition around the disk to the MIC value of the same organism. The serum level that can be achieved in the patient with the usual dose of antibiotic is also considered. For example, if a strain is determined susceptible by statistical analysis, infections caused by that organism should be treatable by the particular antibiotic. The patient's response to treatment should correlate with in vitro data. An MIC value alone means little to the clinician unless he knows the achievable serum level for each antibiotic. Thirdly, the disk test is easier and quicker to perform than the MIC test.

The results of antibiotic testing of anaerobic bacteria are dependent upon several variables: test medium, depth of medium, inoculum size, incubation temperature, incubation atmosphere, and antibiotic deterioration in disks. We have taken into account these variables in our standardized disk method.

STANDARDIZED DISK METHOD FOR ANTIBIOTIC SUSCEPTIBILITY TESTING OF ANAEROBIC BACTERIA

A. Preparation of Media

1. One-half of a No. 1 McFarland standard

   1% (0.36 N) H_2SO_4 (1 ml concentrated H_2SO_4 to 99 ml water)
   1% $BaCl_2$ (1 g $BaCl_2$/100 ml water)
   Add 0.1 ml of 1% $BaCl_2$ to 19.9 ml of 1% H_2SO_4 in screw cap tube.
   Replace once a month as it is not stable for long periods of time.

2. Mueller-Hinton Agar Plates

Mueller-Hinton Agar (Difco)	19 g
Distilled Water	500 ml

   Adjust the medium to pH 7.4. Autoclave at 121 C for 15 min.
   Slow exhaust. Cool to 45-50 C. Add 5 ml Vitamin K_1-Hemin solution and 25 ml defibrinated sheep blood. Recheck the pH of the medium; the final pH should be between 7.4 and 7.6.
   If using 90 mm x 15 mm Petri plates, dispense 30 ml into each plate.
   If using 150 mm x 15 mm Petri plates, dispense 80 ml into each plate.
   Place these plates under anaerobic conditions as soon as they solidify.

3. Mueller-Hinton Broth

Mueller-Hinton Broth (Difco)	10.5 g
Distilled Water	500 ml

Autoclave at 121 C for 15 min. Slow exhaust. Cool broth to 45-50 C. Add 5 ml of Vitamin K_1-Hemin solution. Dispense aseptically with a sterile automatic syringe into sterile 16 x 150 mm tubes with tightly fitting caps. Dispense 5 ml into each tube. Place under anaerobic conditions immediately.

4. Brain Heart Infusion Broth

Brain Heart Infusion Broth (Difco)	37 g
Yeast Extract (Difco)	5 g
Resazurin Solution	4 ml
L (+) Cysteine Hydrochloride	0.5 g
Distilled Water	1000 ml

Autoclave at 121 C for 15 min. Slow exhaust. Add 10 ml Vitamin K_1-Hemin solution.
Dispense aseptically with a sterile automatic syringe into sterile 16 x 150 mm tubes with tightly fitting caps. Dispense 10 ml into each tube. Place under anaerobic conditions immediately.

5. Reagents

a. Vitamin K_1-Hemin Solution (VKH)
   (1) Vitamin K_1 Stock Solution
   Add 0.375 ml of Vitamin K_1 (Sigma Chemical Co.) to 25 ml of ethyl alcohol. Cover flask, stir with magnetic stirrer for 30 min or until Vitamin K_1 is in solution. Filter sterilize. Store at room temperature (RT).
   (2) Hemin Stock Solution
   Dissolve 0.25 g Hemin in 5 ml of 1N NaOH. Add 500 ml distilled water. Autoclave at 121 C for 15 min.
   (3) VKH Solution
   Aseptically add 5 ml of the Vitamin K_1 stock solution to the 500 ml of sterile Hemin solution. Mix. Dispense aseptically in 5 ml amounts into sterile screw cap tubes. Store at RT.
   (4) Add 1 tube (5 ml) of VKH solution to 500 ml of medium requiring VKH.

b. Resazurin Solution
Dissolve 1 tablet (about 11 mg) in 44 ml of distilled water. Add 4 ml of this stock solution to each 1000 ml of medium.

6. Anaerobic Atmosphere:

We use a gas mixture consisting of 80% N_2, 10% H_2, and 10% CO_2 to maintain anaerobic conditions in vented jars and in the anaerobe chamber. A Gas-Pak anaerobe jar has the same atmosphere.

B. Storage of Antibiotic Test Media

1. The media for antibiotic susceptibility testing of anaerobic bacteria include: Mueller-Hinton Broth supplemented with VKH (MHBS); Brain Heart Infusion Broth supplemented with VKH (BHIBS); and Mueller-Hinton Agar supplemented with blood and VKH (MHAS). These media are placed in an anaerobic atmosphere of 80% N_2, 10% H_2, and 10% CO_2 as soon as possible after preparation. Storage in this atmosphere can be in an anaerobe chamber, in a Gas-Pak anaerobe jar or in a vented anaerobe jar.

2. The MHAS plates should be used the same day they are prepared. BHIBS and MHBS may be stored in an anaerobic atmosphere for up to three weeks. We do not recommend use of these two media beyond three weeks.

3. Media stored in an anaerobic atmosphere are classified as reduced media; they are not pre-reduced media.

C. Antibiotic Disk Method

Use MHAS plates on the day of preparation.

1. Inoculum. Inoculate reduced BHIBS with a pure culture; this may be a colony from a plate or a drop from a pre-reduced broth culture. Incubate the BHIBS culture anaerobically at 35 C for 24 h or until good growth is obtained.
2. Add the 24 h BHIBS culture dropwise with a sterile Pasteur pipette to MHBS to obtain a turbidity of one-half that of a No. 1 McFarland nephelometer standard. Mix the diluted culture well on a Vortex mixer or by careful swirling of the tube by hand.
3. Insert a sterile cotton swab into the diluted culture. Press the swab against the tube wall to remove excess inoculum.
4. If the surface of the MHAS plate is wet, remove excess moisture with a sterile swab. Discard swab. With a new swab, inoculate the MHAS plate evenly in three directions.
5. Allow the surface of the medium to dry for 3 to 5 min.
6. Place antibiotic disks on the surface of the medium. Do not use more than 4 or 5 disks per plate; this will help to avoid overlapping zones. Avoid placing penicillin disks

side by side since these zones may be large, especially with the anaerobic cocci.

7. Place the plates in an anaerobic atmosphere for 24 h.
8. Record the zone of inhibition to the nearest mm at 24 h if sufficient growth is obtained. If growth is insufficient, reincubate plates and read zones of inhibition at 48 h. Do not record zones after 48 h. If an inner zone of diminished growth is observed, measure to the inner edge of this zone.
9. Use the interpretive scheme as follows:

ANTIBIOTIC	DISK POTENCY	RESISTANT	INDETERMINANT	SUSCEPTIBLE
Penicillin (2)[a]	10 Units	≤8 mm	9-20 mm	≥21 mm
Carbenicillin (3)[a]	100 ug	≤8 mm	9-12 mm	≥13 mm
Tetracycline (4)[a]	30 ug	≤18 mm	19-20 mm	≥21 mm
Clindamycin	2 ug		6-11 mm	≥12 mm
Chloramphenicol[b]	30 ug		≤24 mm	≥25 mm
Cefoxitin	30 ug	≤8 mm	9-20 mm	≥21 mm

[a] See literature cited.
[b] Lambe and Laslie (unpublished data).

RESULTS AND DISCUSSION

The addition of any components, such as blood, to the medium may affect susceptibility results by decreasing zone sizes by 1 to 2 mm. Since our interpretive values have been obtained on a medium which contains blood, this decrease in zone size has been considered in the interpretive scheme.

One of the most important variables in antimicrobic susceptibility testing is the number of organisms in the inoculum. The inoculum must be large enough to detect high mutation rates to resistance; the inoculum should not be smaller than populations anticipated in significant lesions. The incubation atmosphere is also important. Incubation of test media with antibiotic disks in 5 to 10% CO_2 shifts the pH of the surface of the agar toward the acid range. Some antibiotics are less active in an anaerobic atmosphere than in an aerobic atmosphere. For example, lincomycin and macrolides such as erythromycin will have smaller zone sizes in an anaerobic atmosphere of increased CO_2 than in an aerobic atmosphere of decreased CO_2.

The deterioration of antibiotics, especially penicillins and cephalosporins which lose activity easily, must be monitored. The potency of disks is monitored by the daily use of standard anaerobic

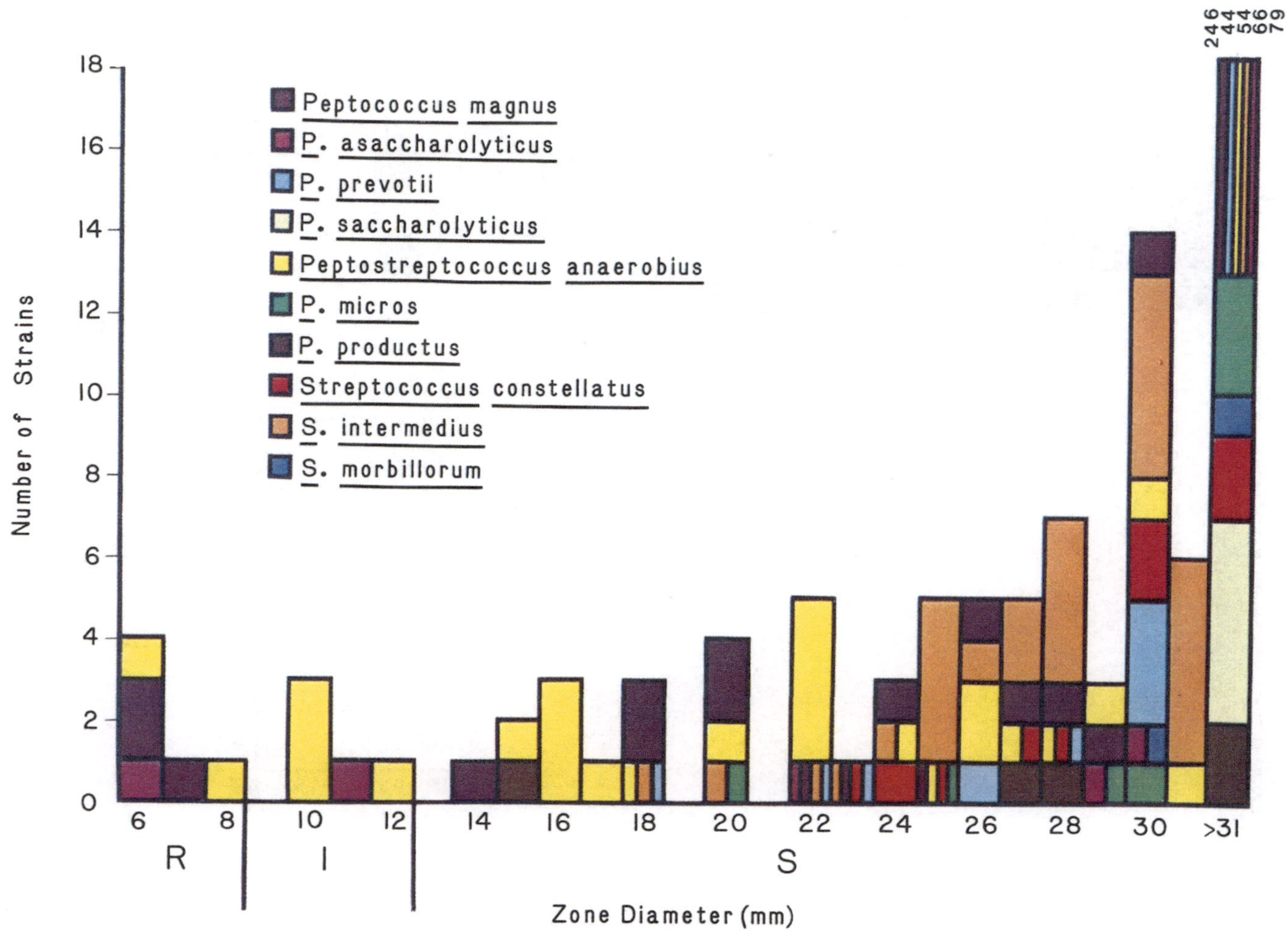

Fig. 1. Distribution of zone diameters of ten anaerobic Gram-positive cocci species with 100 ug carbenicillin disks. Data collected 1974-1977.

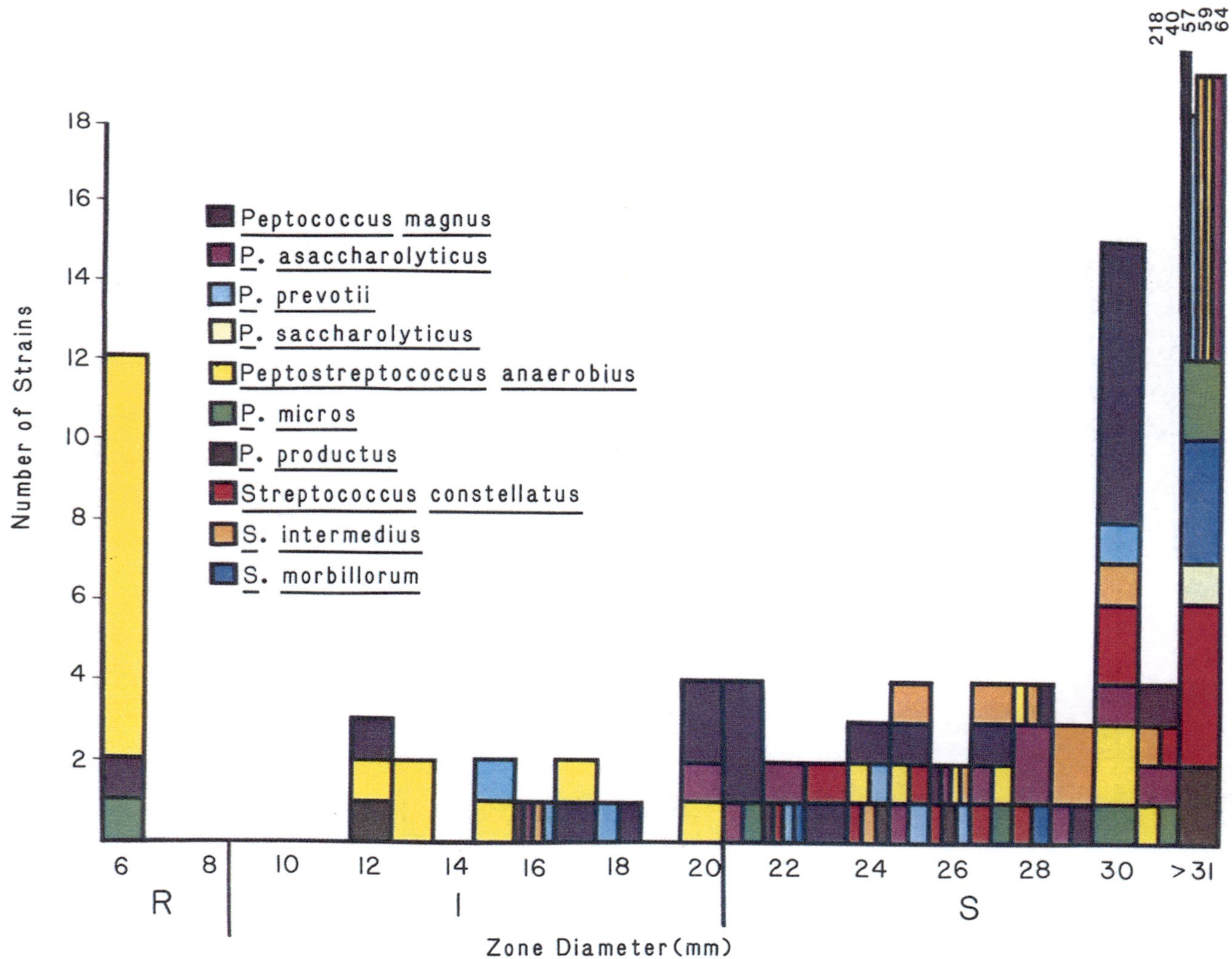

Fig. 2. Distribution of zone diameters of ten anaerobic Gram-positive cocci species with 10 Unit penicillin disks. Data collected 1974-1977.

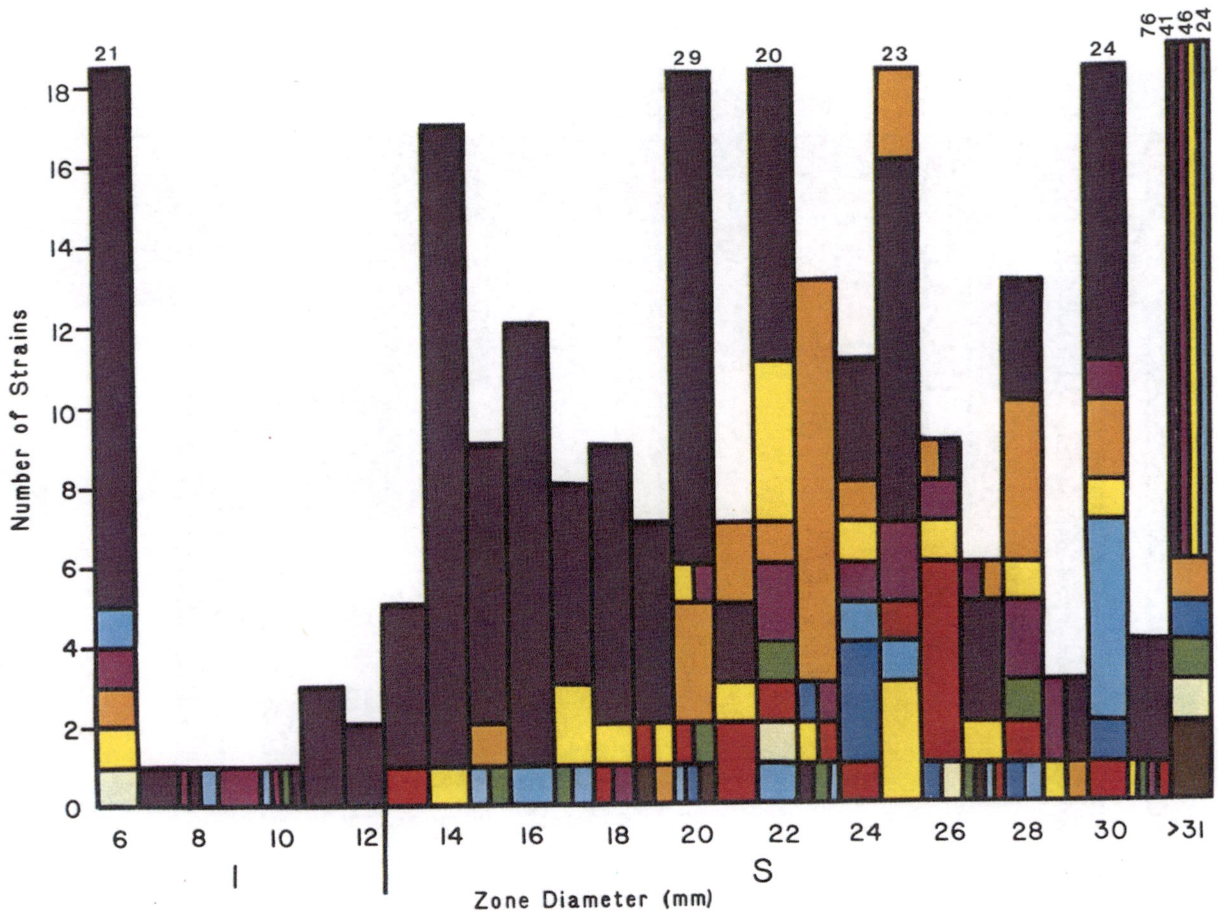

Fig. 3. Distribution of zone diameters of ten anaerobic Gram-positive cocci species with 2 ug clindamycin disks. Data collected 1974-1977.

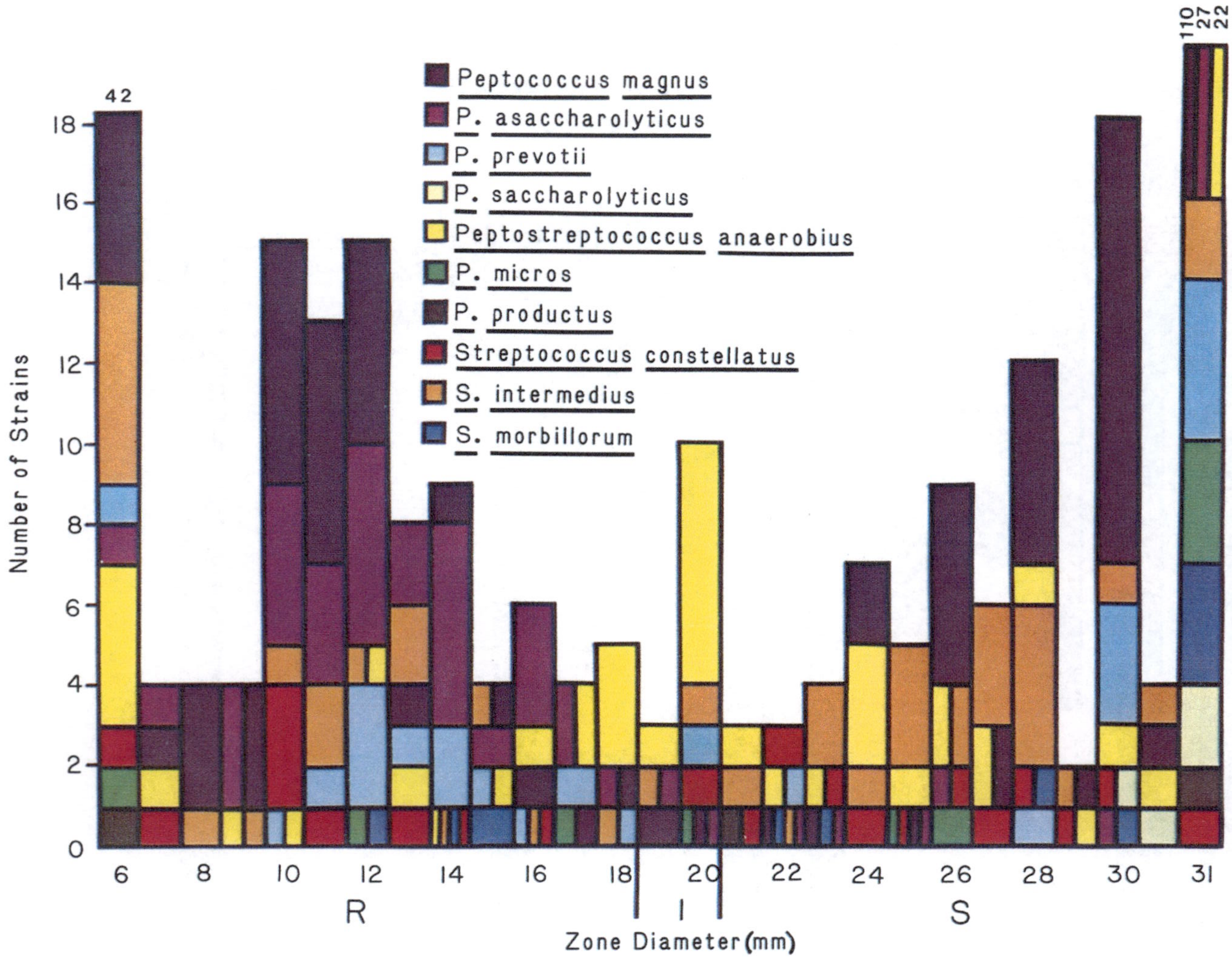

Fig. 4. Distribution of zone diameters of ten anaerobic Gram-positive cocci species with 30 ug tetracycline disks. Data collected 1974-1977.

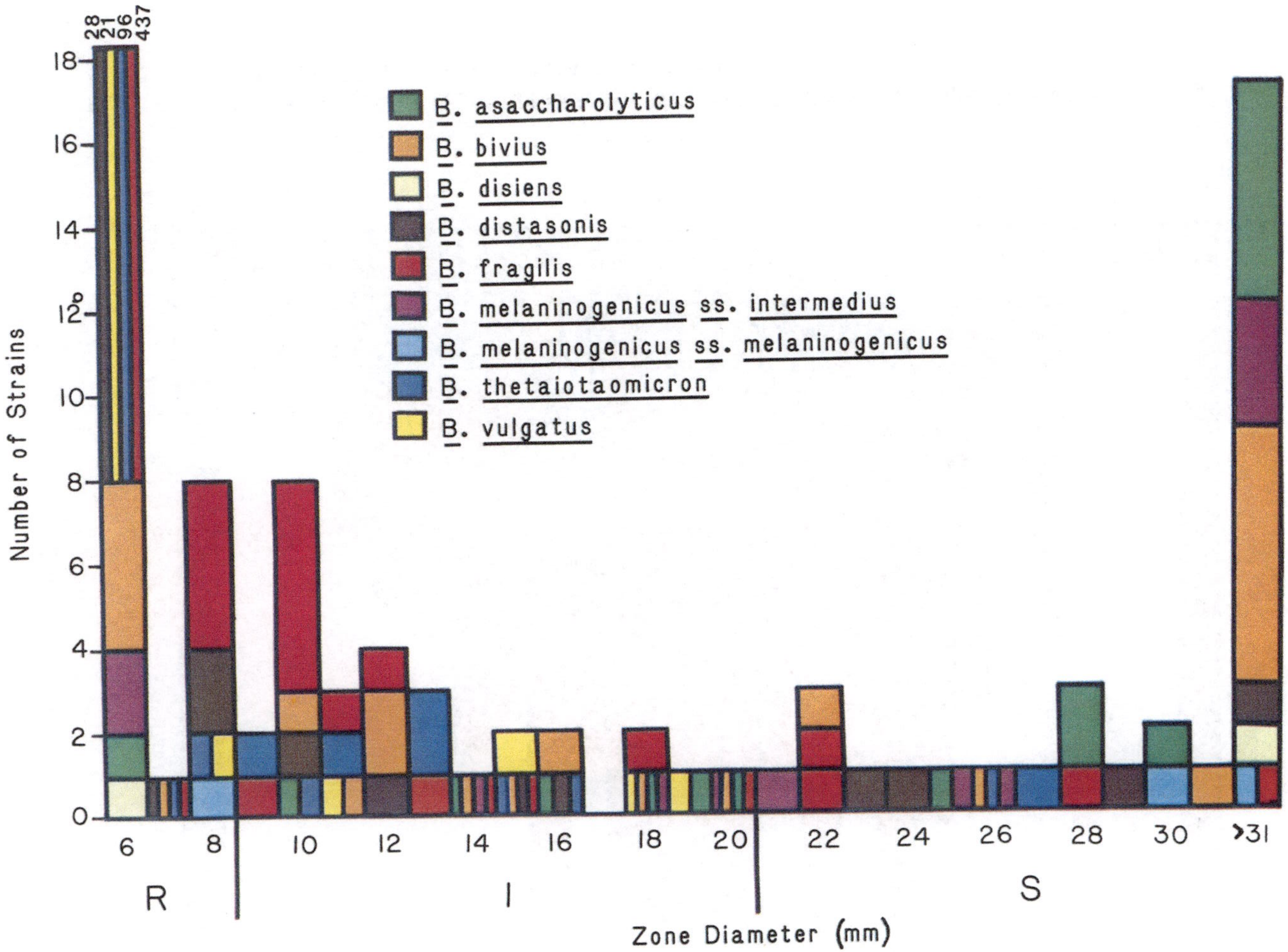

Fig. 5. Distribution of zone diameters of nine Bacteroides species with 10 Unit penicillin disks. Data collected 1974-1977.

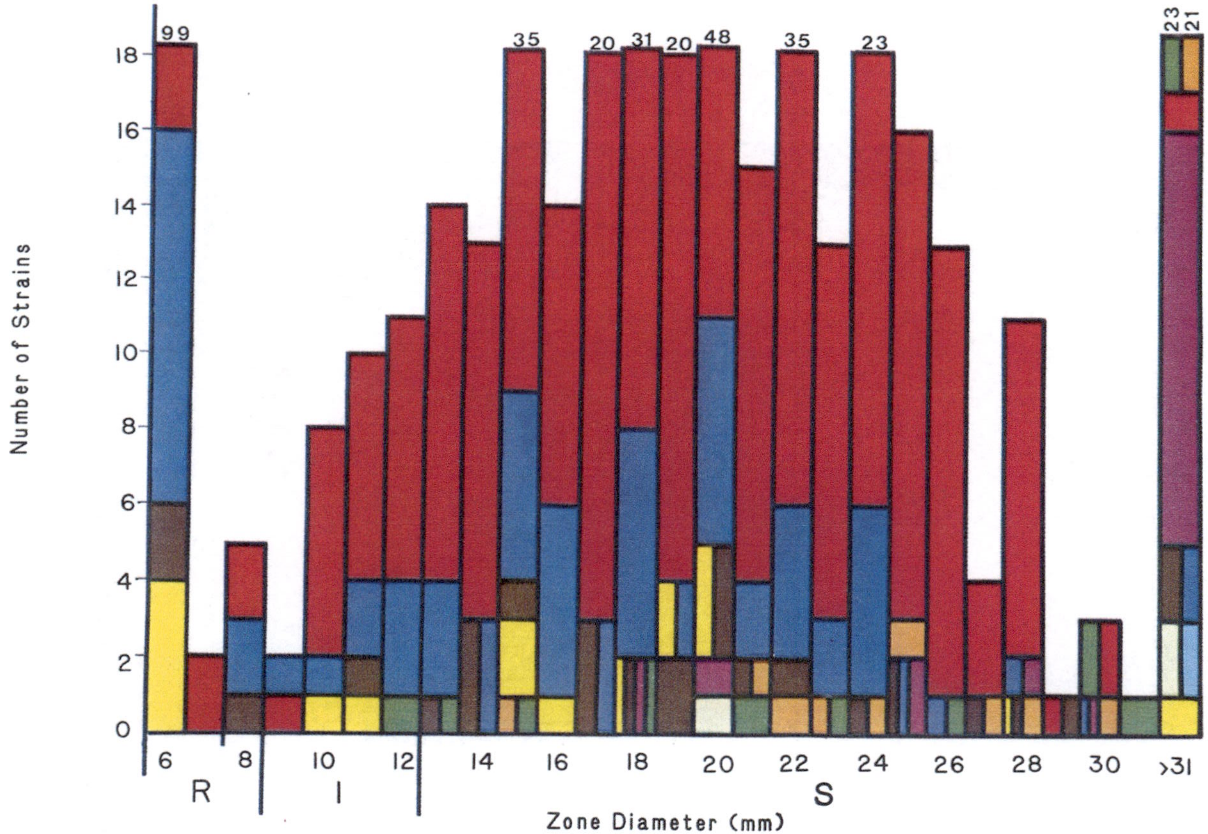

Fig. 6. Distribution of zone diameters of nine Bacteroides species with 100 ug carbenicillin disks. Data collected 1974-1977.

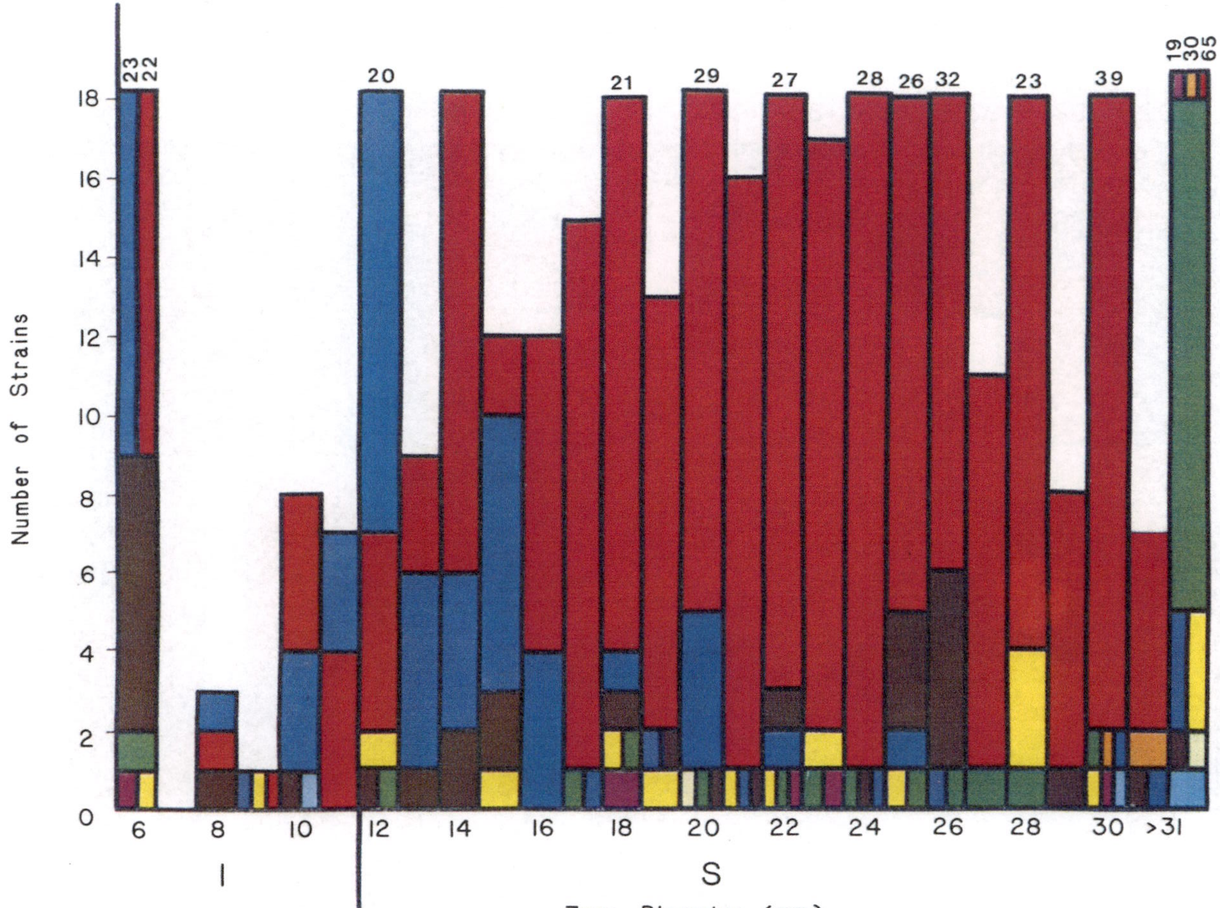

Fig. 7. Distribution of zone diameters of nine Bacteroides species with 2 ug clindamycin disks. Data collected 1974-1977.

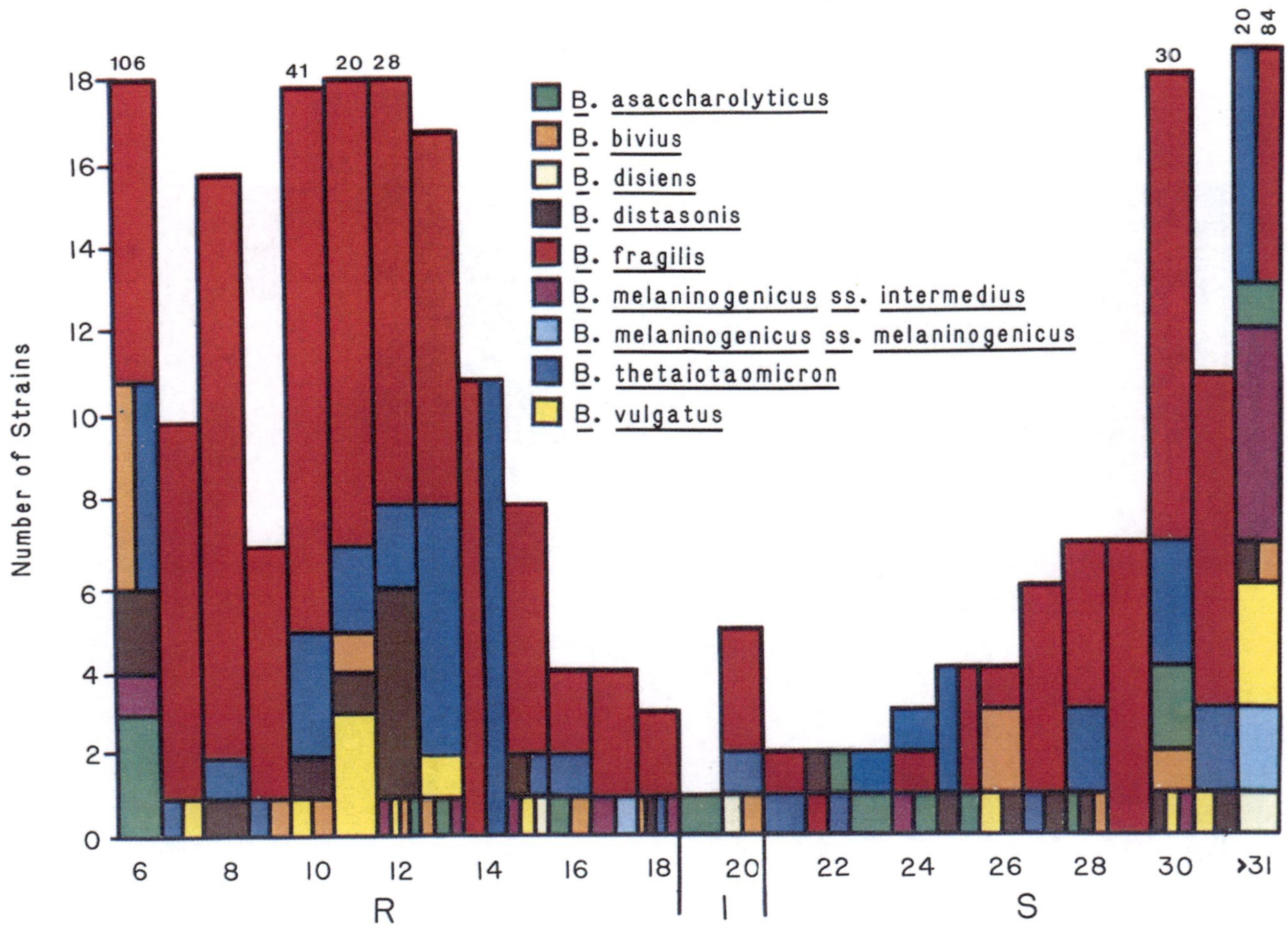

Fig. 8. Distribution of zone diameters of nine Bacteroides species with 30 ug tetracycline disks. Data collected 1974-1977.

control strains which have known inhibition zone diameters with each antibiotic.

Aminoglycosides are inactive under anaerobic conditions and should not be tested.

Some strains of certain anaerobic species such as B. melaninogenicus, Peptococcus prevotii, Peptococcus magnus, and Peptostreptococcus anaerobius grow poorly or not at all on MHAS. Readings of inhibition zones may be made at 24 and 48 h with our test method; readings beyond 48 h are not recommended.

There are no zone diameters given for resistant populations for chloramphenicol and clindamycin. There were no chloramphenicol resistant strains in our collection, thus, we were unable to develop interpretive values for resistant strains. An interim recommendation is to consider strains with a zone diameter of 25 mm or more as susceptible; this zone size corresponds to an MIC of 8 ug/ml, or less, 95% of the time.

We had too few clindamycin resistant strains to develop an interpretive scheme for resistance. Thus, we consider zone diameters of 6-11 mm as indeterminant. The MIC's of strains which produced no inhibition zone around the 2 ug clindamycin disk ranged from 5 ug/ml to 46 ug/ml and would be considered as resistant by our definition. Thus, our data indicate that a strain which fails to produce an inhibition zone around the disk is resistant. Strains producing inhibition zones of 7 to 12 mm had MIC's from 1.6 ug/ml to 5 ug/ml; these strains were considered indeterminant.

The following antibiotic data were collected from 1974 to 1977 at Emory University Hospital, Atlanta, Georgia, and at New England Deaconess Hospital, Boston, Massachusetts. The standardized antibiotic disk test described above was used on hundreds of strains of anaerobic cocci and Bacteroides. The data are presented as the distribution of inhibition zone sizes. The interpretive terms of resistant (R), indeterminant (I) and sensitive (S) were derived from the interpretive scheme shown above.

The anaerobic cocci tested included: species of Peptococcus, Peptostreptococcus, and Streptococcus shown in Fig. 1. Each species is represented by a different color which is indicated in the figure. Note the breakpoints of R, I, and S for carbenicillin. The majority of anaerobic cocci were susceptible to carbenicillin and most strains produced zone diameters of 30 mm or greater. However, about 5% of P. anaerobius strains were resistant to carbenicillin. A few strains of P. magnus and Peptococcus asaccharolyticus were resistant to carbenicillin and a few of these same two species were indeterminant. The species which were susceptible to carbenicillin included: P. prevotii, Peptococcus saccharolyticus, Peptostreptococcus micros,

Peptostreptococcus productus, Streptococcus constellatus, Streptococcus intermedius, and Streptococcus morbillorum. Thus, differences in antibiotic susceptibility to carbenicillin existed depending upon genus and species of anaerobic cocci.

Fig. 2 shows the distribution of the susceptibility of anaerobic cocci to penicillin. There were genus and species differences in susceptibility to penicillin. Approximately 13% (17/95 strains) of P. anaerobius were resistant to penicillin and a small number of P. magnus and P. micros strains were resistant. A number of strains in the indeterminant range included the following species: 8% of P. anaerobius, P. magnus, P. prevotii, P. asaccharolyticus, and S. intermedius; many strains of these species also were susceptible to penicillin. Species that included only susceptible strains were: P. saccharolyticus, S. constellatus, and S. morbillorum. P. anaerobius was the most resistant of the anaerobic cocci to penicillin, which was also true with carbenicillin.

The susceptibility distribution of the anaerobic cocci to clindamycin is shown in Fig. 3. There were a greater number of strains, and species, that were resistant to clindamycin than to carbenicillin or penicillin. For example, about 7% (21/303 strains) of P. magnus plus a number of strains of P. prevotii, P. asaccharolyticus, S. intermedius, P. saccharolyticus, and P. anaerobius produced no zones of inhibition. As mentioned previously, there were too few resistant cocci to calculate statistically an interpretive scheme for resistance to clindamycin. Strains which produced no zones of inhibition around the disk had MIC's of from 5 ug/ml to 46 ug/ml; therefore, such strains would be considered resistant by our definition. A number of strains of the following species which had zone sizes of 7-12 mm and MIC's of 1.6 ug/ml to 5 ug/ml were indeterminant: P. magnus, P. asaccharolyticus, P. prevotii, and P. micros; however, the majority of all of these strains were susceptible. All strains of S. constellatus, P. productus and S. morbillorum were susceptible.

The susceptibility distribution of anaerobic cocci to tetracycline is shown in Fig. 4. There were resistant and susceptible strains of all species tested except one species. All strains of P. saccharolyticus were susceptible to tetracycline.

The next four figures show the susceptibility distribution of nine Bacteroides species to the four antibiotics which were just discussed for the anaerobic cocci. These species include B. asaccharolyticus, Bacteroides bivius, Bacteroides disiens, Bacteroides distasonis, B. fragilis, Bacteroides melaninogenicus subsp. intermedius, Bacteroides melaninogenicus subsp. melaninogenicus, Bacteroides thetaiotaomicron, and Bacteroides vulgatus. The color codes for these species are shown in Fig. 5 which shows the distribution for penicillin. Most strains of B. distasonis, B. fragilis and B. thetaiotaomicron were resistant to penicillin; some strains were also indeterminant. A few strains of these species that were susceptible included: four strains of B. distasonis, four strains of B. fragilis, and one strain of B. thetaiotaomicron. There were no penicillin susceptible strains of B. vulgatus.

Most strains of B. asaccharolyticus, B. melaninogenicus subsp. melaninogenicus, and B. melaninogenicus subsp. intermedius were susceptible to penicillin, although some strains of all three organisms were resistant. Resistance was also noted in B. bivius and B. disiens: 25% (9/36 strains) of B. bivius were resistant to penicillin and one of three strains of B. disiens was resistant. Usually, it is general opinion that B. fragilis is always resistant to penicillin whereas B. asaccharolyticus and B. melaninogenicus are always susceptible. Note that data contrary to both statements is presented.

Fig. 6 shows the susceptibility distribution of Bacteroides species with carbenicillin. All strains of B. melaninogenicus (subsp. melaninogenicus and subsp. intermedius), B. bivius, and B. disiens and all but one strain of B. asaccharolyticus were susceptible to carbenicillin. Species that had susceptible and resistant strains included: B. fragilis, 78% S or I; B. thetaiotaomicron, 83% S or I; B. distasonis, 84% S or I; and B. vulgatus, 87% S or I.

The susceptibility distribution of Bacteroides to clindamycin is shown in Fig. 7. Most strains were susceptible to clindamycin, although a large number of indeterminant strains were found in B. fragilis, B. thetaiotaomicron, B. distasonis, and B. vulgatus. Many strains which produced no inhibition zone were considered resistant; these included 5% of strains of B. fragilis and 21% of B. thetaiotaomicron, as well as strains of B. distasonis, B. vulgatus, B. melaninogenicus subsp. intermedius and B. asaccharolyticus. This distribution again shows differences between species in susceptibility to clindamycin.

Tetracycline susceptibility is shown in Fig. 8. A large number of Bacteroides strains are resistant to tetracycline which has been well documented. Approximately 63% of B. fragilis, 50% of B. melaninogenicus and more than 50% of B. bivius are resistant to tetracycline. However, large numbers of strains are susceptible and this antibiotic may be used in infections of susceptible strains. This, and other data presented above, emphasize the need for routine antibiotic susceptibility testing of anaerobes with a standardized antibiotic disk test.

SUMMARY

A standardized antibiotic disk test for anaerobic bacteria has been described that is practical for a clinical laboratory to perform routinely. The results can be read in 24 to 48 h. Significant differences exist between genus, species, and antibiotic to justify routine testing.

LITERATURE CITED

1. Bennett, J.V, H.M. Camp, and I.C. Eickoff. 1968. Rapid sulfonamide disc sensitivity test for meningococci. Appl. Microbiol. 16: 1056-1060.

2. Lambe, D.W., Jr., A. Curtiss, W.W. Laslie, J. McKie, and J. Seo. 1977. An instrumental system for rapid antimicrobial susceptibility testing of anaerobic bacteria. pp. 254-264. In A.N. Sharpe and D.S. Clark (ed.), Mechanizing microbiology. Charles C. Thomas, Co., Springfield, Ill.

3. Laslie, W.W., and D.W. Lambe, Jr. 1976. Susceptibility testing of anaerobic bacteria with 100-ug carbenicillin disks. Antimicrob. Agents Chemother. 10: 112-118.

4. Overman, S.B., D.W. Lambe, Jr., and J.V. Bennett. 1974. Proposed standardized method for testing and interpreting susceptibility of Bacteroides fragilis to tetracycline. Antimicrob. Agents Chemother. 5: 357-361.

CHANGING TRENDS IN THE ANTIMICROBIAL SUSCEPTIBILITY PATTERN OF ANAEROBIC BACTERIA

Charles V. Sanders, Jr. and A.C. Lewis

School of Medicine, Department of Medicine
Louisiana State University
1542 Tulane Avenue
New Orleans, Louisiana 70112

INTRODUCTION

Within the past few years, the in vitro antimicrobial susceptibility pattern of anaerobic bacteria has undergone a gradual change (1,14,21). For example, some strains of Bacteroides melaninogenicus, other Bacteroides species, and some Clostridium species have become moderately resistant to penicillin G (7,9). Also, many strains of Bacteroides fragilis and other anaerobes are now resistant to tetracycline (21), and in 1976, two strains of Bacteroides fragilis subsp. ovatus (18) resistant to clindamycin were reported. Sutter and Finegold have suggested that specialized centers, nationwide, perform periodic antimicrobial susceptibility tests to monitor changing patterns of resistance of anaerobic bacteria to antimicrobial agents commonly recommended in the treatment of patients with anaerobic infections, and to determine the activity of newer agents against anaerobic bacteria (21). The purpose of this study was to assess the in vitro activity of several antimicrobial agents currently used for therapy of anaerobic infections and to explore the activity of several newer drugs against a variety of recent clinical isolates of anaerobic bacteria.

MATERIALS AND METHODS

Bacteria

A total of 756 strains of anaerobic bacteria were tested; most of these organisms were recovered from clinical specimens submitted to the Louisiana State University Infectious Disease Laboratory from patients hospitalized at Charity Hospital of Louisiana at New

Orleans. Some were collected from patients enrolled in clinical trials of newer antimicrobial agents, and some were from patients seen in consultation by the Infectious Disease Section during the period from February, 1975 to February, 1979. Anaerobic bacteria were isolated and characterized as previously described (10). B. fragilis subspecies and B. melaninogenicus subspecies are referred to as B. fragilis group and B. melaninogenicus group, respectively, because we, like Sutter and Finegold (21), found no difference in the antimicrobial susceptibility of various subspecies of B. fragilis or B. melaninogenicus.

Antimicrobial Agents

Laboratory standard reference powders for susceptibility testing were obtained from the following sources: penicillin G, cephalothin, and cefamandole from Eli Lilly and Co.; Indianapolis, Ind.; carbenicillin from Roerig, New York, N.Y.; ticarcillin sodium from Beecham-Massengill Pharmaceuticals, Bristol, Tenn.; sodium cefoxitin from Merck, Sharp and Dohme, Rahway, N.J.; chloramphenicol from Parke-Davis and Co., Detroit, Mich.; clindamycin from The Upjohn Co., Kalamazoo, Mich.; and metronidazole from G. D. Searle and Co., Chicago, Ill.

Susceptibility Testing

Antimicrobial susceptibility testing was performed as previously described (10).

RESULTS AND DISCUSSION

The activity of the various antimicrobial agents against the anaerobes tested is shown in Table 1. The minimal inhibitory concentration (MIC) breakpoints for determining susceptibility are concentrations easily achieved in vivo during high dose parenteral therapy of the antimicrobial in question.

Penicillins

Only 23% of Bacteroides strains were inhibited by penicillin G whereas Sutter and Finegold (21) reported that 42% of their strains were sensitive to approximately 10 ug/ml. On the other hand, Appelbaum and Chatterton (1) reported that 61% of their isolates were sensitive to $\leq$8 ug/ml. This concentration (8-10 ug/ml) of penicillin can be achieved by giving high doses (10-20 million U) of the drug. Weinrich and DelBene have shown that B. fragilis produces one or more beta-lactamases that can inactivate penicillin G (27). For 25 isolates, the MIC has $\geq$64 ug (107 U/ml). Only 60% of isolates of B. melaninogenicus were inhibited by $\leq$8 ug/ml; Sutter and Finegold (21) demonstrated that 97% of their isolates were sensitive to $\leq$10 ug/ml. Appelbaum and Chatterton (1) noted that 79% of their isolates were

Table 1. Activity of Nine Antimicrobial Agents Against Anaerobic Bacteria

Organism	No. of Strains Tested	Penicillin G (≤8)[a]	Carbenicillin (≤128)	Ticarcillin (≤128)	Cephalothin (≤16)	Cefamandole (≤16)	Cefoxitin (≤16)	Chloramphenicol (≤16)	Clindamycin (≤8)	Metronidazole (≤16)
		Percent of Strains Inhibited								
Bacteroides fragilis[b]	205	23	46	86	11	15	70	96	91	100
Bacteroides melaninogenicus	119	55	85	98	60	70	96	100	100	85
Other Bacteroides	134	60	81	98	55	66	95	96	99	86
Fusobacterium nucleatum	12	67	92	100	83	83	100	100	92	83
Other Fusobacterium	16	75	75	88	81	81	94	100	100	75
Peptococcus	53	96	100	100	94	98	100	100	98	89
Peptostreptococcus	52	82	98	98	88	90	98	100	98	82
Eubacterium	42	83	100	100	74	83	98	100	100	62
Propionibacterium	52	94	98	100	92	94	100	100	100	25
Bifidobacterium	14	71	100	100	64	71	93	100	100	64
Veillonella	19	100	100	100	100	100	100	100	100	95
Clostridium perfringens	14	100	100	100	93	100	100	83	100	100
Other Clostridium	24	83	96	100	92	96	88	100	100	71

[a] ( ) = Minimal inhibitory concentration breakpoints (ug/ml).

[b] Includes all subspecies of B. fragilis.

sensitive to ≤8 ug/ml. Salyers et al. (19) have shown that some strains of B. melaninogenicus can produce a beta-lactamase and this could account for our findings but we have not screened our isolates for beta-lactamase production. Overall, most of the other anaerobes that we tested were less sensitive to penicillin G than reported by previous investigators (1,14,21). Recently, Sutter and Finegold have noted some strains of B. melaninogenicus that were relatively resistant to penicillin G (MIC's as high as 32 U (approximately 18 ug/ml) (8).

Carbenicillin inhibited 46% of B. fragilis strains at ≤128 ug/ml. The MIC's for seven of our isolates was >512 ug/ml. Our strains of B. fragilis were much less sensitive than reported by others (1,21). For example, Sutter and Finegold noted that all but four strains of B. fragilis were inhibited by ≤128 ug/ml; Appelbaum and Chatterton found 93% of their isolates were sensitive at the same concentration. Our strains of Bacteroides species (other than B. fragilis) and Fusobacterium species (other than Fusobacterium nucleatum) had higher MIC's when compared to earlier reports (1,21). Ticarcillin was more active against B. fragilis than carbenicillin; 86% of isolates were inhibited by ≤128 ug/ml. In an earlier report, ticarcillin was effective against all strains tested at ≤128 ug/ml except for two strains of B. fragilis and two strains of Fusobacterium species. Twenty-nine of our B. fragilis isolates required >128 ug/ml and four of these required >512 ug/ml for inhibition. Ticarcillin was shown to be effective in the treatment of serious anaerobic infections (25,26), and in one prospective study, this agent was suggested as an acceptable alternative to clindamycin or chloramphenicol (11).

Cephalosporins and Similar Drugs

Only 11% of B. fragilis strains were sensitive to ≤16 ug/ml of cephalothin; at ≤32 ug/ml only 12% were inhibited. Cephalothin exhibited less activity against B. melaninogenicus, Eubacterium species and Bifidobacterium species than previously reported (21). One of 14 strains of Clostridium species had an MIC >64 ug/ml. In general, most Gram-positive anaerobes were more sensitive to cephalothin than Gram-negative anaerobes. Cefamandole at ≤16 ug/ml inhibited only 15% of isolates; at ≤32 ug/ml only 17% of isolates were inhibited. The activity of cefamandole against all other anaerobes tested was no different from cephalothin. Cefamandole has been shown to be a safe and effective agent for the treatment of anaerobic infections but should not be used when B. fragilis is suspected or proven to be the cause of the infection (10). Overall, cefoxitin, a new beta-lactamase resistant cephamycin, was considerably more active against all anaerobes tested when compared to cefamandole and cephalothin. Seventy percent of our B. fragilis strains were inhibited by cefoxitin at ≤16 ug/ml; at ≤32 ug/ml 86% were inhibited. The MIC for nine isolates was >64 ug/ml. Several clinical studies have established that cefoxitin is a safe, effective drug for the therapy of serious noncentral nervous system infections caused by anaerobic or mixed anaerobic/aerobic bacteria (13,15,22). Two recent studies have compared cefoxitin to other antimicrobials in the treatment of serious anaerobic infections. The first study compared cefoxitin ± amikacin to clindamycin + amikacin (23) and the second study compared cefoxitin to clindamycin + gentamicin (6). In both studies, cefoxitin was as efficacious as clindamycin in the treatment of these infections.

Chloramphenicol

Chloramphenicol was the most active agent tested; at a level of ≤16 ug/ml (a serum level readily achievable), all but 14 of 756 anaerobes were inhibited. The MIC of four isolates of *B*. fragilis was >64 ug/ml. These results were similar to previous reports (1,21) except for slightly higher MIC's for four *B*. fragilis isolates. Britz and Wilkinson have recently isolated some strains of *B*. fragilis moderately resistant to chloramphenicol due to a chloramphenicol acetyltransferase (3).

Clindamycin

This agent was almost as active as chloramphenicol; 91% of strains of *B*. fragilis were inhibited by ≤8 ug/ml. The MIC of 10 isolates was ≥8 ug/ml. In two previous studies, all strains of *B*. fragilis were inhibited by ≤8 ug/ml (1,21). A plasmid-mediated transferable resistance to clindamycin and erythromycin in *B*. fragilis (24) and transfer of multiple antibiotic resistance (including clindamycin) between subspecies of *B*. fragilis (16) has recently been reported.

Metronidazole

At <16 ug/ml 100% of *B*. fragilis strains were inhibited. The MIC for 23 strains of *B*. fragilis was >64 ug/ml. This is similar to an earlier report (21) which found that all strains of *B*. fragilis were inhibited by ≤64 ug/ml and another report (1) which found that all strains of *B*. fragilis were inhibited by ≤16 ug/ml. Metronidazole exhibited only fair activity against Eubacterium species and Bifidobacterium species and poor activity against Propionibacterium species. This antimicrobial agent has activity only against obligate anaerobes and is the only agent that demonstrates consistently bactericidal activity against *B*. fragilis (17). This agent is not approved for the treatment of anaerobic infections but both intravenous and oral metronidazole has been shown to be effective in the treatment of many different types of anaerobic infections (2,4). Metronidazole passes readily into the cerebrospinal fluid and brain; several cases of anaerobic meningitis and brain abscess have been successfully treated with this compound, in some cases, even after the patient has failed to respond to chloramphenicol (5,12). However, metronidazole is not recommended as a single agent in the therapy of anaerobic pleuropulmonary infection (20).

SUMMARY

This report has documented that antimicrobial susceptibility of anaerobic bacteria is changing and that now some anaerobic bacteria are more resistant than previously reported. Additional prospective studies will be necessary to monitor future changing trends in susceptibility patterns of anaerobic bacteria.

LITERATURE CITED

1. Appelbaum, P.C., and S.A. Chatterton. 1978. Susceptibility of anaerobic bacteria to ten antimicrobial agents. Antimicrob. Agents Chemother. 14:371-376.

2. Baines, E.J. 1978. Metronidazole: its past, present and future. J. Antimicrob. Chemother. 4 (Suppl. C): 97-111.

3. Britz, M.L., and R.G. Wilkinson. 1978. Chloramphenicol acetyltransferase of Bacteroides fragilis. Antimicrob. Agents Chemother. 14:105-111.

4. Brogden, R.N., R.C. Heel, T.M. Speight, and G.S. Avery. 1978. Metronidazole in anaerobic infections. A review of its activity, pharmacokinetics and therapeutic use. Drugs 16:387-417.

5. Bryan, C.S., L.J. Huffman, V.E. DelBene, C.V. Sanders, and M. C. Scalcini. 1979. Intravenous metronidazole therapy for Bacteroides fragilis meningitis. South Med. J. 72:494-497.

6. Drusano, G., J. Warren, A. Saah, J. Tenney, E. Caplan, S. Hansen, J. Granados, and T. Eisenstat. Cefoxitin vs clindamycin/gentamicin for penicillin-resistant anaerobic infections; abstracted in Abstracts of the 19th Interscience Conference on Antimicrobial Agents and Chemotherapy, Boston, Mass., October 1-5, 1979, Abstract #823.

7. Finegold, S.M. 1977. Anaerobic bacteria in human disease. Academic Press, Inc., New York.

8. Finegold, S.M. 1977. Therapy for infections due to anaerobic bacteria: an overview. J. Infect. Dis. 135 (Suppl): S25-S29.

9. Finegold, S.M. 1979. Anaerobic infections. Arch. Int. Med. 129:144-145.

10. Greenberg, R.N., M.C. Scalcini, C.V. Sanders, and A.C. Lewis. 1979. Cefamandole therapy in anaerobic infections. Antimicrob. Agents Chemother. 15:337-341.

11. Harding, G.K., T.J. Marrie, F. Buckwold, P. Muir, J. Koss, M.J. Gurwith, G. Stiver, and W. Albritton: A controlled comparison of ticarcillin, clindamycin and chloramphenicol in the therapy of anaerobic infections, abstracted in Abstracts of the 17th Interscience Conference on Antimicrobial Agents and Chemotherapy, New York, N.Y., October 12-14, 1977, Abstract #178.

12. Ingham, H.R., J.B. Seklon, and C.M. Roxby. 1978. The bacteriology and chemotherapy of otogenic cerebral abscesses. J. Antimicrob. Chemother. 4 (Suppl. C):63-69.

13. Kirby, B.D., D.F. Busch, D.M. Citron, and S.M. Finegold. 1979. Cefoxitin for treatment of infections due to anaerobic bacteria. Rev. Infect. Dis. 1:113-116.

14. Martin, W.J., M. Gardner, and J.A. Washington, II. 1972. In vitro antimicrobial susceptibility of anaerobic bacteria isolated from clinical specimens. Antimicrob. Agents Chemother. 1:148-158.

15. Nair, S.R., and C.E. Cherubin. 1978. Use of cefoxitin, a new cephalosporin-like antibiotic, in the treatment of aerobic and anaerobic infection. Antimicrob. Agents Chemother. 14:866-875.

16. Privitera, G., A. Dublanchet, and M. Sebald. 1979. Transfer of multiple antibiotic resistance between subspecies of Bacteroides fragilis. J. Infect. Dis. 139:97-101.

17. Ralph, E.D., and W.M.M. Kirby. 1975. Unique bactericidal action of metronidazole against Bacteroides fragilis and Clostridium perfringens. Antimicrob. Agents Chemother. 8:409-414.

18. Salaki, J.S., R. Black, F.P. Tally, and J.W. Kislak. 1976. Bacteroides fragilis resistant to the administration of clindamycin. Am. J. Med. 60:426-428.

19. Salyers, A.A., J. Wong, and T.D. Wilkins. 1977. Beta-lactamase activity in strains of Bacteroides melaninogenicus and Bacteroides oralis. Antimicrob. Agents Chemother. 11:142-146.

20. Sanders, C.V., B.J. Hanna, and A.C. Lewis. 1979. Metronidazole in the treatment of anaerobic infections. Am. Rev. Resp. Dis. 120:337-343.

21. Sutter, V.L., and S.M. Finegold. 1976. Susceptibility of anaerobic bacteria to 23 antimicrobial agents. Antimicrob. Agents Chemother. 10:736-752.

22. Tally, F., P.V.W. Miao, J.P. O'Keefe, and S.L. Gorbach. 1979. Cefoxitin therapy of anaerobic and aerobic infections. J. Antimicrob. Chemother. 5:101-108.

23. Tally, F.P., K. McGowan, T. O'Donnell, J.J. Kelly, J. Kellum, and S.L. Gorbach. Randomized comparison of cefoxitin and clindamycin in suspected anaerobic sepsis, abstracted in Abstracts of the 19th Interscience Conference on Antimicrobial Agents and Chemotherapy, Boston, Mass., October 1-5, 1979, Abstract #822.

24. Tally, F.P., D.R. Snydam, S.L. Gorbach, and M.H. Malamy. 1979. Plasmid-mediated transferable resistance to clindamycin and erythromycin in Bacteroides fragilis. J. Infect. Dis. 139: 83-88.

25. Torres, J.R., B. Lorbes, B. Hanna, R.M. Swenson, C.V. Sanders, and A.C. Lewis: Treatment of anaerobic infections with ticarcillin, clinical and laboratory aspects, abstracted in Abstracts of the 18th Interscience Conference on Antimicrobial Agents and Chemotherapy, Atlanta, Ga., October 2-4, 1978, Abstract #361.

26. Webb, D., H. Thadepalli, I. Roy, and V.T. Bach. 1978. Ticarcillin disodium in anaerobic infections. Arch. Int. Med. 138: 1618-1620.

27. Weinrich, A.E., and V.E. DelBene. 1976. Characterization of β-lactamase activity in anaerobic bacteria. Clin. Res. 24:27A.

CAMPYLOBACTER ENTERITIS AND SEPTICEMIA

Sabine Lauwers

Department of Microbiology
A.Z. Vrije Universiteit Brussel
Laarbeeklaan 101, 1090 Brussels, Belgium

INTRODUCTION

Campylobacter enteritis is a relatively new disease that went unrecognized for a long time. Since Butzler stressed the importance of the organism now known as Campylobacter as an etiologic agent in enteritis in 1974 (3), several other workers in Britain, the United States, Canada, the Netherlands, Sweden, Australia and Africa confirmed Butzler's findings (2,7,8,11,14,15).

Campylobacter was known by veterinary microbiologists since the beginning of the century. In 1909 MacFadyean and Stockman (12) described a vibrio-shaped organism isolated from sheep-abortion material. In 1918, in a study of abortion in cattle, Smith and Taylor (18) recovered a microaerophilic spirillum, which proved to be identical to MacFadyean's organism, and they named it Vibrio fetus.

Since V. fetus differs greatly from the other vibrios (Vibrio cholera and Vibrio parahemolyticus), notably in the G + C content of their DNA, Sebald and Veron (13) proposed a new genus, Campylobacter, with Campylobacter fetus as the type species.

Campylobacter is a Gram-negative rod, comma- or S-shaped, sometimes forming a spirillum. They are very motile with a flagellum at one or both poles of the cell. They can be encapsulated but never form spores. They do not ferment sugars; nitrates are reduced; and oxidase is positive. They do not possess a urease, gelatinase or lipase. Citrate, methyl red and Voges-Proskauer reactions are negative. The catalase production varies with the species: Campylobacter sputorum and Campylobacter bubulus are catalase negative, whereas

C. fetus, Campylobacter jejuni and Campylobacter coli are catalase positive.

C. sputorum and C. bubulus have no place in human disease. C. fetus is well known to veterinarians (17) (it causes sterility and abortion in cattle and sheep), but it is not very pathogenic for humans: as an opportunistic organism it can cause septicemia in debilitated patients with cirrhosis, diabetes, cancer, or immunosuppressive therapy (1). Campylobacter jejuni/coli is an important causative agent of diarrhea and septicemia in healthy children and adults.

Smibert (16) considers Campylobacter causing enteritis as a subspecies of C. fetus, but Veron (20) recognizes two species, C. jejuni and C. coli.

C. jejuni/coli formerly went unrecognized because of inappropriate isolation techniques used in clinical laboratories. In 1957, King (9) described a Campylobacter, different from C. fetus, as a causative agent of enteritis in infants and children. But these "related" vibrios, as she called them, were isolated from blood and not from stool specimens. Blood culture is an uncommon diagnostic procedure in enteritis, especially in infants and young children. This explains why Campylobacter enteritis remained almost unrecognized in humans for more than ten years since the original reports of King.

ISOLATION AND BIOCHEMICAL CHARACTERISTICS OF C. JEJUNI/COLI

In the first isolations from human stools, Butzler used a filtration technique, based on the ability of Campylobacter to pass through a 0.65 um filter, whereas other enteric bacteria do not (6). Later, the technique (10) was simplified by adding antibiotics to the medium as follows: thioglycollate broth, 1,000 ml; agar, 30 g; defibrinated sheep blood, 100 ml; bacitracin, 25,000 I.U.; novobiocin, 5 mg; actidione, 50 mg; cephalothin, 15 mg; and colistin, 10,000 U.

Campylobacter also requires special growth conditions: they must be cultivated in an atmosphere with less O_2 and more CO_2 than is present in air. This can be achieved by partial replacement of the normal atmosphere of the incubator with a mixture of N_2 and CO_2. The plates are incubated at 37 C, or better at 42 C which is the optimum temperature for C. jejuni/coli. The colonies appear in one to two days, sometimes later. Different types of colonies can be seen: colonies a few mm in diameter, round and raised, shiny, grey, exceptionally pink; other colonies are very flat, often irregular, becoming 5 to even 10 mm in diameter, sometimes with a white center. Colonies often have a tendency to spread along the streaks of the inoculating loop or swab. A stained smear of a young culture shows the characteristic S-shaped forms. As cultures grow older, the organisms are gradually transformed into coccoid forms which stain very poorly. These coccoid organisms have also lost motility.

We studied the biochemical characteristics of over 100 strains of C. jejuni/coli and of a few strains of C. fetus. They were all catalase and oxidase positive and did not grow on 3.5% NaCl. With a few exceptions they tolerated glycine, reduced sodium selenite and grew in 8% glucose. All C. jejuni/coli strains tolerated tetrazolium in the medium, whereas C. fetus did not. An easy and reliable way to distinguish C. fetus from C. jejuni/coli is the tetrazolium test and their ability to grow at different temperatures (Table 1).

CLINICAL PICTURE AND TREATMENT

The incubation period usually varies between two and five days. The first symptoms are often non-specific: about one-half of the patients show a febrile prodromal period with malaise, dizziness, headache, backache, and myalgia that lasts from a few hours to a few days. In most cases the patient suffers from central abdominal pain which occurs during the prodromal period. The intensity of the abdominal pain can become so distressing that a diagnosis of acute peritonitis can be suspected in a few cases. The stools become liquid, foul smelling, often bile stained and contain fresh blood. The diarrhea lasts for a few days, but abdominal pain may persist much longer. Vomiting is not a very common feature in adults, although many patients have nausea.

Young children often are less severely ill than adults. They sometimes show only a few loose stools with or without a febrile episode. However, they may suffer from persistent diarrhea which lasts for weeks. Vomiting, more common in children than in adults,

Table 1. Identification of Campylobacter fetus and Campylobacter jejuni/coli

Characteristic	C. fetus	C. jejuni/coli
Growth at 25 C	+	-
Growth at 42 C	-	+
Growth on TTC[a]	-	+

[a] Growth on medium containing 0.4 mg/ml triphenyltetrazolium chloride.

appears one or two days after onset of diarrhea. In infants, we have seen cases of acute enteritis with dehydration and a need for intravenous fluids.

Karmali and Fleming (8) studied 37 cases of Campylobacter enteritis in children. Typically, the patients presented with fever, intermittent colic, central abdominal pain and diarrhea. A few days later, 90% of the children showed blood in their stools. In our series, 25% of Belgian children have bloody stools, whereas in North African children living in Brussels, blood was only seen in two patients out of over 120 patients.

Karmali found that direct phase contrast microscopy of a fresh stool specimen is useful in establishing a rapid diagnosis of Campylobacter enteritis. Campylobacter can be recognized by the spiral form of the cells and their rapid oscillating motility.

Specific chemotherapy for Campylobacter enteritis can be started immediately. However, in enteritis cases caused by other pathogens such as Salmonella and Escherichia coli, antibiotics are not always needed. Many patients do well without chemotherapy: indeed, we often see that the patient has recovered at the moment of the bacteriological diagnosis. Nevertheless, appropriate chemotherapy is needed in severe cases with septicemia. The aminoglycosides, erythromycin, tetracyclines and chloramphenicol are the most active antibiotics (19). Our treatment of choice is erythromycin. In cases with septicemia gentamycin can be used.

The serological response to the infection can be investigated with a tube agglutination technique using formalinized antigen. As this test is very specific, only the patient's Campylobacter strain should be used. Antibodies appear by about the fifth day of the disease and quickly rise to a maximum level which can be very high. Titers then gradually decline over the ensuing few months.

PATHOGENESIS

There is now significant evidence about the pathogenic role of C. jejuni/coli in the human enteritis: (i) although healthy carriers exist, and although Campylobacter is occasionally isolated with other pathogens, there is a good correlation between the presence of the organisms in feces and the occurrence of diarrhea and enteritis; (ii) in patients with enteritis and septicemia, the same Campylobacter was isolated from both feces and blood; (iii) erythromycin therapy specifically active against Campylobacter and not against other enteric pathogens such as Enterobacteriaceae and viruses gives a rapid regression of symptomatology in many cases. The high specific antibody titers the patients develop to their own Campylobacter strains tend to disappear more quickly after erythromycin treatment; and (iv) the invasive power of Campylobacter in chickens was shown by Butzler (4).

After oral ingestion Campylobacter was isolated from blood, liver and feces of 50% of the birds.

Tests for demonstration of thermolabile and thermostable enterotoxins remain negative. Thus, the main pathogenicity of Campylobacter seems to be the ability to penetrate the intestinal wall and eventually enter the blood stream. The principal sites of infection are the jejunum and ileum (5) but the colon could be involved as well.

EPIDEMIOLOGY

The disease seems to occur all over the world. It may be particularly common in the tropics. Seasonal variations are seen. Both in Brussels and Britain infections were more prevalent in summer months. It is difficult to measure the true incidence of infection in different age groups since oversampling in certain groups may distort the figures, but it seems that children under five years of age are more frequently affected.

How do people get infected? The organisms are found in a wide variety of animals, and strains identical to human strains have been isolated from animals. Dogs suffering from Campylobacter enteritis may pass on the infection to humans (2). The chicken intestine often contains C. jejuni/coli and unhygienic handling of the birds can lead to infection. Unpasteurized cows' milk may be a source of infection, and recently there have been a few outbreaks of this kind in Britain. Probably the organisms are not introduced into the milk through the cow's udder, but by fecal contamination.

C. jejuni/coli has been isolated from several natural waters and several water-borne outbreaks have already occurred notably in Britain, but also in Vermont where about 2,000 people were infected. In this outbreak, Campylobacter was isolated from only 15 patients.

Cross-infection between humans does not occur very frequently. Family studies have shown that infectivity is low. However, spread is possible, notably in nurseries. Butzler described five outbreaks in infant day nurseries. In one outbreak, cross-infection occurred through the use of an insufficiently cleaned communal bath.

A good serologic typing scheme of these organisms would aid in a better understanding of the Campylobacter enteritis. The antigenic structure of Campylobacter is very complex. In Brussels, we are working on a reliable and simple serotyping technique. Live suspensions which probably reflect superficial heat-labile antigens have been tested in the slide agglutination test, but results were not reliable. Many problems with autoagglutinating strains were encountered and too many different serotypes were found. In the tube agglutination technique with formalinized suspensions the antigen-antibody reactions are very specific; all strains were agglutinated to a titer of 640 or more by their homologous sera, but almost no cross-reactions occurred.

Heated suspensions, probably corresponding to somatic O-antigens were used in a complement fixation test which was insensitive. Alternative techniques are fluorescent antibody tests, indirect hemagglutination tests, ELISA-techniques, but these are difficult to perform or to read. We are now working with a direct hemagglutination test which seems to be very promising.

LITERATURE CITED

1. Bejot, J. 1973. La campylobactériose humaine ou vibriose à Campylobacter foetus. Méd. et Mal. Infectieuses. 3: 281.

2. Blaser, M.J., J. Cravens, B.W. Powers, and W.L. Wang. 1978. Campylobacter enteritis associated with canine infection. Lancet ii: 979.

3. Butzler, J.P., P. Dekeyser, M. Detrain, and F. Dehaen. 1973. Related vibrio in stools. J. Pediat. 82: 318.

4. Butzler, J.P., D. Dekegel, J.M. Hubrechts, S. Lauwers, and G. Zissis. Mode of transmission of human campylobacteriosis, p. 174-175. In W. Siegenthaler and R. Lüthy (ed.), Current Chemotherapy. Proceedings of the 10th International Congress of Chemotherapy, Vol. I. American Society for Microbiology, Washington, D.C.

5. Cadranel, S., P. Rodesch, J.P. Butzler, and P. Dekeyser. 1973. Enteritis due to "related vibrio" in children. Amer. J. Dis. Child. 126: 152.

6. Dekeyser, P., M. Gossuin-Detrain, J.P. Butzler, and J. Sternon. 1972. Acute enteritis due to related vibrio: first positive stool culture. J. Infect. Dis. 125: 390.

7. Demol, P. and E. Bosmans. 1978. Campylobacter enteritis in Central Africa. Lancet i: 604.

8. Karmali, M.A. and P.C. Fleming. 1979. Campylobacter enteritis in children. J. Pediat. 94: 527.

9. King, E.O. 1957. Human infection with Vibrio foetus and a closely related vibrio. J. Infect. Dis. 101: 119.

10. Lauwers, S., M. De Boeck, and J.P. Butzler. 1978. Campylobacter enteritis in Brussels. Lancet ii: 604.

11. Linquist, B., J. Kjellander, and T. Kosunen. 1978. Campylobacter enteritis in Sweden. Br. Med. J. 1: 303.

12. MacFadyean, J. and S. Stockman. 1914. Report of the Departmental Committee appointed by the Board of Agriculture and Fisheries to inquire into epizootic abortion. Appendix to part 3: abortion in sheep, London 1913, House of Commons Sessional Paper, 12.

13. Sebald, M. and M. Veron. 1963. Teneur en bases de l' ADN et classification des vibrions. Ann. Inst. Pasteur. 105: 897.

14. Severin, W.P.J. 1978. Campylobacter en enteritis. Ned. T. Geneesk. 122: 15.

15. Skirrow, M.B. 1977. Campylobacter enteritis: a "new" disease. Br. Med. J. 2: 9.

16. Smibert, R.M. 1974. Campylobacter, p. 207. In R.E. Buchanan, and N.E. Gibbons (ed.), Bergey's Manual of Determinative Bacteriology, 8th ed. The Williams & Wilkins Company, Baltimore.

17. Smith, T. 1918. Spirilla associated with disease to the fetal membranes in cattle (infectious abortion). J. Exp. Med. 28: 701.

18. Smith, T. and M.S. Taylor. 1919. Some morphological and biological characters of spirilla (Vibrio foetus n.s.p.) associated with disease of fetal membranes in cattle. J. Exp. Med. 30: 299.

19. Vanhoof, R., M.P.Vanderlinden, R. Dierickx, S. Lauwers, E. Yourassowsky, and J.P. Butzler. 1978. Susceptibility of Campylobacter fetus subsp. jejuni to twenty-nine antimicrobial agents. Antim. Agents and Chemoth. 14: 553.

20. Veron, M. and R. Chatelain. 1973. Taxonomic study of the genus Campylobacter Sebald and Veron and designation of the neotype strain for the type species, C. fetus (Smith and Taylor) Sebald and Veron. Int. J. Syst. Bact. 23: 122.

ROLE OF ANAEROBES IN CROHN'S DISEASE

Dan Danielsson

Department of Clinical Bacteriology and Immunology
Central County Hospital
S-701 85 Örebro, Sweden

INTRODUCTION

Crohn's disease is an idiopathic chronic inflammatory disease of the bowel. Ulcerative colitis is the other main disease of this group. Crohn et al. (4) described this syndrome as regional or terminal ileitis. They recognized an acute type of short duration usually followed by spontaneous recovery; and a chronic type of longer duration. This basic definition is valid today. It has been convincingly shown that the acute type is an entirely separate entity from the chronic form (14). Yersinia enterocolitica is the etiologic agent in at least 50-60% of the acute cases in Sweden (14).

Patients with chronic Crohn's disease usually have a history of the symptoms which accompany intestinal obstruction and/or diarrhea, including an elevated erythrocyte sedimentation rate, elevated concentration of orosomucoid, weight loss, and anemia; as well as other non-characteristic symptoms. When located in the terminal ileum, which is usual, X-rays show a very narrow lumen. A stiff and thickened wall of the terminal ileum is found upon operation. Histopathologic examination reveals a heavy inflammatory reaction with large numbers of plasma cells, polymorphonuclear cells, granuloma formation, so-called skip lesions in the mucosa, sometimes fissures and micro-abscesses.

The etiology of the chronic form of Crohn's disease is unknown. It was originally described as regional ileitis; the terminal ileum is the most common location of this disease, but any part of the gastrointestinal tract may be involved. Therefore, the modern terminology is chronic granulomatous enteritis or enterocolitis. Crohn's disease may be difficult to differentiate from ulcerative colitis when the predominant symptoms are those of a colitis.

Since Crohn's original description a large number of endogenous and exogenous etiopathogenetic factors have been related to the disease. Endogenous factors include: (i) vascular disorders, (ii) abnormal reactions to mental stress, and (iii) immunologic and genetic factors discussed below. Exogenous agents include chemicals, viruses, and bacteria or bacterial products.

In our laboratory, we have been interested in three aspects of Crohn's disease: the immune state of diseased intestinal tissue, the role of intestinal bacteria with emphasis upon the immune response to anaerobes, and the ability of two compounds, azathioprine (Imuran^{R}, Imurel^{R}) and metronidazole (Flagyl^{R}) which have been used to treat Crohn's disease to inhibit anaerobic bacteria.

DISCUSSION

Immune Mechanisms Involved in Crohn's Disease

Some observations indicate that immunologic and genetic factors might be involved in the immune response of patients with Crohn's disease. There is an increased incidence of allergic and autoimmune diseases among both Crohn patients and their relatives (8). These patients often show manifestations associated with immune complex diseases; uveitis, iritis, arthritis, erythema nodosum and erythema multiforme (8). Anticolonic antibodies cross-reacting with phenol extractable antigens from Escherichia coli 0:14, a common enterobacterial antigen, have been demonstrated (16,17). Lymphocytes from patients with active Crohn's disease are cytotoxic to colon epithelial cells. This cytotoxicity can be induced in "normal" lymphocytes with IgM from patients with active Crohn's disease and with phenol extracted antigens from E. coli 0119:B14 (21). Persson and Danielsson (13) have demonstrated an increase in IgG-, IgA- and IgM-producing plasma cells in diseased tissue of the terminal ileum of Crohn patients as compared to subjects with no inflammatory intestinal disease. The ratio of IgA to IgG was usually above 5 to 15 in the control subjects while it was below 1 in the Crohn patients. Similar findings have been reported by others (2). Since IgA is regarded as the first line of specific mucosal defense and IgG-IgM as the second, our observations indicate that the second line of specific mucosal defense has been activated in Crohn patients typical of a booster response of IgG.

Immune Response to Bacteroides and E. Coli

The large increase of immunoglobulin-producing plasma cells (2,13), the presence of antibodies against antigens of colon epithelial cells which cross-react with antigens of E. coli (10,17,19), and the induction of lymphocytes, cytotoxic to colon epithelial cells with E. coli antigens (21), indicate that the immune system, probably the gastrointestinal associated lymphoid tissue, of patients with Crohn's disease has been activated or sensitized by intestinal bacterial flora. Our data support this view. We have found that patients with Crohn's disease have high titers of circulating antibodies against strains of certain Bacteroides species. This was in contrast to subjects with no evidence of gastrointestinal disease (6,15). In a similar investigation with antigens from eight different serotypes of E. coli we showed that Crohn patients had statistically higher serum titers than control patients (15). The antibodies of the healthy individuals against different Bacteroides species were sensitive to treatment with beta-mercaptoethanol while those of Crohn patients were resistant (6).

Antibacterial Activity of Azathioprine (Imurel^{R}, Imuran^{R}) Against Anaerobic Intestinal Bacteria

Autoimmunity is one theory of the etiopathogenesis of Crohn's disease. In the 1960's treatment with azathioprine, the most commonly used immunosuppressive drug, was examined. Although reports conflict, results of some controlled trials indicate clinical improvement during treatment with this drug (11,12,22). Some of our patients, especially those with intestinal fistulas, showed rapid improvement within one or two days which was probably not due to immunosuppression alone. We found azathioprine had a definite antibacterial activity against anaerobic, but not against aerobic, intestinal bacteria isolated from patients with Crohn's disease as well as from healthy persons. Anaerobic Gram-positive cocci, Gram-positive rods, and Gram-negative rods were inhibited by azathioprine with minimal inhibitory concentration (MIC) ranging from 37.5 ug/ml to 300 ug/ml. None of the aerobic enterobacteria or Pseudomonas species investigated were inhibited. Nonpathogenic and pathogenic Neisseria and Haemophilus species were also inhibited with MIC's ranging from 37.5 ug/ml to 150 ug/ml (5). These concentrations cannot be achieved in serum with the current dosage used. However, we demonstrated the antibacterial activity of azathioprine in the secretion of an intestinal (jejunal) fistula of a Crohn patient being treated with this drug. The secretion contained approximately 4 to 10 mg/ml of azathioprine which was ten times the MIC of the anaerobes.

Azathioprine is split in vivo to 6-mercaptopurine (7), but in parallel experiments no antibacterial effect was demonstrated with 6-mercaptopurine. It is reasonable to assume that the demonstrated antibacterial activity of azathioprine is due to an unsplit molecule for which the mechanism of action is not yet understood.

The improvement in some patients with Crohn's disease treated with azathioprine has been ascribed to its immunosuppressive and/or anti-inflammatory effect. It is reasonable to suggest that improvement is also due to the antibacterial activity of azathioprine.

Ursing and Kamme (20) have reported rapid and prompt improvement of Crohn patients treated with metronidazole. This drug, besides its antiparasitic effect, also has a strong growth-inhibiting effect on various anaerobic bacteria.

We recently reported a radical change of the anaerobic intestinal flora in Crohn patients who responded well during treatment with metronidazole. No such changes were noted in the patients who did not respond, nor in healthy individuals (9). In our study in patients with Crohn's disease who responded well to metronidazole therapy, Bacteroides species could not be isolated during therapy, while these bacteria remained in the patients who did not respond during the treatment period. Recently, Belsheim et al. (1) reported a significant decreased migratory activity of polymorphonuclear leucocytes in patients with active Crohn's disease. The migratory activity of these cells significantly increased during treatment with metronidazole, or with timidazole, which has similar antiparasitic and antibacterial activity. At the same time the patients showed a clinical improvement (1). The therapeutic effect of metronidazole on patients with Crohn's disease could therefore be ascribed to its inhibitory activity of anaerobes, especially Bacteroides species, as well as its stimulatory effect on the migration of polymorphonuclear cells.

SUMMARY

There is an increase of immunoglobulin-producing plasma cells in the diseased intestinal tissue of patients with Crohn's disease with a reversed ratio of IgA:IgG (2,3). Patients with Crohn's disease make antibodies against colon epithelial cell antigens which are cross-reactive with a common enterobacterial antigen (10,16,19). Lymphocytes of Crohn patients have a cytotoxic effect on colon epithelial cells and normal lymphocytes can be made cytotoxic with antigens from *E.* coli (21). Patients with Crohn's disease have significantly higher serum titers than healthy individuals against Bacteroides and *E.* coli antigens (6,15). Azathioprine, besides its immunosuppressive and anti-inflammatory activity, has an inhibitory effect against anaerobes (5). Metronidazole significantly reduces anaerobic bacteria, especially Bacteroides species, and increases the migratory activity of polymorphonuclear cells in patients who respond to therapy with this drug (1,9).

What are the implications of these observations on Crohn's disease? Watson and Shorter et al. (18,21) proposed that a blocked, impaired mucosa due to recurrent intestinal infections, permits an abnormal diffusion or resorption of enterobacterial antigens that can sensitize lymphocytes. When these cells are sensitized with enterobacterial antigens cross-reacting with colon epithelial cell antigens, lymphocytes cytotoxic to colon epithelial cells are developed. Such lymphocytes might be responsible for the lesions known

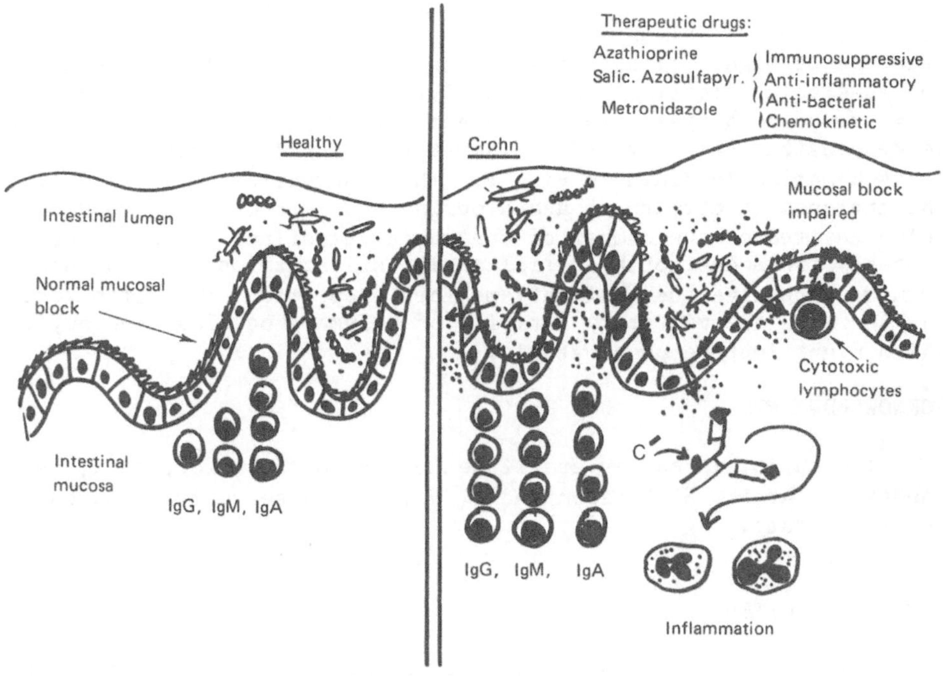

Fig. 1. A diagrammatic representation of the bacteriological and immunological events in the intestinal mucosa of healthy individuals and patients with Crohn's disease.

as skip lesions (21). The sensitized lymphocytes may also react with enterobacterial antigens absorbed because of impaired mucosa, resulting in an inflammatory reaction which is the typical histopathological finding in Crohn's disease.

The presence of antibodies to colon epithelial cell antigens which cross-react with a common enterobacterial antigen further supports Watson and Shorter's hypothesis (10,16,17). The increased number of immunoglobulin-producing plasma cells in diseased intestinal tissue (13) could result from stimulation of lymphoid cells with enterobacterial antigens. This is further supported by the presence of higher titers of serum antibodies against both aerobic and anaerobic intestinal bacteria (6,15). These antibodies could form immune complexes with complement fixing properties which could be responsible for a type-3 inflammatory reaction. These hypotheses are schematically drawn in Fig. 1. The observations might explain the therapeutic effects of azathioprine and metronidazole, both of which may reduce the number of anaerobic intestinal bacteria and probably the amount of bacterial antigens. Azathioprine also has immunosuppressive and anti-inflammatory properties, and metronidazole can increase the migratory activity of polymorphonuclear leucocytes which might improve phagocytosis.

ACKNOWLEDGMENTS

I wish to express my gratitude to Drs. G. Järnerot, J. Kjellander, A. Krook, S. Persson and S. Wallensten for permission to use their data.

LITERATURE CITED

1. Belsheim, J., H. Gnarpe, and S. Persson. 1978. Influence of metronidazole and timidazole on leucocyte chemotaxis in Crohn's disease. Infection 6 (Suppl. 1): 107.

2. Brandtzaeg, P., and K. Baklien. 1976. Immunohistochemical studies on the formation and epithelial transport of immunoglobulins in normal and diseased human intestinal mucosa. Scand. J. Gastroent. 11 (Suppl. 36): 1-45.

3. Campbell, D.E.S. 1973. New findings on the pharmacokinetics and pharmacology of sulfasalazine. Läkartidningen 70: 3068-3071.

4. Crohn, B.B., L. Ginzburg, and G.D. Oppenheimer. 1932. Regional ileitis. A pathologic and clinical entity. JAMA 99: 1323-1329.

5. Danielsson, D., and S. Persson. 1978. Antibacterial activity of Azathioprine (Imuran) against anaerobic intestinal bacteria: implications in Crohn's disease. Curr. Chemother. 295-298.

6. Danielsson, D., J. Kjellander, S. Persson, and S. Wallensten. 1979. Investigation of the immune response to aerobic and anaerobic intestinal bacteria in a patient with Crohn's disease. Scand. J. Infect. Dis. (Suppl. 19): 52-60.

7. Elion, G.B., S.W. Callahan, G.H. Hitchings, R.W. Rundles, and J. Laszlo. 1962. Experimental, clinical and metabolic studies of thiopurines. Cancer Chemother. Rep. 16: 167-202.

8. Kraft, S.C., and J.B. Kirsner. 1975. The immunology of ulcerative colitis and Crohn's disease: clinical and humoral aspects, p. 60-80. In J.B. Kirsner and R.G. Shorter (ed.), Inflammatory bowel disease. Lea and Febiger, Philadelphia.

9. Krook, A., D. Danielsson, J. Kjellander, and G. Järnerot. 1979. Changes in the fecal flora of patients with Crohn's disease during treatment with metronidazole. Scand. J. Gastroent. (In press).

10. Lagercrantz, R., S. Hammarström, P. Perlmann, and B.E. Gustavsson. 1966. Immunological studies in ulcerative colitis. III. Incidence of antibodies to colon-antigen in ulcerative colitis and other gastro-intestinal disease. Clin. Exp. Immunol. 1: 263-276.

11. O'Donoghue, D.P., A.M. Dawson, J. Powell-Tuck, and R.L. Brown. 1978. Double-blind withdrawal trial of azathioprine as maintenance treatment for Crohn's disease. Lancet ii: 955-957.

12. Rosenberg, J.L., B. Levin, A.J. Wall, and J.B. Kirsner. 1975. A controlled trial of azathioprine in Crohn's disease. Am. J. Dig. Dis. 20: 721-726.

13. Persson, S., and D. Danielsson. 1973. Studies on Crohn's disease II. Immunoglobulin-containing cells in the terminal ileum. Acta. Chir. Scand. 139: 735-738.

14. Persson, S., D. Danielsson, J. Kjellander, and S. Wallensten. 1976. Studies on Crohn's disease. I. The relationship between Yersinia enterocolitica infection and terminal ileitis. Acta. Chir. Scand. 142: 84-90.

15. Persson, S., and D. Danielsson. 1979. On the occurrence of serum antibodies to Bacteroides fragilis and serogroups of E. coli in patients with Crohn's disease. Scand. J. Infect. Dis. (Suppl. 19): 61-67.

16. Perlmann, P., S. Hammarström, R. Lagercrantz, and D. Campbell. 1967. Autoantibodies to colon in rats and human ulcerative colitis: Cross reactivity with Escherichia coli 0:14 antigen. Proc. Soc. Exp. Biol. Med. 125: 975-980.

17. Perlmann, P., and O. Broberger. 1969. Lower gastrointestinal system, p. 551-561. In P.A. Miescher and H.J. Müller-Eberhard (ed.), Textbook of immunopathology, Vol. 2. Grune and Stratton, New York.

18. Shorter, R.G., K.A. Huizenga, and R.J. Spencer. 1972. A working hypothesis for the etiology and pathogenesis of nonspecific inflammatory bowel disease. Am. J. Dig. Dis. 17: 1024-1032.

19. Thayer, W.R., M. Brown, M.H. Sangree, J. Katz, and T. Hersh. 1969. Escherichia coli 0:14 and colon hemagglutinating antibodies in inflammatory bowel disease. Gastroenterology 57: 311-318.

20. Ursing, B., and C. Kamme. 1975. Metronidazole in Crohn's disease. Lancet 1: 775-777.

21. Watson, D.W., and R.G. Shorter. 1975. The immunology of ulcerative colitis and Crohn's disease: Cell-mediated immune response, p. 81-89. In J.B. Kirsner and R.G. Shorter (ed.), Inflammatory bowel disease. Lea and Febiger, Philadelphia.

22. Willoughby, J.M.T., P.J. Kumar, J. Beckett, and A.M. Dawson. 1971. A controlled trial of azathioprine in Crohn's disease. Lancet ii: 944-946.

INFECTIONS FOLLOWING GASTRODUODENAL OPERATIONS

Ronald Lee Nichols and Joseph LoCicero III*

Henderson Professor of Surgery
Professor of Microbiology and Immunology
Department of Surgery
Tulane University School of Medicine
New Orleans, Louisiana

*Resident in Surgery
Tulane University School of Medicine
New Orleans, Louisiana

ENDOGENOUS GASTRIC MICROFLORA IN HEALTH

The stomach in a normal, fasting individual contains very low concentrations, if any, of both aerobic and/or anaerobic bacteria (15). This finding is of interest if one considers the large variety and numbers of bacteria that transiently enter the stomach primarily in swallowed saliva from the oral pharynx and to a lesser degree from small bowel contents that have refluxed through the pylorus. A review of each of these microfloras follows.

Oral Microflora In Health and Disease

The mouth and pharynx normally harbor a luxuriant microflora composed of both aerobic and anaerobic microorganisms. Saliva contains approximately 10^6 organisms per ml of a mixed flora which includes the following anaerobic oral bacteria: Bacteroides oralis, Bacteroides melaninogenicus, Peptostreptococcus, Bifidobacterium, and Fusobacterium. These anaerobes are generally sensitive to penicillin and are referred to as oral anaerobes. The oral pharynx also normally harbors fungi as well as aerobic bacteria such as Neisseria, streptococci, Haemophilus and occasionally staphylococci.

Studies have shown that extremely anaerobic conditions (Eh below -300 mV) exist in the dental plaque and around the gingival sulcus, providing an ideal environment for the growth of obligate oral anaerobes (8). Good dental hygiene and adequate nutrition are contributing factors to the prevention of an overgrowth of these organisms which are frequently found in patients with periodontal disease. Chronic alcoholics with poor dental hygiene who are prone to aspiration frequently develop pulmonary infections from these oral anaerobic microorganisms (4).

Proximal Small Intestinal Microflora in Health and Disease

This zone includes duodenum, jejunum, and most of the ileum. In health the sparse microflora consists chiefly of aerobic enteric bacteria: Escherichia coli, Klebsiella species, Enterobacter species, enterococci, and streptococci. Occasional anaerobes are isolated and are generally of the penicillin sensitive oral type, which appear to pass down the gastrointestinal tract after meals. Colonic anaerobes, such as Bacteroides fragilis, are rarely isolated from unobstructed proximal intestinal contents.

In the presence of mechanical small bowel obstruction, there is luxuriant overgrowth of microorganisms. Generally, above a high small intestinal obstruction, the flora is profuse; but below it the the flora is scant. The concentration of bacteria recovered from the small bowel progressively increases as the point of obstruction is located more distally in the jejunum or upper ileum (5). The microflora recovered in obstruction is a mixture of both oral and fecal flora. The source of fecal microorganisms in the upper small bowel in the presence of obstruction has not been clearly delineated. It would seem unlikely that retrograde contamination is the only mechanism involved (9).

THE INFLUENCE OF GASTRIC BACTERIAL INHIBITORY FACTORS ON THE ORGANISMS ENTERING THE STOMACH

The association of the intragastric acid-base balance and the bacterial flora of the stomach, duodenum and jejunum was stressed as early as 1926 (2). In a series of animal experiments the authors demonstrated the bacteriostatic action of the gastric acid (2,3). Subsequent studies by others, employing a variety of sample collection techniques, showed that individuals with normal gastric acid output and motility harbored few if any bacteria in the stomach or proximal intestine (6,7,10). Bacterial overgrowth in the stomach, however, was routinely reported in patients with either decreased gastric acid output (the elderly or patients with pernicious anemia) or altered gastric motility (duodenal or jejunal diverticuli) or both (following peptic ulcer surgery) (11,12,13).

INTRAGASTRIC MICROBIAL COLONIZATION IN COMMON DISEASE STATES OF THE STOMACH AND DUODENUM

We have examined the qualitative nature of the gastric microflora at the time of operation in patients undergoing elective or emergent gastric operations (Table 1) (16). A needle aspirated specimen of intragastric contents was taken after the peritoneal cavity was opened in each case. We also observed whether the presence of gastric microflora was related to postoperative wound infections or intraabdominal abscesses. None of the patients studied was given preoperative or intraoperative antibiotics.

Patients who underwent elective operation for chronic nonobstructing duodenal ulcer all had high preoperative gastric acid levels in a 12 h overnight study, and normal gastric motility as determined by barium study. In this group of patients, the gastric aspirate was sterile in 84% of cases. The remaining 16% demonstrated purely aerobic growth representative of the endogenous aerobes of the oropharynx and proximal intestine (Table 2).

In another group of patients undergoing emergent surgical procedures for acutely-bleeding duodenal ulcer, acid studies could not be done. Presumably, however, blood present in the stomach in these patients neutralized gastric acid and also impaired gastric motility. The gastric aspirates from all of these patients showed growth of microorganisms (Table 3). Sixty-seven percent exhibited a mixed aerobic-anaerobic microflora; 25% had pure anaerobic, and eight percent had pure aerobic flora.

The majority of patients with obstructing duodenal ulcer (89%) and gastric ulcer (83%) also had bacteria in the stomach at the time of surgery. Also, all patients with gastric cancer were found to have a mixed aerobic-anaerobic microflora. The postoperative infection rates ranged from 0 to 33% in these groups of patients (Table 4). The highest infection rates were observed in patients with

Table 1. Indications for Operation

Stomach or Duodenal Pathology	Number of Patients
Chronic duodenal ulcer	18
Bleeding duodenal ulcer	12
Obstructing duodenal ulcer	9
Gastric ulcer	6
Gastric carcinoma	4
Total	49

Table 2. Microflora of Stomach in Patients with Chronic Nonobstructing Duodenal Ulcer

Organisms		Number of Patients
No growth		15
Aerobic growth		3
Alpha streptococci, enterococci	(1)	
Klebsiella species, Candida species	(1)	
alpha streptococci, Neisseria species	(1)	
Anaerobic growth		0
Mixed (aerobic-anaerobic) growth		0
Total patients		18

bleeding duodenal ulcer (33%) and gastric malignancy (25%). The patients in these groups with high infection rates had a gastric microflora, due to compromise of the gastric inhibitory factors at the time of surgery, usually of a mixed aerobic-anaerobic nature. None of the patients in the chronic duodenal ulcer group, those with functioning acid, normal motility, and sparse intragastric microflora

Table 3. Microflora of Stomach in Patients with Bleeding Duodenal Ulcer

Organisms		Number of Patients
No growth		0
Aerobic growth		1
Escherichia coli, alpha streptococci, Neisseria species	(1)	
Anaerobic growth		3
Peptostreptococcus	(1)	
Bacteroides oralis, Bacteroides melaninogenicus	(2)	
Mixed (aerobic-anaerobic) growth		8
Alpha streptococci, *B*. oralis	(2)	
E. coli, *B*. oralis, Peptostreptococcus	(2)	
Alpha streptococci, Neisseria species, *B*. oralis, *B*. melaninogenicus	(2)	
Klebsiella species, *B*. melaninogenicus	(1)	
E. coli, Klebsiella species, Bifidobacterium	(1)	
Total patients		12

Table 4. Postoperative Wound Infections in Patients Undergoing Gastric Surgery

Indication for Operation	Number of Infections
Chronic duodenal ulcer	0/18-0%
Bleeding duodenal ulcer	4/12-33%
Obstructing duodenal ulcer	1/9 -11%
Gastric ulcer	1/6 -16%
Carcinoma of stomach	1/4 -25%
	7/49-14%

were infected postoperatively. All but one of these postoperative infections was due to one or more of the organisms isolated from the original intragastric needle aspiration. We therefore feel that, when present, the gastric microflora is the prime source of postoperative infections after gastric surgery. The organisms causing these infections were usually the oral anaerobes or the intestinal aerobic coliforms.

ANTIBIOTIC THERAPY IN GASTRIC SURGERY

Prophylaxis Before Gastric Surgery

There is no adequate double blind, prospective, random study to show the efficacy of prophylactic antibiotics in gastroduodenal surgery. The authoritative committees who have concerned themselves with surgical prophylaxis have therefore not recommended the use of prophylactic antibiotics in gastric surgery (1,19). However, recent studies have shown significantly lower infection rates in those patients treated with antibiotic prophylaxis before elective gastroduodenal operations (14,18).

It is apparent from our study that gastric bacterial colonization occurs almost uniformly in patients undergoing operation for bleeding or obstructing duodenal ulcer or for gastric ulcer or malignancy (29 of 31 patients). The reason for the gastric colonization in these groups of patients can best be explained by a compromise of the normal inhibitory effects of gastric acid and/or gastric motility. When present, this gastric microflora is usually equally divided between oral or proximal intestinal aerobes and oral penicillin-sensitive anaerobes. Only one penicillin-resistant anaerobe, B. fragilis, was isolated in our study. However, clostridial infections occur not infrequently after gastric surgery in the compromised host.

A double blind, prospective, random study is presently underway to determine if the administration of an appropriate parenteral antibiotic (a second generation cephalosporin) decreases this infection rate in the high risk groups of patients undergoing gastric surgery. The antibiotic is started preoperatively, so that tissue levels are present at the time of abdominal incision, and is continued for only a 12 h period thereafter, similar to the approach advocated by Polk (17) in patients undergoing colon resection.

Based on our experience as well as others advocating antibiotic prophylaxis in gastric surgery, this practice is indeed indicated in all patients undergoing gastric operation except those with uncomplicated chronic duodenal ulcer. The antibiotics chosen should be effective in controlling the usual organisms isolated in the gastric microflora (Table 5). Our preferences are either a second generation cephalosporin or a combination of penicillin and aminoglycoside.

Table 5. Antibiotic Susceptibilities of Commonly Isolated Upper Gastrointestinal Bacteria

Organisms	Penicillin[a]	Ampicillin	Cephalasporins[b]	Aminoglycosides[c]	Carbenicillin[d]
Aerobes					
Coliforms	-[e]	+[f]	++[g]	++	+
Streptococci	++	+	+	-	+
Anaerobes					
Oral Bacteroides	++	+	++	-	++
Clostridia	++	+	+	-	+
Peptostreptococci	++	+	++	-	++

[a] Aqueous.

[b] Second generation agents (cefoxitin, cefamandole).

[c] Gentamicin, tobramycin or amikacin.

[d] Carbenicillin or ticarcillin.

[e] Ineffective drugs or agents less useful because of irregular clinical responses.

[f] Other agents clinically useful.

[g] Drug of choice.

Therapy of Infections After Gastric Surgery

Early infections occurring within 48 h of operation are usually caused by streptococci or clostridia. Gram stains help to easily differentiate these organisms. As in any postsurgical infection adequate debridement and drainage of localized exudate remain the cardinal feature of therapy. The antibiotic of choice is penicillin which should be started preoperatively and continued six to 10 days.

Late infections limited to the operative incision require adequate drainage. Rarely are parenteral antimicrobials indicated. Intraperitoneal abscesses require both drainage and parenteral antibiotics. The initial agents employed should be similar to those used in prophylaxis. Alteration of these agents can be accomplished when culture and sensitivity results are available.

LITERATURE CITED

1. Antimicrobial Prophylaxis. 1977. Prevention of wound infection and sepsis after surgery. Medical Letter 19:37.

2. Arnold, L., and L. Brody. 1926. Bacterial flora and hydrogen ion concentration of the duodenum. J. Infect. Dis. 38:249.

3. Arnold, L. 1933. The bacterial flora within the stomach and small intestine. Am. J. Med. Sci. 186:471.

4. Bartlett, J.G., and S.M. Finegold. 1972. Anaerobic pleuropulmonary infections. Medicine 51:413.

5. Bishop, R.F., and E.A. Allcock. 1960. Bacterial flora of the small bowel in acute intestinal obstruction. Br. Med. J. 1: 766.

6. Bornside, G.H., and I. Cohn, Jr. 1965. The normal microbial flora. Am. J. Dig. 10:844.

7. Brooks, J.R., H.F. Smith, and F. B. Pease, Jr. 1974. Bacteriology of the stomach immediately following vagotomy: the growth of Candida albicans. Ann. Surg. 179:859.

8. Burnett, G.W., and H.W. Scherp. 1968. Oral microbiology and infectious disease, 3rd ed. Williams and Wilkins, Baltimore.

9. Condon, R.E., and R.L. Nichols. 1975. Antimicrobial therapy for surgical gastrointestinal disease. In B. M. Kagan (ed.), Antimicrobial therapy, 2nd ed. Saunders, Philadelphia.

10. Cregan, J., and N.J. Hayward. 1953. The bacterial content of the healthy human small intestine. Br. Med. J. 1:356.

11. Dellipiani, A.W., and R.H. Girdwood. 1964. Bacterial changes in the small intestine in malabsorptive states and in pernicious anemia. Clin. Sci. 26:359.

12. Giannella, R.A., S.A. Brottman, and N. Zamcheck. 1972. Gastric acid barrier to ingested microorganisms in man: studies in vivo and in vitro. Gut 13:251.

13. Gray, J.D.A., and M. Shiner. 1967. Influence of gastric pH on gastric and jejunal flora. Gut 8:574.

14. Lewis, R.I. 1977. Wound infection after gastric duodenal operation: a 10 year review. Can. J. Surg. 29:435.

15. Nichols, R.L., and R.E. Condon. 1975. Role of the endogenous gastrointestinal microflora in postoperative wound sepsis. In L.M. Nyhus (ed.). Surgery Annual. Appleton-Century-Crofts, New York.

16. Nichols, R.L., and J.W. Smith. 1975. Intragastric microbial colonization in common disease states of the stomach and duodenum. Ann. Surg. 182:557.

17. Polk, H.C., Jr., and J.F. Lopez-Mayor. 1969. Postoperative wound infection: a prospective study of determinant factors in prevention. Surgery 67: 97.

18. Stone, H.H., C.A. Hooper, L.D. Kolb, C.E. Geheber, and E.J. Dawkins. 1976. Antibiotic prophylaxis in gastric, billiary and colonic surgery. Ann. Surg. 181:443.

19. Veterans Administration Ad Hoc Interdisciplinary Advisory Committee on Antimicrobial Drug Usage. 1977. 1. Prophylaxis in surgery. J.A.M.A. 237:1003.

THE ANAEROBIC MICROFLORA ASSOCIATED WITH PERIODONTAL DISEASE

B.L. Williams

Department of Periodontics
University of Washington
Seattle, Washington 98195

INTRODUCTION

The human oral cavity supports dense populations of microbes associated with the surfaces and crevices afforded by various oral structures. Tooth surfaces above and below the gingiva, the dorsum of the tongue and the buccal surfaces are the major oral habitats amenable to colonization by bacteria. In recent years an impressive body of information has accumulated on many members of the oral microbiota, largely as a result of a quest for etiologic agents, pathogenic mechanisms and eventual control of oral disease. The purpose of this report is to relate the complexity of the oral flora associated with the periodontium in health and disease and to emphasize the role of the oral cavity as an important reservoir for systemic infections.

MICROBIAL SUCCESSION ON DENTAL SURFACES

Both the composition of the microbial plaque and the state of gingival or periodontal health associated with any portion of an individual's dentition are related to the frequency and efficiency of dental hygiene. The influence of good oral hygiene on periodontal health has been demonstrated most graphically by light and electron microscope studies of the development of dental plaque on unbrushed surfaces (5) and of the microbes which are present in association with periodontal health or various disease states (6). The microbial complexity of dental plaque is illustrated in Fig. 1 and Fig. 2.

Within minutes of thoroughly cleaning a tooth, as many as 10^5 bacteria become reattached per cm^2 of enamel surface (19). This bacterial adherence is mediated, in part, by salivary components,

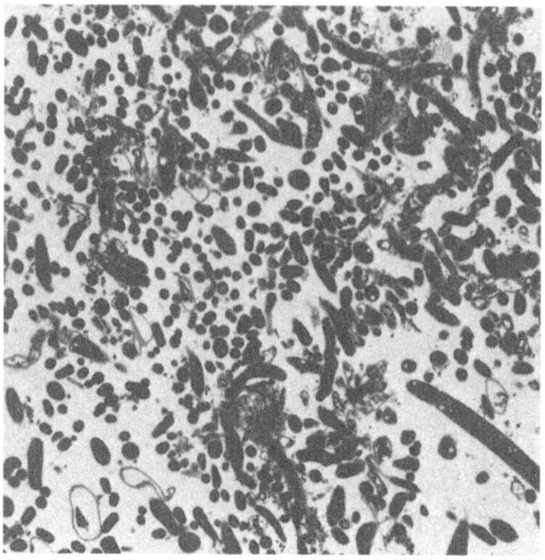

Fig. 1. Electron micrograph of dental plaque microorganisms located at the gingival margin in a clinically healthy mouth. (Photographed by B.B. Gallucci).

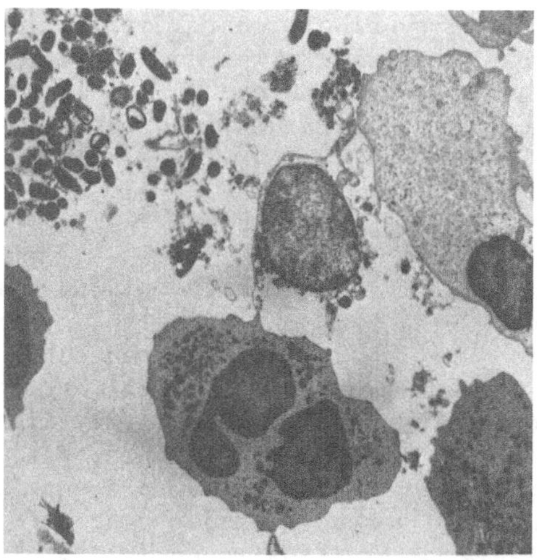

Fig. 2. Electron micrograph of plaque bacteria in close proximity to polymorphonuclear leukocytes in the same plaque sample as Fig. 1. (Photographed by B.B. Gallucci).

including a number of acidic and basic glycoproteins. Organisms accumulating within the first day or two consist primarily of alpha-hemolytic streptococci and the facultative Actinomyces, Actinomyces viscosus and Actinomyces naeslundii. These often appear as micro-colonies perpendicular to the enamel surface.

Metabolic processes of several organisms, particularly Streptococcus species and Veillonella parvula, reduce the oxidation-reduction potential of the microenvironments which surround developing plaques, creating habitats suitable for the survival of the more fastidious anaerobes. Thus, protected areas, such as between teeth and beneath the gingiva of individuals with a healthy dentition may contain a complex bacterial flora. Although subgingival plaque associated with a healthy periodontium is quantitatively less than that associated with most forms of periodontal disease, juvenile periodontitis is the exception, the organisms isolated from healthy subgingival sites reflect the diversity in the flora which constitute dental plaque (Table 1). Established plaques on clinically normal teeth are composed primarily of streptococci but these plaques may contain numerous anaerobes, including Gram-negative Veillonella, Fusobacterium, and Bacteroides as well as a diverse population of Gram-positive cocci and rods.

Table 1. Organisms Commonly Cultured from the Normal Gingival Sulcus

Gram Positive	Gram Negative
Staphylococcus epidermidis	Veillonella parvula
Micrococcus spp.	Capnocytophaga ochracea
Streptococcus sanguis	Capnocytophaga gingivalis
Streptococcus mitis	Bacteroides oralis
Streptococcus intermedius	Bacteroides melaninogenicus
Streptococcus morbillorum	subsp. melaninogenicus
Streptococcus constellatus	subsp. intermedius
Peptostreptococcus micros	Fusobacterium nucleatum
Lactobacillus casei	Eikenella corrodens
Lactobacillus acidophilus	"corroding" Bacteroides species
Eubacterium lentum	Anaerobic Vibrio species
Propionibacterium acnes	Campylobacter species
Rothia dentocariosa	
Actinomyces viscosus	
Actinomyces naeslundii	
Actinomyces odontolyticus	
Actinomyces israelii	

PLAQUE AND PERIODONTAL DISEASES

Gingivitis

When microbial masses are allowed to accumulate by cessation of dental hygiene measures, as in experimental gingivitis studies on healthy individuals, the time of onset of gingival inflammation can be correlated with increased proportions of Actinomyces in plaque formed along the gingival margins (8). Actinomyces, especially the facultative A. viscosus and A. naeslundii (23), are also prominent in the subgingival plaques surrounding teeth in cases of chronic gingivitis with loss of several millimeters of supporting alveolar bone; the latter is the hallmark of periodontitis. Another filamentous organism found on the external surface of "aged" plaque is Bacterionema which is often covered with a coccoid flora in specific aggregations known as "corncob" formations (Fig. 3 and Fig. 4). Fusobacterium, Veillonella and Campylobacter are additional Gram-negative species isolated from plaques associated with chronic gingival inflammation.

Periodontitis

It appears appropriate to digress with a brief review of clinical and histological features that characterize periodontal disease. The normal periodontium is a functional and dynamic association of the tooth root surface (cementum) with the gingival epithelium and subjacent connective tissues. The integrity of an individual's dentition depends on the status of the alveolar bone in which the

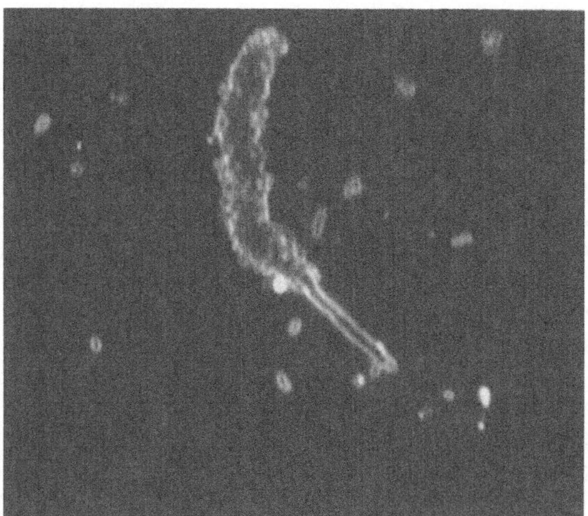

Fig. 3. Microbial association of a filament and cocci ("corn-cob" formation) from supragingival plaque by darkfield microscopy.

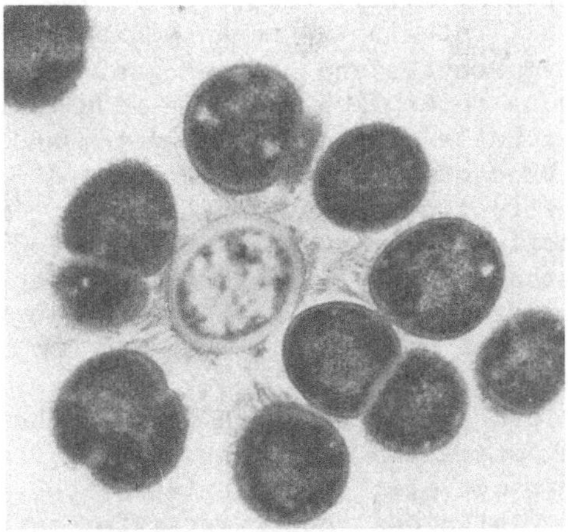

Fig. 4. Electron micrograph demonstrating a cross-sectional view of the central filament and surrounding cocci of a "corncob" formation. The morphology of the cell wall of the filament is consistent with that of Bacterionema. (Photographed by B.B. Gallucci).

teeth are embedded as well as on the bundles of collagen fibers which function to "lace" the teeth together by connecting and surrounding them. Fibroblasts and macrophages are the most common cell types in the clinically normal periodontal connective tissue.

In response to the accumulation of microbial plaque, inflammation which is first observed clinically in the gingiva as gingivitis extends to the underlying periodontal structures, resulting in the loss of attachment between these structures and the tooth. If the microbial insult is allowed to continue unimpeded, the end result is the loss of the teeth, as the collagen fibers and alveolar bone virtually disappear. The entire process takes place in the absence of microbial penetration into the gingival tissues. It is mediated by direct tissue destroying effects of bacterial products and by the response of humoral and cellular components of the immune system to antigens and other molecular species of plaque which gain access to the connective tissue.

Prior to the appearance of clinically visible signs of disease, the development of periodontitis and gingivitis begins with increasing numbers of neutrophils and loss of collagen in the gingiva. Neutrophil chemotaxis, presumably in response to microbial components of plaque, appears to be an important feature from the onset of the disease. During the sequence of changes which leads to the advanced periodontal lesion, large numbers of lymphocytes and an acute inflammatory exudate infiltrate the tissues. The depth of the gingival sulcus increases by several millimeters, reflecting these inflammatory changes. The infiltrate in the advanced lesion includes numerous plasma cells, lymphocytes and macrophages. By mechanisms not clearly understood, bone resorption probably results from complex interactions among the cells of the immune system and by direct effects of bacterial products such as endotoxin and lipoteichoic acid. Periodontal destruction appears to occur as periods of accelerated osteoclastic activity interspersed with periods of remission. Such periods of exacerbation and remission may reflect changes in the subgingival microflora or in the host's immunologic responsiveness, or both.

The microbial etiology of periodontal disease has been the subject of intense investigation in recent years. Progress has been relatively slow as a result of the complexity of the subgingival flora (Fig. 5), their fastidious requirements for nutrients and anaerobic atmospheres and, finally, the preponderance of microbial species that have been poorly defined taxonomically. The potential periodontal pathogens implicated to date are the spirochetes and a variety of Gram-negative bacteria, including Fusobacterium nucleatum capnophilic fusiform rods of the recently designated genus of Capnocytophaga, Selenomonas sputigenum, "corroding" species of Vibrio, Bacteroides and Eikenella, and Bacteroides asaccharolyticus as well as a number of unidentified organisms. These associations have been recently reviewed by Socransky (18), Slots (17), and Newman (13).

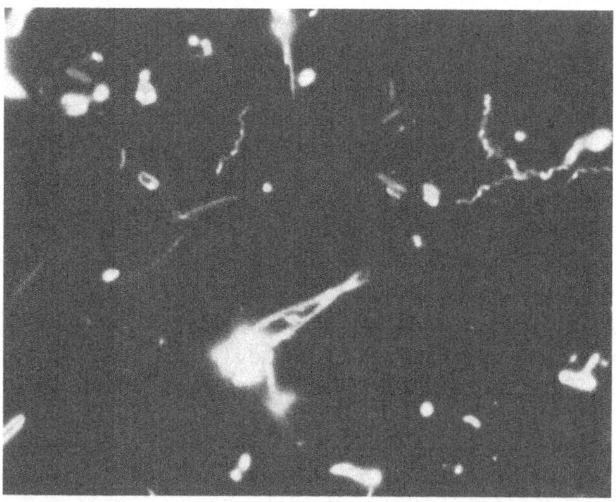

Fig. 5. Darkfield microscopy of subgingival plaque from rapidly advancing periodontitis. The small slender rods exhibited gliding motility characteristic of Capnocytophaga. Several spirochetes, Selenomonas and vibrio-like organisms can also be distinguished.

The role played by these and other specific members of the oral microbiota in periodontal pathology is often obscured by (i) the variable nature of dental plaque and (ii) the fact that alveolar bone loss appears in a spectrum of periodontal diseases. Bacterial populations in dental plaque have been observed to differ in supragingival to subgingival locations, from tooth to tooth and from patient to patient.

Different bacterial plaques have been isolated from patients exhibiting current bone loss accompanied by minimal inflammation than from those with moderate to severe inflammation. In a recent study by Tanner et al. (21), the proportion of B. asaccharolyticus isolated showed a positive correlation with the degree of inflammation. Samples of subgingival plaque from the most inflamed sites contained B. asaccharolyticus as 40-45% of the prominent cultivable flora. F. nucleatum, in contrast, often comprised 30% of the flora from sites with current or recent bone loss but the proportions of the latter organism showed no relation to the degree of inflammation surrounding the site investigated.

Juvenile Periodontitis

Periodontal disease most often is considered as a disease of the aging adult. Rapid loss of alveolar bone may, however, occur in the adolescent and, less frequently, in the pre-school child. Depressed neutrophil chemotaxis has been observed in affected individuals. The destruction may be generalized or it may be localized around first molars and incisors. Tooth loss occurs within two to six years.

In many cases of the juvenile disease, there has been no obvious accumulation of plaque although subgingival accumulation of organisms occurs. Lesions may progress rapidly in the absence of marked clinical signs of inflammation. Clear patterns of microbial etiology and pathogenic mechanisms among juvenile cases have not evolved. Microbial studies of the flora associated with such lesions (10,11,16) indicate the predominance of anaerobic Gram-negative rods. In contrast to the microbiota cultured from most adult periodontitis, the isolates from juveniles have frequently been saccharolytic. Again, much of this flora has been difficult to classify taxonomically.

Among five groups of unique Gram-negative rods isolated from cases of localized juvenile periodontitis, the most numerous were surface-translocating (gliding) Gram-negative bacilli (Fig. 6). Preliminary characterization of these isolates by Newman et al. (10) indicated that their taxonomic features were intermediate between those of the genera Bacteroides and Cytophaga. As a result of further collaborative studies, a new genus Capnocytophaga has been proposed to include gliding, anaerobic to microaerophilic, Gram-negative rods producing acetate and succinate as major metabolic end products and requiring carbon dioxide for growth (2,3,20,22). In DNA homology studies (22) 27 of 28 oral isolates of Capnocytophaga formed three mutually exclusive homology groups. DNA sequence homology of 77% was demonstrated between Bacteroides ochraceus ATCC 27872 and one of the homology groups of Capnocytophaga. They were, therefore, considered the same species and the new combination Capnocytophaga ochracea was proposed. New species Capnocytophaga sputigena and Capnocytophaga gingivalis were proposed for the other two phenotypically and genotypically distinct groups (20,22).

Acute Necrotizing Ulcerative Gingivitis (ANUG, Vincent's Infection)

This is an acute and painful infection occurring most commonly in teenagers and young adults. ANUG is recognized clinically by the ulcerated interdental papillae which have a characteristic "punched-out" appearance. The disease is associated with nutritional, physical or psychological stress as predisposing factors. Spirochetes and fusiforms have long been observed in the lesions. This so-called fusospirochetal complex does invade the gingival tissue (4). Although the precise ecologic role of microbial and other factors involved remains unclear, the disease is resolved with antimicrobial therapy. The anaerobic spectrum of metronidazole was accidently discovered by Shinn (15) when an unusually rapid improvement in ANUG infections was observed in patients taking metronidazole for the treatment of trichomonas infections.

Odontogenic Abscesses

Abscess formation beneath the gums often complicates periodontal disease. Such periodontal abscesses cause an exacerbation of bone

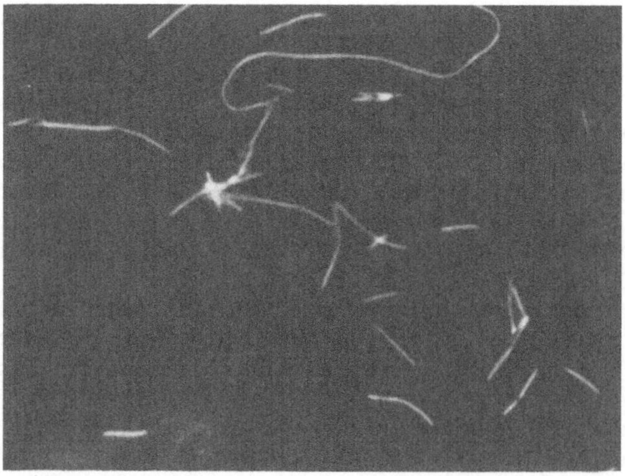

Fig. 6. Darkfield microscopy of Capnocytophaga ochracea ATCC 27872 after 18 h in Todd-Hewitt broth.

resorption and periodontal destruction. Periodontal abscesses may be superimposed on pre-existing periodontitis and are often recurrent. They may also develop in clinically healthy subgingival sites. Occlusion of the gingival sulcus at the gingival margin by food impaction or shrinkage due to localized reduction of gingival inflammation may be followed by abscess formation. These are mixed infections in which 60 to 75% of the cultivable flora consists of anaerobic Gram-negative rods (12). The most numerous isolates from purulent exudates are B. asaccharolyticus, the anaerobic peptococci and peptostreptococci, Capnocytophaga and Fusobacterium species as well as streptococci and staphylococci (Table 2).

Abscesses which arise beneath the root of the tooth are termed periapical abscesses. The microbial flora of periapical abscesses similarly is mixed, 75% of the isolates being anaerobic or microaerophilic. In recent cultivation studies by Williams, McCann and Schoenknecht (Table 2) one of 10 abscesses yielded a pure culture of a viridans streptococcus, Streptococcus milleri. Staphylococcus epidermidis was prominent in another abscess. Other isolates common to these lesions were F. nucleatum, Bacteroides melaninogenicus, Bacteroides oralis, Bacteroides ruminicola, Peptostreptococcus micros, and Streptococcus intermedius (Table 2). In addition to bacteria found in the pulp chambers of endodontically involved teeth, the source of infecting organisms and their entry to the site of abscess initiation is potentially via hematogenous routes. Once the infection is established at the apex of the tooth, the lesion must progress

Table 2. Relative Proportions (%) of Bacteria Isolated from Exudates of Ten Periapical Abscesses (Williams, McCann and Schoenknecht, Unpublished Results) and Nine Periodontal Abscesses (Newman and Sims, 1979)

Organism	Periapical	Periodontal
Anaerobic Gram-negative rods	36.9	61.5
Bacteroides asaccharolyticus		19.3
Bacteroides melaninogenicus	4.1	2.5
Bacteroides oralis/ruminicola	4.9	
Other Bacteroides species	11.7	0.4
Capnocytophaga	0.6	12.0
Fusobacterium species	15.6	10.1
"Vibrio corrodens"		8.0
Anaerobic Gram-positive cocci	30.3	13.5
Facultative Gram-positive cocci	16.4	9.7
Anaerobic Gram-negative cocci		9.5
Anaerobic/facultative Gram-positive rods	7.1	4.4

through the alveolar bone to produce the pathognostic fluctuant swellings.

ANTIMICROBIALS AND PERIODONTAL THERAPY

Early observations on the effectiveness of chemotherapeutic agents in controlling the destructive processes in acute forms of periodontal disease led to the acceptance of a microbial component in the etiology of the disease. The multiplicity as well as the ubiquitous occurrence of potential oral pathogens have complicated the application of antimicrobials against these mixed anaerobic infections. However, as with acute infections in general, antibiotics do have a significant therapeutic potential in the treatment of advanced and rapidly progressing periodontal lesions. Their role is that of an adjunct to mechanical debridement of microbial accumulations and necrotic tissues from the subgingival area.

Antimicrobial approaches to plaque-related diseases have been reviewed by Loesche (9). Broad-spectrum antibiotics generally have been employed because of the complexity of the flora and our inability to delineate the target pathogens. Antibiotics are administered systemically due to the inaccessability of subgingival plaque to agents applied topically.

The application of tetracycline to periodontal therapy has been the subject of a growing interest and debate among periodontitis in the United States. Although tetracycline is not the optimum agent for systemic use against a disease as common as periodontitis, remarkable success in reversing the destructive processes has been achieved by Socransky et al. at the Forsyth Dental Center in Boston (personal communication). The therapeutic effects of tetracycline administered in a dose of 1000 mg per day for two weeks may last from one to several years. Scaling and root planing without adjunctive antibiotic therapy may be similarly effective, at least over time intervals of up to six months, provided that very high levels of efficiency in oral hygiene measures are maintained (1,7). However, the systemically administered antibiotic provides the greatest long-term benefits by the more effective elimination of the causative microorganisms from niches which, in the absence of the antibiotic, would serve as intraoral reservoirs for future reinfection.

Dental plaques of individuals who are on tetracycline at a dose of 1000 mg per day are comprised predominantly of oral Streptococcus species and the branching, filamentous Gram-positive rods, Actinomyces and Rothia (24). Streptococcus, Veillonella and Neisseria are the oral genera which are consistently resistant to tetracycline when isolated during treatment; minimum inhibitory concentrations (MIC) of 128 ug/ml are commonly observed. Actinomyces, in contrast, seldom exhibit MIC's greater than 4 ug/ml (an exception is Actinomyces odontolyticus which always showed MIC's of 16 ug/ml or greater).

Prolonged doses of 250 mg of tetracycline per day, commonly used in the treatment of acne vulgaris, promotes the growth of a heterogeneous plaque containing antibiotic-resistant derivatives of many potential Gram-negative pathogens.

Socransky (18) has proposed the examination of microbial specificity in periodontal disease by eliminating the pathogenic flora with antimicrobial agents and monitoring disease activity. In a case reported by our laboratory (14), removal of the complex, predominantly asaccharolytic anaerobic periodontal pocket flora, by the administration of tetracycline was correlated with improved clinical status which was measured by decreased pocket depth as well as decreased gingival inflammation. "Corroding" anaerobic rods and B. asaccharolyticus failed to recolonize during the 12 months of surveillance; the implied etiologic significance of these organisms is consistent with the results of studies cited previously. The overgrowth by F. nucleatum, accompanied by P. micros, within six to eight weeks following therapy (Table 3) may reflect the relative

Table 3. Examples of Changes in Subgingival Flora of a Single Periodontal Pocket in Response to Tetracycline Therapy (Osterberg, Williams and Jorgensen, 1979)

Flora	Sample		
	A[a]	B[b]	C[c]
Peptostreptococcus micros	7[d]	--	19
Streptococcus mutans	--	45	--
Streptococcus sanguis	--	37	--
Actinomyces viscosus	--	17	--
Actinomyces, unidentified species	1	--	25
Eubacterium lentum	5	5	--
Bacteroides asaccharolyticus	31	--	--
Bacteroides melaninogenicus subsp. intermedius	2	--	--
Capnocytophaga species	--	--	1
Fusobacterium nucleatum	6	--	45
"Corroding" anaerobic Gram-negative rods	8	--	--
Unidentified non-fermentative anaerobic Gram-negative rods	35	--	--

[a] Periodontal pocket flora before treatment.

[b] Pocket flora after two weeks of 1000 mg tetracycline per day.

[c] 14 weeks after discontinuing tetracycline.

[d] Per cent of total flora isolated.

ability of these organisms to dominate the subgingival flora under conditions of ecological stress. They are prominent in odontogenic abscesses. Indeed, periapical abscess formation is not an uncommon complication following termination of tetracycline therapy. However, these observations together with the data of Tanner et al. (21) indicate that the proportions of F. nucleatum in subgingival plaque may not have a significant role in periodontal destruction but that their numbers reflect an adaptation and competitive advantage in this highly proteinaceous niche.

PERSPECTIVES AND SUMMARY

The human oral cavity is an active area of microbiological investigation. In this report, I have sketched some of the recent attempts at characterizing dental plaques and their constituent organisms in the initiation and progression of periodontal lesions. Major progress has been made in the ability to identify these organisms taxonomically. The interactions that occur between microbes and immune cells to precipitate periodontal destruction is an interesting problem which has recently come into focus.

The inclusion of aspects of oral bacteriology in numerous microbiology symposia such as this has disseminated much of our knowledge of normal and pathogenic oral bacteria from the microcosm of a relatively few investigators to the periphery of a world of medical microbiologists and clinical laboratories. This point is perhaps best illustrated by the new subject category of "Oral Microbiology and Immunology" in Infection and Immunity. An appreciation of oral microbes is an important advance medically, as one need not spend but a day in most hospital laboratories to recognize the oral cavity as a significant reservoir for infections occurring in many locations in the human host.

From an infectious disease point of view, periodontitis must be recognized as an ulceration of a major integument, the epithelial lining of the gingival sulcus. As individuals with advanced or chronic periodontitis characteristically have an involvement of half to two-thirds of their dentition, with periodontal pockets extending from 6 to 12 mm in depth, the ulceration of the apical regions of these pockets may be comparable to an exposed wound the size of a quarter. Considering the grams of anaerobic bacteria harbored in such sites, the profuse vasculature of the gingival tissues and the mechanical pressures applied by mastication, bacteremias must continually tax the host defenses of these compromised individuals.

LITERATURE CITED

1. Helldèn, L.B., M.A. Listgarten, and J. Lindhe. 1979. The effect of tetracycline and/or scaling on human periodontal disease. J. Clin. Periodont. 6: 222-230.

2. Holt, S.C., E.R. Leadbetter, J.L. Simpson, E.D. Savitt, and S.S. Socransky. 1979. Capnocytophaga: new genus of Gram-negative gliding bacteria. II. Morphology and ultrastructure. Arch. Microbiol. 122: 17-27.

3. Leadbetter, E.R., S.C. Holt, and S.S. Socransky. 1979. Capnocytophaga: new genus of Gram-negative gliding bacteria. I. General characteristics, taxonomic considerations and significance. Arch. Microbiol. 122: 9-16.

4. Listgarten, M.A. 1965. Electron microscopic observations on the bacterial flora of acute necrotizing ulcerative gingivitis. J. Periodont. 36: 328.

5. Listgarten, M.A., H.E. Mayo, and R. Tremblay. 1975. Development of dental plaque on epoxyresin crowns in man. A light and electron microscopic study. J. Periodont. 46: 10-26.

6. Listgarten, M.A. 1976. Structure of the microbial flora associated with periodontal health and disease in man. J. Periodont. 47: 1-18.

7. Listgarten, M.A., J. Lindhe, and L. Helldèn. 1978. The effect of tetracycline and/or scaling on human periodontal disease--clinical, microbiological and histological observation. J. Clin. Periodont. 5: 246-271.

8. Loesche, W.J. 1975. Bacterial succession in dental plaque: role in dental disease, p. 132-136. In. D. Schlessinger (ed.), Microbiology - 1975. American Society for Microbiology, Washington, D.C.

9. Loesche, W.J. 1976. Chemotherapy of dental plaque infections. Oral Sci. Rev. 9: 65-107.

10. Newman, M.G., S.S. Socransky, E.D. Savitt, D.A. Propas, and A. Crawford. 1976. Studies on the microbiology of periodontosis. J. Periodont. 47: 373-379.

11. Newman, M.G., and S.S. Socransky. 1977. Predominant cultivable microbiota in periodontosis. J. Periodont. Res. 12: 120-128.

12. Newman, M.G., and T.N. Sims. 1979. The predominant cultivable microbiota of the periodontal abscess. J. Periondont. 50: 350-354.

13. Newman, M.G. 1979. The role of Bacteroides melaninogenicus and other anaerobes in periodontal infections. Rev. Infect. Dis. 1: 313-323.

14. Österberg, S.K.-Å, B.L. Williams, and J. Jorgensen. 1979. Long-term effects of tetracycline on the subgingival microflora. J. Clin. Periodont. 6: 133-140.

15. Shinn, D.L.S. 1962. Metronidazole in acute ulcerative gingivitis. Lancet 1: 1191.

16. Slots, J. 1976. The predominant cultivable microbiota of periodontosis. Scand. J. Dent. Res. 84: 1-10.

17. Slots, J. 1979. Subgingival microflora and periodontal disease. J. Clin. Periodont. 6: 351-382.

18. Socransky, S.S. 1977. Microbiology of periodontal disease-present status and future consideration. J. Periodont. 48: 497-504.

19. Socransky, S.S., A.D. Manganiello, D. Propas, V. Oram, and J. van Houte. 1977. Bacteriological studies of developing supragingival dental plaque. J. Periodont. Res. 12: 90-106.

20. Socransky, S.S., S.C. Holt, E.R. Leadbetter, and A.C.R. Tanner. 1979. Capnocytophaga: new genus of Gram-negative gliding bacteria. III. Physiological characterization. Arch. Microbiol. 122: 29-33.

21. Tanner, A.C.R., C. Haffer, G.T. Bratthall, R.A. Visconti, and S.S. Socransky. 1979. A study of the bacteria associated with advancing periodontitis in man. J. Clin. Periodont. 6: 278-307.

22. Williams, B.L., and B.F. Hammond. 1979. Capnocytophaga: new genus of Gram-negative gliding bacteria. IV. DNA base composition and sequence homology. Arch. Microbiol. 122: 35-39.

23. Williams, B.L., R.M. Pantalone, and J.C. Sherris. 1976. Subgingival microflora and periodontitis. J. Periodont. Res. 11: 1-18.

24. Williams, B.L., S.K.-Å Österberg, and J. Jorgensen. 1979. Subgingival microflora of periodontal patients on tetracycline therapy. J. Clin. Periodont. 6: 210-221.

THE RELATIONSHIP BETWEEN THE PERIODONTAL MICROFLORA AND ALVEOLAR BONE LOSS IN MACACA ARCTOIDES

Jørgen Slots, Ernest Hausmann, Christian Mouton,
Lance F. Ortman, Paulette G. Hammond and Robert J. Genco

Department of Oral Biology and Periodontal Disease
Clinical Research Center, State University of New York
at Buffalo, Buffalo, New York 14226

INTRODUCTION

Several investigators have studied intensively for the last five years the subgingival microflora associated with various clinical entities of human periodontal disease (13,16). These studies have all been cross-sectional in nature. Although of considerable interest, the available data cannot provide information as to whether an organism initiates, contributes to the progression of, or is secondary to the pathological changes.

Longitudinal investigations of destructive periodontal disease cannot be readily carried out in humans because of the potential risk of irreversibility of the periodontal defects. Therefore, development of an animal model is desirable. The feasibility of using the stump-tailed macaque, Macaca arctoides (Macaca speciosa) as a model for the study of human periodontal disease has recently been evaluated in our department. This monkey species closely resembles humans in several important aspects: (i) gingivitis is readily induced using the experimental gingivitis model (8); (ii) the gingivitis histopathology is similar (8); (iii) diphenylhydantoin administration results in gingival hyperplasia in the presence of bacterial dental plaque (17); (iv) the gingivitis microflora is closely related (10); (v) major salivary secretions appear identical (9). In M. arctoides, as shown for other animal models (7,11), a stable established gingivitis lesion can be converted into a progressive periodontal lesion with loss of tooth-supporting tissues by the insertion of a ligature in the periodontal pocket area. This ligature technique permits study of alveolar bone loss in a relatively short period of time.

This report describes (i) the effect of a subgingival ligature on the alveolar bone of M. arctoides, (ii) the relationship between the subgingival microbial composition and the clinical status of the periodontal tissues, and (iii) biochemical and immunological properties of M. arctoides isolates of the Bacteroides melaninogenicus/Bacteroides asaccharolyticus group. Portions of this report appear elsewhere (4,14,15).

MATERIALS AND METHODS

Animals

Six adult M. arctoides females (6-9 kg in weight) were used in this study. They were fed Purina Monkey Chow and housed individually in a room with other monkeys.

Design

Prior to the present study, the monkeys received the primate diet in its original hard form. During the experimental period, the diet was moisture-softened to enhance dental plaque formation. For all six monkeys, base-line alveolar bone mass measurements were made over a period of one to three weeks, afterwards a 3-0 silk ligature was placed subgingivally on the mesial surface of the left lateral maxillary incisor. Bone mass measurements were carried out during a period of two to four weeks following the ligature placement. In three monkeys, a ligature was also placed around the right lateral maxillary incisor at a time when the animals received a daily dose of 250 mg tetracycline in the drinking water and a daily rinsing of the ligated area with 0.2% solution of chlorhexidine gluconate. For two monkeys, representative of the six monkeys, microbiological analysis of the periodontal microflora was carried out prior to the experimental period (week 0), after one week with the soft diet regimen and immediately before the insertion of the ligature (week 1), after three weeks with ligature (week four), and one week following the termination of a two to three week antibacterial therapy (week eight). Routine clinical measurements were performed to evaluate the periodontal conditions. In addition, the Henrikson ^{125}I absorptiometric technique was used to quantitate the alveolar bone mass. This technique measures the bone mass at the same localized alveolar bone site with a precision of 1 to 3% (5).

Bacteriological Processing, Isolation, and Identification

Bacteriological specimens were collected by insertion of six sterile paperpoints into the periodontal pocket, each being retained therein for 10 s. The paperpoints were transferred to a tube containing 1.5 ml of PRAS Ringer solution and the sample material was mixed by a Vortex mixer for 60 s. Plating of portions (0.1 ml) of appropriate dilutions were performed on Trypticase soy agar (BBL) supplemented with 10% sheep blood, 5 ug of hemin per ml, and 0.5 ug of menadione per ml. Following seven days of incubation, a total of 24-52 isolates from each periodontal pocket sample was subcultured and characterized according to established microbiological procedures. Sample collecting and processing were done under anaerobic conditions by flushing with a mixture of 85% Ar, 10% H_2, and 5% CO_2. The bacterial cultivation took place in an anaerobic glove box (Coy Manufacturing Co., Ann Arbor, Mich.). An average of 45% of the total monkey subgingival bacterial cells were cultivated with the present microbiological techniques. Comparison between culture results and direct phase-contrast microscopic counts revealed that spirochetes and Vibrio/Selenomonas-like organisms made up approximately 75% of the noncultivable microflora.

Indirect Immunofluorescent-Technique

An immunological study of monkey B. melaninogenicus and B. asaccharolyticus isolates was carried out using an indirect fluorescent antibody staining procedure routinely performed in our laboratory. Briefly, heat fixed smears of formalinized broth or plate cultures were reacted with the highest dilution of specific rabbit antiserum giving a 4+ reaction when tested with the immunizing strain. The antisera against the monkey strains 7724-3-5 and MD1-17 and against the human strains 381 (immunosorbed with strain 20-3) and 20-3/4127 (immunosorbed with strain 381) were used at a dilution 1:800. The antiserum to monkey strain MC1-9 was diluted 1:400.

After reacting the antisera with the bacterial cells, the slides were washed and dried. A drop of a 1:100 dilution of goat antibodies monospecific for rabbit IgG conjugated with fluorescein isothiocyanate was added to each smear, and the smears were incubated, washed, and dried as before. The smears were read with a Leitz Orthoplan microscope equipped for phase-contrast illumination and for incident light fluorescence. A moderate (3+) to brilliant (4+) fluorescence with a good cell envelope definition was considered serologically significant.

RESULTS

Alveolar Bone Mass

The alveolar bone mass was measured in six monkeys using the ^{125}I absorptiometric technique at a localized site immediately below the alveolar crest (Fig. 1). In general, only small fluctuations in alveolar bone mass were observed during the base-line period. Subgingival placement of silk ligatures on the left lateral maxillary incisors, however, resulted within two-three weeks in a distinct inflammatory response at the ligated site (Fig. 2) and a significant

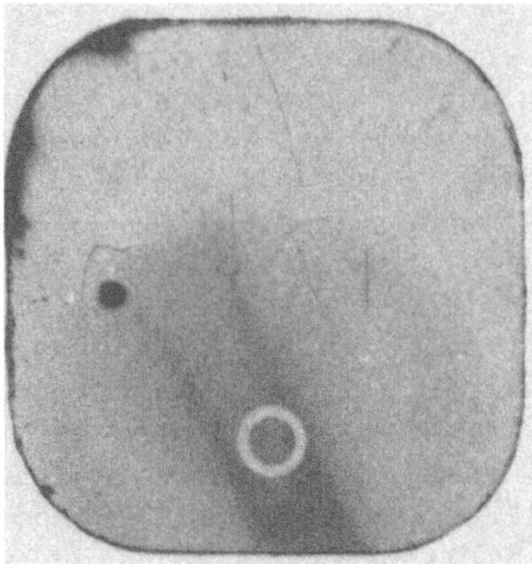

Fig. 1. X ray of an interproximal area at which ^{125}I absorptiometric measurements were taken. The circle (diameter of 1 mm) shows the area where bone mass measurements were made.

bone loss at the localized test site (Fig. 3). This bone loss was demonstrated to be reversible (at sites in monkeys 7397 and 7444) when antibacterial therapy was started several weeks after placement of ligatures (Table 1). Also, ligatures placed around the right lateral maxillary incisors of three monkeys concomitant with antibacterial therapy induced no significant local inflammatory response and loss of alveolar bone (Fig. 3). These data indicate that the alveolar bone loss observed was due to bacterial action and not to a mechanical trauma of the ligature.

Monkey Periodontopathic Microflora

The microbial variation between multiple subgingival samples was examined in one female M. arctoides (7511) during a period of six weeks when no net alveolar bone loss was observed using the 125I absorptiometric technique. This monkey was fed a soft diet 10 weeks prior to and during the six weeks test period which resulted in the development of a significant amount of dental plaque on most tooth surfaces. The bacteriological samples originated from the mesial surfaces of the left and right lateral maxillary incisors, which showed moderate gingival inflammation during the six week experiment. The subgingival microbial composition varied relatively little both qualitatively and quantitatively during the six week period of study (Table 2). Gram-positive facultative organisms comprised more than 60% of the cultivable microflora in eight of the nine samples investigated and the same bacterial genera and species tend to predominate through the study.

By contrast, the subgingival microflora in the experiment with a

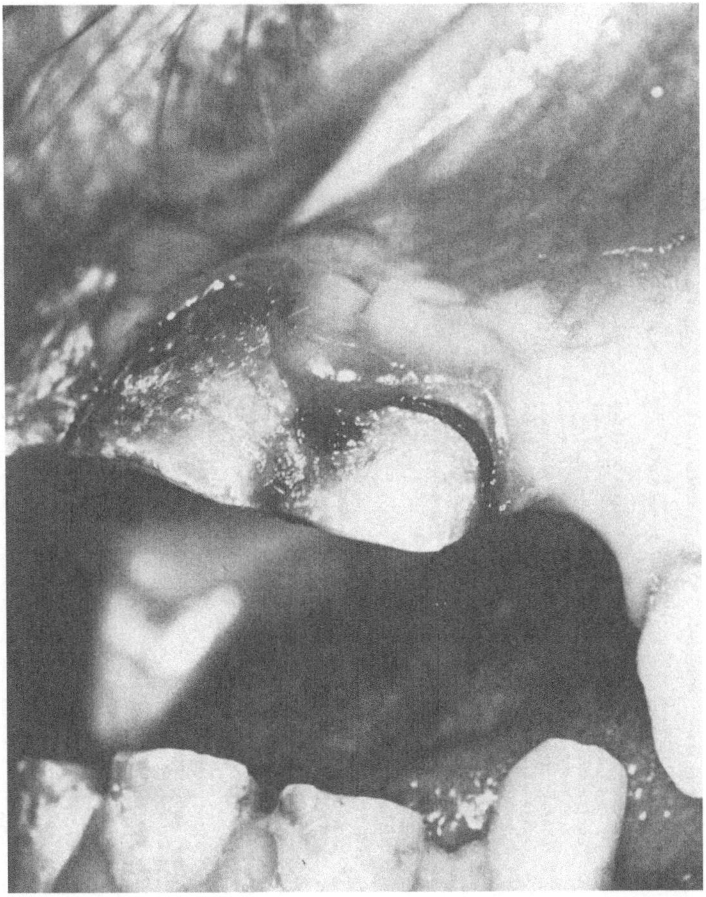

Fig. 2. Ligature placed around maxillary lateral incisor. Note the edema in the papilla between the central and lateral incisor.

subgingivally inserted ligature exhibited marked quantitative changes during the eight week experimental period (Table 1).

At week zero, Gram-positive organisms constituted approximately 3/4 of the subgingival microflora. Asaccharolytic Eubacterium species and Peptostreptococcus/Peptococcus species predominated in monkey 7397 and Streptococcus species were the predominant isolates in monkey 7444 (Table 1).

The institution of a soft diet regimen resulted in the development of a more severe gingivitis and a major shift in the subgingival

Table 1. A Longitudinal Study of Experimentally Induced Periodontitis in two Macaca arctoides Females; Changes in the Predominant Subgingival Microflora and the Alveolar Bone Mass

Monkey	Hard Diet	Week 0	Soft Diet Started	Week 1	Ligature Inserted	Week 4	Ligature; Chemotherapy Started	Week 8
7397		6% Streptococcus sanguis 2% Streptococcus milleri 19% Peptostreptococcus/ Peptococcus spp. 8% Facultative actinomycetes 36% Eubacterium spp. 11% Haemophilus spp. 2% Vibrios 4% Bacteroides spp. 11% Bacteroides melaninogenicus subsp. macacae 19% Vibrios[a] 8% Spirochetes[a]		4% S. sanguis 2% S. milleri 6% Peptostreptococcus/ Peptococcus spp. 8% Facultative actinomycetes 17% Eubacterium spp. 4% Veillonella parvula 45% Haemophilus spp. 4% Vibrios 4% Fusobacterium nucleatum 8% Bacteroides spp. 2% B. melaninogenicus subsp. macacae 57% Vibrios 5% Spirochetes		2% S. sanguis 5% Facultative actinomycetes 7% Eubacterium spp. 15% F. nucleatum 2% Bacteroides spp. 2% B. melaninogenicus subsp. intermedius 15% B. melaninogenicus subsp. macacae 51% B. asaccharolyticus 18% Vibrios 13% Spirochetes		4% Peptostreptococcus/ Peptococcus spp. 13% Facultative actinomycetes 21% Haemophilus spp. 29% F. nucleatum 12% Bacteroides spp. 13% B. melaninogenicus subsp. intermedius 8% B. melaninogenicus subsp. macacae 20% Vibrios 10% Spirochetes
% Change in Bone Mass		0		-2		-11 (-21 at week 5)		+3
7444		52% S. sanguis 19% S. milleri 2% Streptococcus mitior 2% Staphylococcus/ Micrococcus spp. 23% Haemophilus spp. 2% F. nucleatum 23% Vibrios 10% Spirochetes		2% S. sanguis 7% Staphylococcus/ Micrococcus spp. 7% Peptostreptococcus productus 13% Facultative actinomycetes 11% Eubacterium spp. 24% Haemophilus spp. 13% Vibrios 4% F. nucleatum 9% Bacteroides spp. 11% B. asaccharolyticus 18% Vibrios 10% Spirochetes		15% Facultative actinomycetes 3% Propionibacterium acnes 3% Haemophilus spp. 3% Vibrios 3% F. nucleatum 8% Bacteroides spp. 63% B. melaninogenicus subsp. macacae 5% B. asaccharolyticus 3% Vibrios 7% Spirochetes		4% Facultative actinomycetes 36% Haemophilus spp. 4% F. nucleatum 52% B. melaninogenicus subsp. macacae 4% B. asaccharolyticus 26% Vibrios
% Change in Bone Mass		0		-10		-38 (+8 at week 7)		-28

[a] The vibrios and the spirochetal data originate from direct phase-contrast microscopic examination.

Table 2. A Longitudinal Study of the Predominant Gingivitis Microflora in a Macaca arctoides Female during a Six Week Experimental Period

Monkey	Week 0	Week 1	Week 2	Week 3	Week 4	Week 6
7411 Left lateral maxillary incisor	18% Streptococcus spp. 6% Actinomyces viscosus 36% Actinomyces naeslundii 9% Campylobacter spp. 12% Fusobacterium spp. 12% Bacteroides spp. 6% Bacteroides melaninogenicus subsp. macacae 32% Vibrios[a] 5% Spirochetes[a]	24% Streptococcus spp. 30% Staphylococcus/ Micrococcus spp. 21% A. viscosus 14% Catalase +, anaerobic Actinomyces spp. 10% Veillonella parvula 3% Fusobacterium spp. 44% Vibrios 8% Spirochetes	19% Streptococcus spp. 23% A. viscosus 23% A. naeslundii 10% Actinomyces israelii 6% V. parvula 6% Fusobacterium spp. 9% Bacteroides spp. 3% B. melaninogenicus subsp. intermedius 50% Vibrios 33% Spirochetes			
7511 Right lateral maxillary incisor	28% Streptococcus spp. 34% A. naeslundii 10% Catalase +, anaerobic Actinomyces spp. 3% A. israelii 17% Vibrio succinogenes 7% Fusobacterium spp. 53% Vibrios 6% Spirochetes	36% Streptococcus spp. 4% A. viscosus 50% V. parvula 11% Fusobacterium spp. 15% Vibrios 7% Spirochetes	46% Streptococcus spp. 4% Peptostreptococcus/ Peptococcus spp. 14% A. viscosus 11% A. israelii 4% V. parvula 4% Haemophilus spp. 18% Fusobacterium spp. 50% Vibrios 6% Spirochetes	3% Streptococcus spp. 53% A. viscosus 6% A. naeslundii 6% A. israelii 6% Campylobacter spp. 18% Fusobacterium spp. 9% Bacteroides spp. 27% Vibrios 18% Spirochetes	33% Streptococcus spp. 29% A. viscosus 8% A. israelii 8% Campylobacter spp. 4% Fusobacterium spp. 13% Bacteroides spp. 4% B. melanino- genicus subsp. intermedius 50% Vibrios 40% Spirochetes	22% Streptococcus spp. 59% A. viscosus 6% A. naeslundii 3% A. israelii 9% Fusobacterium spp. 13% Vibrios 30% Spirochetes

[a] The vibrios and the spirochetal data originate from direct phase-contrast microscopic examination.

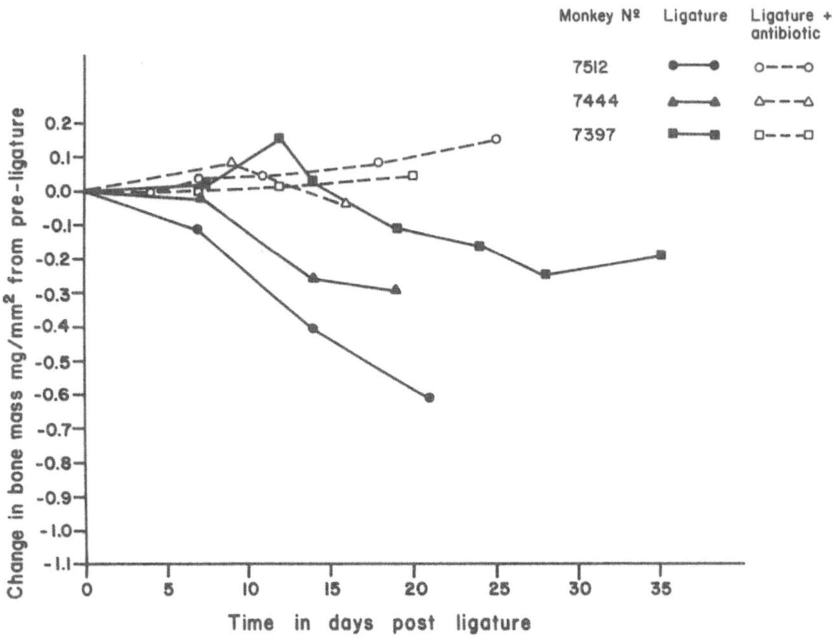

Fig. 3. Change in alveolar bone mass in three monkeys in response to placement of a ligature. , ligature without antibacterial therapy; -----, ligature plus antibacterial therapy.

microflora. At week one, Gram-negative isolates made up almost 2/3 of the total microflora; the predominant isolates were Haemophilus-like organisms in monkey 7397 and various Gram-negative anaerobic rods in monkey 7444 (Table 1).

The placement of subgingival ligatures induced a bone resorption of up to 38% at the localized site beneath the alveolar crest studied and also significantly altered the subgingival microflora (Table 1). At week four, Gram-negative bacteria comprised more than 80% of the microflora in both monkeys and approximately 66% of the total isolates were strains of B. asaccharolyticus and Bacteroides melaninogenicus subsp. macacae (Table 1).

The chemotherapy again changed the subgingival microflora. In monkey 7397, B. asaccharolyticus was not isolated and B. melaninogenicus subsp. macacae comprised only 8% of the total isolates one week following the termination of the antibacterial therapy (Table 1). The clinical data for monkey 7397 at week eight revealed that the bone loss had stopped and that a remineralization of the alveolar bone was taking place (Table 1). In monkey 7444, at week eight the subgingival microflora sampled closely resembled that of week four with a strong predominance of B. melaninogenicus subsp. macacae (Table 1). Bone breakdown reappeared in this monkey after a period of bone regeneration at the time of antibacterial therapy (Table 1).

Monkey Isolates of the B. melaninogenicus/B. asaccharolyticus Group

The demonstration of a close relationship between the number of B. melaninogenicus-like isolates and the amount of alveolar bone loss led to a study of these organisms' biochemical properties. Their antigenic characteristics were also studied by an indirect fluorescent antibody procedure. Monkey and human oral isolates of B. asaccharolyticus and Bacteroides melaninogenicus subsp. intermedius appeared biochemically (data not presented) and immunologically (Table 3) identical. The monkey periodontopathic microflora, however, also contained a significant number of a H_2O_2-splitting B. melaninogenicus species termed B. melaninogenicus subsp. macacae (subsp. nov.) which previously has not been isolated from humans. These organisms, in addition to being catalase positive, produced indole and H_2S, hydrolyzed gelatin, but not esculin and starch, and weakly fermented galactose, glucose, lactose, and mannose (a pH decrease of 0.6-1.0 unit compared to inoculated PY broth) (6). No fermentation took place of 24 other carbohydrates tested. The organisms formed approximately 6.0 meq/100 ml acetic and propionic acids and less than 1.0 meq/100 ml isobutyric, butyric, isovaleric, and succinic acids in PYG cultures. Furthermore, antiserum to B. melaninogenicus subsp. macacae exhibited no positive fluorescent reaction with monkey and human strains of B. asaccharolyticus and B. melaninogenicus subsp. intermedius, Bacteroides melaninogenicus subsp. melaninogenicus, and Bacteroides melaninogenicus subsp. levii (Table 3) indicating that B. melaninogenicus subsp. macacae possesses a distinct surface antigen composition.

DISCUSSION

The ^{125}I absorptiometric technique permits precise measurements of alveolar bone loss observed longitudinally. All six monkeys studied exhibited a significant decrease in alveolar bone mass after the application of a subgingival ligature. However, variation in the magnitude of bone loss was also observed. Differences in alveolar bone breakdown may reflect variations in the pathogenicity of the periodontal microflora and/or variations in host response to the bacterial insults.

The present study revealed that strains of B. asaccharolyticus and B. melaninogenicus subsp. macacae together increased in proportion from a few percent to about 66% of the total subgingival isolates concomitant with the development of a significant alveolar bone loss.

Table 3. Immunological Relationship between Monkey and Human Strains of B. asaccharolyticus and B. melaninogenicus Determined by Indirect Fluorescent Antibody Technique

Organisms and Strain Number[a]	Antisera to Monkey Strains			Antisera to Human Strains	
	MC1-9	7724-3-5	MD1-17	381	20-3/4127
Human oral B. asaccharolyticus 381, 1021, 1432, K110	+[b]	-[c]	-	+	-
Human non-oral B. asaccharolyticus 536, 27067, 207-72	-	-	-	-	-
Human B. melaninogenicus subsp. intermedius oral: 20-3, 4127, AB1-10, I(2516) non-oral: 2845,25261,532-70,275-70A	-	+	-	-	+
Human B. melaninogenicus subsp. melaninogenicus oral: 25845 non-oral: 2721	-	+	-	-	+
Non-oral B. melaninogenicus subsp. levii human: 9644-1A, 10458A bovine: 12466,10450 (ATCC 29147)	-	-	-	-	-
Monkey oral B. asaccharolyticus MC1-9, MC1-11, MC1-14, MC1-16	+	-	-	(+) to +	-
Monkey oral B. melaninogenicus subsp. intermedius 7724-3-5, 7724-3-1, 7728-L-1-1, MM2	-	+	-	-	+
Monkey oral B. melaninogenicus subsp. macacae MD1-17, MC1-3, MD1-1, 7511L-2-2	-	-	+	-	-

[a] Source of strains: S.S. Socransky (381), R.J. Gibbons (K110), J.M. Hardie (19069), S.M. Finegold (536, 2721, 2845), D.W. Lambe (207-72, 532-70, 275-70A), L.V. Holdeman (9644-1A, 10450, 10458A, 12466), ATCC (25261, 25845, 27067). The remaining strains were isolated in our laboratory.

[b] +: 3+ or 4+ fluorescence

[c] -: 0,1+, or 2+ fluorescence

These data along with the finding that B. asaccharolyticus is a prevalent organism in advanced adult periodontitis in humans (12), incriminate greatly B. asaccharolyticus as an important pathogen in certain types of actively progressing periodontal disease. That B. asaccharolyticus is a potential pathogenic organism has also repeatedly been indicated from studies of non-oral infections (1).

The mechanism(s) whereby strains of the B. asaccharolyticus and B. melaninogenicus group contribute to the pathology associated with them is not well understood. Synergistic anaerobic infection is the most extensively studied model system of the pathogenicity of B. melaninogenicus (2). Several studies have demonstrated that the addition of a strain of B. melaninogenicus to an avirulent mixture of oral bacteria can make the bacterial complex uniformly infective, resulting in abscess formation in experimental animals. Periodontal disease is only exceptionally associated with development of abscesses; however, it is tempting to speculate that similarities exist in the pathologic processes of abscess formation and active periodontal disease, the important difference being that in periodontal disease a constant drainage can take place through the orifice of the periodontal pocket. The specific molecular biology of the relationship between bacterial products and alveolar bone resorption has been examined in recent studies. Endotoxin and other bacterial amphophiles, prostaglandins whose concentration in inflamed human gingival tissues may be increased more than ten-fold, and osteoclast activating factor released by sensitized lymphocytes can stimulate bone resorption in bone organ cultures (3). Several potential mechanisms thus exist by which periodontal bacteria can cause alveolar destruction. Whether a multiplicity of pathogenic mechanisms or only a few are operative in periodontal disease remains to be established. The use of the M. arctoides model in the study of the molecular biology of periodontal disease may prove to be advantageous.

SUMMARY

The present results obtained by the use of a monkey periodontitis model point to the importance of the bacterial-host interaction in the loss of alveolar bone. In two monkeys examined, representative of a group of six monkeys, B. asaccharolyticus and B. melaninogenicus subsp. macacae (subsp. nov.) constituted about 66% of the cultivable subgingival microflora associated with rapidly progressing alveolar bone breakdown. The present studies therefore strongly implicate B. asaccharolyticus and closely related strains as important pathogens in actively destructive periodontal disease.

ACKNOWLEDGEMENTS

This study was supported in part by Public Health Service Grants DE 01932 and DE 04898 from the National Institute of Dental Research.

The authors express appreciation to Phyllis M. Lobbins, Judith E. Wolf, and Homer S. Reynolds for their competent technical assistance.

LITERATURE CITED

1. Finegold, S.M. 1977. Anaerobic bacteria in human disease. Academic Press Inc., New York.

2. Gibbons, R.J. 1974. Aspects of the pathogenicity and ecology of the indigenous oral flora of man, p. 268-285. In A. Balows, R.D. Dehann, V.R. Dowell, and L.B. Guze (ed.). Anaerobic bacteria: role in disease. International Conference on Anaerobic Bacteria, Center for Disease Control, 1972. Charles C. Thomas, Springfield, Ill.

3. Hausmann, E., and L. Ortman. 1979. Present status of bone resportion in human periodontal disease. Special issue: The proceedings of the James A. English symposium on oral perspectives on bone biology. J. Periodontol. 50: 7-10.

4. Hausmann, E., L.F. Ortman, and N. Sedransk. 1979. Experimental alveolar bone loss in the monkey evaluated by ^{125}I absorptiometry. Calcif. Tiss. Int. 29: 133-139.

5. Henrikson, C.O., and J. Bergström. 1974. Quantitative long-term determinations of the alveolar bone mineral mass in man by the ^{125}I absorptiometry. I. Accuracy and precision of the method. Acta Radiol. Ther. Phys. Biol. 13: 377-392.

6. Holdeman, L.V., E.P. Cato, and W.E.C. Moore (ed.). 1977. Anaerobe laboratory manual, 4th ed. Virginia Polytechnic Institute and State University, Blacksburg.

7. Kennedy, J.E., and A.M. Polson. 1973. Experimental marginal periodontitis in squirrel monkeys. J. Periodontol. 44: 140-144.

8. Krygier, G., R.J. Genco, P.A. Mashimo, and E. Hausmann. 1973. Experimental gingivitis in Macaca speciosa monkeys: clinical, bacteriologic and histologic similarities of human gingivitis. J. Periodontol. 44: 454-463.

9. Levine, M.J., M.C. Herzberg, S.A. Ellison, J.P. Shomers, and G.A. Sadowski. 1978. Biochemical and immunological comparison of monkey (Macaca arctoides) and human salivary secretions. Comp. Biochem. Physiol. 60B: 423-431.

10. Mashimo, P.A., S.A. Ellison, and J. Slots. 1979. Microbial composition of monkey dental plaque (Macaca arctoides and Macaca fascicularis). Scand. J. Dent. Res. 87: 24-31.

11. Schroeder, H.E., and J. Lindhe. 1975. Conversion of stable established gingivitis in the dog into destructive periodontitis. Arch. Oral Biol. 20: 775-782.

12. Slots, J. 1977. The predominant cultivable microflora of advanced periodontitis. Scand. J. Dent. Res. 85: 114-121.

13. Slots, J. 1979. Subgingival microflora and periodontal disease. J. Clin. Periodontol. 6: 351-382.

14. Slots, J., and E. Hausmann. 1979. Longitudinal study of experimentally induced periodontal disease in Macaca arctoides: relationship between microflora and alveolar bone loss. Infect. Immun. 23: 260-269.

15. Slots, J., and R.J. Genco. 1980. Bacteroides melaninogenicus subsp. macacae, a new subspecies from monkey periodontopathic indigenous microflora. Int. J. Syst. Bacteriol. 30: 82-85

16. Socransky, S.S. 1977. Microbiology of periodontal disease-present status and future considerations. J. Periodontol. 48: 497-504.

17. Staple, P.H., M.J. Reed, P.A. Mashimo, N. Sedransk, and T. Umemoto. 1978. Diphenylhydantoin gingival hyperplasia in Macaca arctoides: prevention by inhibition of dental plaque deposition. J. Periodontol. 49: 310-325.

EXPERIMENTAL ANIMAL MODELS FOR ANAEROBIC INFECTIONS

A.B. Onderdonk, D.L. Kasper,* B.J. Mansheim,
T.J. Louie, S.L. Gorbach and J.G. Bartlett

Infectious Disease Research Laboratory, Veterans Administration Hospital, Boston; Department of Medicine, Tufts University School of Medicine; the Channing Laboratory and the Department of Medicine, Harvard Medical School, Boston, Massachusetts

INTRODUCTION

The role of obligate anaerobes in serious infection has received increasing attention over the past several years. Initially, little was known about many of these microbes except that they were commonly found in certain infections and that they were the dominant components of the colonic microflora. Clinical studies often failed to document the pathogenic role of anaerobes because they were usually found in combination with aerobes at infected sites. Subsequent research has employed animal models to determine the pathogenic potential of anaerobic bacteria. This approach is particularly attractive because, unlike clinical studies, the investigations can be conducted under controlled conditions.

Development of an Animal Model of Intraabdominal Sepsis

Our initial studies were designed to develop an animal model simulating intraabdominal sepsis as seen in patients. The goal of this work was to evaluate the role of various microbes in infections involving the colonic microflora. Wistar rats were implanted intraperitoneally with gelatin capsules containing an inoculum of pooled cecal contents and barium sulfate (22). Sequential anatomical and bacteriological studies showed two distinct stages in the ensuing infection. During the initial five day period there was an acute

*Recipient of Research Career Development Award No. 1K04A100126 from the National Institute of Allergy and Infectious Diseases.

peritonitis in all animals associated with a mortality rate of approximately 40%. Surviving recipients of this inoculum uniformly developed the second stage characterized by intraabdominal abscess formation.

Bacteriologically, the experimental infection also revealed two distinct phases. During the initial peritonitis stage, Escherichia coli and enterococci were the numerically dominant species (17). Additionally, blood cultures performed during the first 72 hours following implantation yielded E. coli. In contrast, the numerically dominant bacteria in abscess contents were obligate anaerobes, a Bacteroides species (formerly Bacteroides fragilis subsp. other) and Fusobacterium varium. E. coli and enterococci were also found in these abscesses but they were present in lesser concentrations. These data suggested that facultative species, and E. coli in particular, were important to the initial, often lethal peritonitis phase of disease, while anaerobes were the principal pathogens during abscess formation. One additional observation made during these studies concerned simplification of the infecting microflora. The cecal contents used for implantation contained at least 23 identifiable species in numbers exceeding 10^3 CFU/ml, yet peritoneal fluids and abscess pus consistently yielded only four bacterial species.

Antimicrobial Trials

To further define the role of coliforms and obligate anaerobes during the experimental infection, these two bacterial components were selectively suppressed with antimicrobials (23). It was found that treatment with gentamicin reduced mortality rates in this model but had no effect on the incidence of abscess. On the other hand, clindamycin failed to decrease mortality rates but only 5% of the surviving animals had abscesses. If both antimicrobials were given simultaneously there was a decrease in both mortality and abscess rates. These data supported the previous impression regarding the role of coliforms in the early lethal peritonitis stage of disease and the importance of anaerobes in abscess formation.

Implantation of Pure and Mixed Cultures

Additional studies were performed using inocula of the four bacterial species which were consistently present at infected sites: E. coli, enterococcus, Bacteroides species (formerly B. fragilis subsp. other), and F. varium. These species were implanted alone, in all possible combinations of two and as a combination of all four. In each experiment there were a comparable number of total organisms as well as 50% sterile cecal contents and 10% (w/v) barium sulfate (18). It was found that early lethality was associated exclusively with inocula containing E. coli and that mortality rates were directly correlated with the number of E. coli in the challenge. Abscesses were not produced by any single species, but were found in nearly all animals which were challenged with the combination of a facultative species and an anaerobe. These data suggested that coliforms were responsible for the early lethality and that abscesses resulted from a synergistic interaction of an anaerobe and a facultative organism.

Studies of Bacteroides fragilis

The role of B. fragilis in intraabdominal infections is of particular interest due to its prevalence in clinical specimens as well as resistance to many commonly used antimicrobials (5). There are three important recent observations which provide background information for our studies of this microbe. First, B. fragilis previously included five closely related organisms which were designated as subspecies; based on DNA homology studies these five subspecies have recently been reclassified as species (4). The second relevant observation concerns studies by Kasper et al. showing that one of the former subspecies (B. fragilis subsp. fragilis) has an antigenically distinct polysaccharide external to the outer membrane (10,11). The third point is that clinical studies indicate that encapsulated strains, e.g., the organism previously classified as B. fragilis subsp. fragilis, are the predominant isolates from the "B. fragilis group" found at infected sites. Our experience which supports this contention is summarized (Table 1). These observations suggest that some unique property of this organism may represent a virulence factor.

The animal model has been used to compare the pathogenic potential of encapsulated and unencapsulated strains from the "B. fragilis group" (20). These studies showed that inocula of encapsulated strains in pure culture produced abscesses in 95% of recipient animals whereas unencapsulated strains consistently failed to produce detectable disease. Additionally, it was noted that heat-killed encapsulated organisms also produced abscesses despite the absence of viable bacteria. This suggested that a heat stable factor which promoted abscess formation was present in encapsulated strains and absent in unencapsulated strains. Additional animals were challenged with the various components of the outer membrane of B. fragilis to determine which fraction was responsible for abscess formation. Four distinct fractions were tested in this manner including the entire outer membrane, a protein polysaccharide fraction, a lipopolysaccharide fraction and purified capsular polysaccharide. The results of this experiment showed that the capsular polysaccharide component was the responsible fraction.

Summary of Previous Studies

The previously summarized studies indicate that rats challenged

Table 1. Isolation Rates of Organisms Previously Classified as Bacteroides fragilis in Clinical Specimens

Organism According to Current Taxonomic Schema	Blood Culture (56 patients)	Exudate Culture (227 patients)
B. fragilis	43 (77%)	144 (63%)
B. thetaiotaomicron	4 (7%)	53 (23%)
B. distasonis	5 (9%)	26 (11%)
B. vulgatus	2 (2%)	26 (11%)
B. ovatus	1 (2%)	24 (11%)
Bacteroides "others"[a]	1 (2%)	18 (8%)

[a] Previously classified as B. fragilis but failed to conform to criteria for subspeciation.

with an inoculum of cecal contents results in an infection which simulates intraabdominal sepsis as it is encountered in clinical practice according to both bacteriological and pathological criteria. This work indicates that both coliforms and anaerobes are pathogens in this model. However, these organisms appear to have distinctive roles in the pathogenic events as the infection evolves from generalized peritonitis to abscess formation. Of particular interest are the studies with B. fragilis which show that pure cultures of encapsulated strains of this organism produce intraabdominal abscesses. This work forms the background for our more recent studies which will be described in greater detail.

METHODS OF PROCEDURE

Source of Bacterial Strains

All bacterial strains were grown in pre-reduced peptone yeast glucose broth (Scott Laboratories, Fiskeville, RI) within an anaerobic chamber. Aliquots of each culture were placed into sterile glass vials following 48 h of incubation at 35 C. The vials of culture were frozen in liquid nitrogen and stored at -40 C until used. B. fragilis (ATCC 23745 and 44198), Bacteroides thetaiotaomicron (43172), Bacteroides vulgatus (2242), Bacteroides distasonis (ATCC 8503), Bacteroides asaccharolyticus (382,536), and Bacteroides melaninogenicus subsp. intermedius (10946), B. melaninogenicus subsp. intermedius (BVA 1-121) and E. coli (BVA 1-13) were obtained from the stock culture collection of the Infectious Disease Research Laboratory, Boston VA Hospital or the Channing Laboratory. Clostridium perfringens (249) was obtained from the Infectious Disease Service, Tufts-New England Medical Center.

Antimicrobial Trials in Experimental Intraabdominal Sepsis

The details for implanting rats, administering antimicrobials and assessing results have been published elsewhere (17,22,23). In general, these studies showed results which could be predicted on the basis of in vitro susceptibility patterns and the data summarized previously for the results with clindamycin and gentamicin. A brief description of these techniques is provided since two antimicrobial regimens yielded results which were not anticipated and warranted further studies which are reported here. Chloramphenicol was chosen for additional testing since this agent failed to protect animals from abscess formation despite in vitro activity of this antimicrobial versus anaerobes. In contrast, metronidazole was selected for study due to its reduction of mortality in this model even though in vitro testing showed little activity versus coliforms.

Male Wistar rats weighing 180-200 grams were used for all studies. Animals were implanted with either a cecal inoculum or combinations of bacterial species as previously described (18,22). Four hours following surgery, antimicrobial treatment was initiated and continued by intramuscular injection at 8 h intervals for 10 days. Chloramphenicol and metronidazole were given at a dose of 16 mg/animal. Surviving animals were sacrificed on the 12th postoperative day for necropsy examination to detect intraabdominal abscesses. Blood cultures using pour plate techniques were obtained in some animals by percutaneous transthoracic cardiac puncture. All plates were incubated within an anaerobic chamber at 35 C for 3-5 days. Following incubation, colonies were enumerated and identified by established procedures (3,8).

Assay of Chloramphenicol and Related Compounds

Biologically active chloramphenicol was measured by the hemolysis inhibition assay (14) using C. perfringens (249) as an indicator strain. Since this assay measures only biologically active antimicrobials, a gas liquid chromatographic procedure was also used. Aliquots of 0.5 ml of each sample to be tested were extracted with 1 ml of ethyl acetate. The solvent was removed from the tube following centrifugation and the ethyl acetate fraction dried under N at 60 C in a sand bath. The residue was dissolved in 0.2 ml of pyridine (Applied Science Laboratories, Inc., State College, PA) and silylated with 0.2 ml of trimethyl silylimidizole (Supelco, Inc., Bellefonte,

PA). The mixture was incubated at 40 C for 20 min and the reaction stopped by addition of 0.5 ml of phosphate buffered saline. Silyl derivatives of chloramphenicol and related compounds were extracted with 0.5 ml of N-hexane. Detection of silyl esters was accomplished by injecting 2 ul samples onto a 2m x 3mm glass column packed with 3% OV101 (Supelco, Bellefonte, PA). The column was housed within a Shimadzu 6-AM gas chromatograph (Shimadzu Instruments Inc., Columbia, MD) at a temperature of 220 C. The flow rate was 30 ml/min and peaks were detected by a flame ionization detector. Quantitative estimates of chloramphenicol (D-threo-1-p-nitrophenyl-2-dichloroacetamido-1,3-propanediol) was accomplished by the addition of 10 ug/ml of D-threo-1-p-nitrophenyl-2-monochloroacetamido-1,3-propanediol to each sample. A comparison of the integration ratio of the monochloro derivative and unknown amounts of chloramphenicol or the aryl amine to known concentrations of each compound was used to obtain a quantitative estimate. Preliminary trials had shown this method to give a linear response from concentrations of 1 to 100 ug/ml.

Effect of Metronidazole on E. coli in vitro

The effects of metronidazole on E. coli growth were tested in a chemostat. Pure cultures of E. coli (BVA 1-13) or mixed cultures of E. coli and B. fragilis (ATCC 23745) were established in a chemostat (model C-30, New Brunswick Scientific, New Brunswick, NJ) modified to maintain an anaerobic environment (19). A minimal medium (25) containing glucose was used for all experiments. Cultures were grown at 37 C at a dilution rate of 0.16 hr^{-1}. Eh, pH and viable cell density were monitored as described previously (19). Following establishment of the steady state, cultures were exposed to antimicrobial via addition of metronidazole to the media reservoir in a concentration of 30 ug/ml. Samples were removed from the fermentation vessel periodically for assay of viable cell density and biologically active antimicrobial (as determined by the hemolysis inhibition assay). Samples were placed in an anaerobic chamber and aliquots removed for filtration through a 0.45 micron filter for antimicrobial assay, or for viable counts. Colony counts were made in duplicate on Trypticase soy blood agar incubated under 5% CO_2 and Brucella base blood agar incubated within the anaerobic chamber. Viable cell density was expressed as $\log_{10}$ colony forming units/ml.

Animal Model for Wound Abscess

An animal model simulating human wound infection was developed since anaerobic bacteria are often involved in these infections and the host defenses in the subcutaneous tissues may be considerably different than those present in the peritoneal cavity. In addition, a subcutaneous infection would allow daily inspection of developing lesions.

Male Wistar rats weighing 200-250 grams were used for all experiments. Animals were anesthetized with 0.15 ml of nembutol (50 mg/ml) and the back was shaved and prepped with iodine. A one cm incision through the skin and underlying fascia was made on either side of the midline approximately 1 cm from the thoracic spine. The incisions were closed with two sutures using 3-0 silk. Inocula consisting of either broth cultures alone, cecal contents or sterile cecal contents plus bacterial cultures were injected through the closed incision using an 18 gauge needle. Details for preparation of inocula have been described elsewhere (17,18). Aliquots of 0.25 ml of each inoculum were injected through each incision.

Wounds were examined daily for evidence of infection. Each wound was cultured at seven day intervals using needle aspirates of 0.05 ml. Blood cultures were obtained from animals as described previously and bacterial strains isolated from blood or wounds were identified by established criteria (3,8).

RESULTS

Inactivation of Chloramphenicol by Obligate Anaerobes

Chloramphenicol administration to 60 implanted rats resulted in a 3% mortality as compared to 37% in 157 untreated animals. At necropsy, 100% of untreated animals and 59% (34/58) of chloramphenicol recipients had intraabdominal abscesses. These results were unexpected since chloramphenicol showed excellent in vitro activity against the major isolates recovered from infections in untreated animals receiving the same challenge. Minimum inhibitory concentrations for these organisms with chloramphenicol were: _B_. fragilis, 8 ug/ml; _F_. varium, 4 ug/ml and _E_. coli, 4 ug/ml. The mean peak serum concentration of chloramphenicol with the dose utilized in rats was 22 ug/ml indicating levels well above the MIC values. The discrepancy between in vivo and in vitro results suggested the possibility that obligate anaerobes might inactivate the antimicrobial in vivo.

Preliminary tests of the ability of obligate anaerobes to inactivate chloramphenicol were made by adding known concentrations of this antimicrobial to 18 h broth cultures of the test microorganisms diluted to approximately 10^8 CFU/ml. The results (Table 2) indicate that both _B_. fragilis (ATCC 23745) and _C_. perfringens (249) were capable of inactivating chloramphenicol over a six hour incubation period. _B_. fragilis decreased the concentration of biologically active chloramphenicol from 97 ug/ml to 39 ug/ml over this interval while _C_. perfringens decreased the concentration from 100 ug/ml to 2 ug/ml over the same time frame. Additional testing showed that culture filtrates of these strains also inactivated chloramphenicol. The strains used in these studies did not develop in vitro resistance

Table 2. Detection of Chloramphenicol and Its Aminophenyl Derivative

Species/Time[a]		Chloramphenicol	D-threo-1-p-aminophenyl-2-dichloroacetamido-1,3-propanediol
B. fragilis	0 h	97[b]	0[b]
	3 h	72	25
	6 h	39	50
C. perfringens	0 h	100	0
	3 h	65	35
	6 h	2	63

[a] Hours after addition of chloramphenicol to the culture.

[b] ug/ml.

to the antimicrobial after exposure. The inactivation of chloramphenicol proved to be dependent on inoculum size, since similar tests using 10^6 CFU/ml of bacteria failed to decrease the concentration of active drug. The ability of B. fragilis to inactivate chloramphenicol was tested using 19 additional strains obtained from clinical sources. All 19 strains inactivated antimicrobial, with a mean decrease in active drug over 6 h of incubation of 60%. Since in vitro resistance did not develop in these strains, it was considered unlikely that acetylation was responsible for antimicrobial inactivation. A quantitative assay for other inactive derivatives of chloramphenicol was necessary to define the mechanism of inactivation.

The results of gas liquid chromatographic analysis of silyl derivatives of chloramphenicol and related compounds revealed the presence of the aminophenyl derivative of chloramphenicol in bacterial cultures exposed to antimicrobials (Table 2). Quantitative determinations of the concentration of the inactive aminophenyl compound, as well as the absence of other derivatives, suggests a direct reduction of the nitro group to the corresponding amine. Recent data also indicates that the inactive aminophenyl derivative can be detected in the purulent exudate obtained from infected rats given chloramphenicol. The results suggest that reduction of chloramphenicol by anaerobes may explain the discrepancy between in vivo and in vitro results.

Reduction of Mortality by Metronidazole

Metronidazole was administered to 50 rats implanted with the cecal inoculum. The results showed a significant reduction in early lethality with a mortality rate of only 10% compared to 37% in untreated control animals (Table 3). This was unexpected since our previous studies with this model showed that coliforms were primarily responsible for bacteremia and lethality in the initial stages of this infection. In vitro susceptibility studies showed the MIC of E. coli recovered from blood culture of untreated animals was 1024 ug/ml for metronidazole, well above the peak serum level in rats of 30 ug/ml. As expected, there was also a reduction in the incidence of abscesses at necropsy studies and the B. fragilis strain used in this experiment was highly susceptible to metronidazole (MIC = 0.5 ug/ml). These results suggested two possibilities: metronidazole had some effect on E. coli in vivo not consistent with in vitro susceptibility data, or anaerobes made a more significant contribution to early lethality in this model than previously realized.

Additional animals were implanted with either E. coli (BVA 1-13) alone, or a combination of E. coli and B. fragilis (ATCC 23745). All inocula contained a total of 1 x 10^8 CFU/ml, with equal numbers of E. coli and B. fragilis used in mixed inocula. It was found that recipients of E. coli alone, with and without metronidazole treatment, had mortality rates of 85% and 100%, respectively (Table 3). All animals tested had positive blood cultures for E. coli 24 h post-operatively. It should be noted that blood culture data were obtained from animals not included in the previously noted mortality data, since transthoracic puncture might contribute to lethal outcome. In contrast to the data obtained with E. coli alone, recipients of a combination of E. coli and B. fragilis showed marked differences when the metronidazole treatment group was compared to untreated animals. Metronidazole treated animals showed a mortality of 20% with none of 10 blood cultures being positive. Untreated recipients of the combination of E. coli and B. fragilis had a 100% mortality rate and all ten blood cultures were positive for E. coli. These data suggest that metronidazole has an effect on mortality only when anaerobes were part of the infecting inoculum. To exclude the possibility that anaerobes contribute to lethality in this model, animals were challenged with combinations of B. fragilis and E. coli in various concentrations. These studies showed mortality rates were directly correlated with the inoculum size of E. coli and the addition of B. fragilis to the inoculum had no apparent effect.

Chemostat cultures of E. coli alone and E. coli combined with B. fragilis were employed to determine the effect of metronidazole on E. coli growth which could not be detected by other in vitro systems. It was found that exposure of E. coli to a continuously increasing concentration of metronidazole had no effect on population density (Table 4). Additionally, the measured concentrations of metronidazole in the fermentation vessel corresponded closely to the calculated amounts which had been added via the nutrient reservoir. Since metronidazole is reduced by sensitive bacterial cells to a biologically active, but labile compound which then can no

Table 3. Results of Metronidazole Treatment of Rats Implanted with Various Inocula

Antimicrobial	Inoculum	Mortality	Abscess	Positive Blood Culture at 24 h
Untreated controls	Cecal contents	58/157(37)[a]	99/99(100)[b]	20/20
Metronidazole	Cecal contents	5/50 (10)	6/45(13)	1/10
Untreated controls	*E. coli*	10/10(100)	-	10/10
Metronidazole	*E. coli*	17/20(85)	0/3	10/10
Untreated controls	*E. coli* + *B. fragilis*	10/10(100)	-	10/10
Metronidazole	*E. coli* + *B. fragilis*	2/10(20)	0/8	0/10

[a] No. died/no. tested (%).
[b] No. with abscesses/no. of survivors tested (%).

longer be detected by bioassay, the accumulation of metronidazole indicates it has not been reduced at the nitro group on the imidazole ring and therefore was not activated by *E. coli* alone. In contrast, mixed cultures of *E. coli* and *B. fragilis* show a much different effect. When metronidazole is added to these cultures, the *E. coli* population decreases from $10^{9.0}$ to $10^{7.8}$ CFU/ml over a five h period. During this same time, *B. fragilis* populations decreased from $10^{8.4}$ to $10^{6.1}$ CFU/ml. Unlike the previous experiment, metronidazole could not be detected in the fermenter until the *B. fragilis* population had decreased over 100-fold. These data suggest that metronidazole is reduced in the presence of *B. fragilis* and this form of the drug is active against *E. coli*. Once *B. fragilis* has been eliminated from the fermenter, metronidazole is no longer reduced and concentrations of *E. coli* return to their previous levels. Since the rapid decrease in *B. fragilis* levels could conceivably effect the *E. coli* population by mechanisms which are independent of antimicrobial activity, a similar experiment was performed using clindamycin instead of metronidazole. No decrease in *E. coli* populations were seen despite a rapid decrease in concentrations of *B. fragilis*.

Development of a Model Simulating Wound Abscess

Initial experiments employed the subcutaneous injection of the

Table 4. Effect of Metronidazole on Pure and Mixed Continuous Cultures of E. coli and B. fragilis

Culture	Time (h)	Log CFU/ml E. coli	Log CFU/ml B. fragilis	Concentration of Metronidazole
E. coli	0[a]	8.4	-	0[b]
	1	8.3	-	1.5
	3	8.4	-	6.0
	5	8.4	-	11.0
	7	8.4	-	14.5
	12	8.3	-	22.5
E. coli + B. fragilis	0	9.0	8.4	0
	1	8.6	7.5	0
	3	8.3	6.9	0
	5	7.8	6.1	0.2
	7	7.9	5.7	0.8
	12	8.3	5.5	2.0

[a] Hours after starting metronidazole exposure via the nutrient reservoir.
[b] ug/ml of biologically active antimicrobial.

cecal inoculum and barium sulfate into rats directly beneath a surgical incision. It was found that animals implanted in this manner developed discrete abscesses within five days which became progressively larger until the 14th to 17th day (Table 5). The mean Eh of the purulent material measured in situ at seven days was -113 mv in six animals tested, indicating the presence of a reduced environment. The abscess drained spontaneously through the site of the incision between the 14th to 17th day after challenge and, in some cases, drainage occurred through sinus tracts 2 to 3 cm from the incision. In contrast to the previously described intraabdominal sepsis model, no mortality was noted in these animals. Blood cultures at 24 h were positive in only one of 10 animals, with E. coli being the single bacterial isolate. Cultures of abscess pus were uniformly positive for E. coli, enterococci and B. fragilis. Another difference compared to the intraabdominal sepsis model was the observation that cecal contents implanted without barium sulfate produced abscesses in all 10 recipients.

Implants composed of pure cultures of B. fragilis (ATCC 23745), Bacteroides melaninogenicus (10946), and E. coli (BVA 1-13), each at a concentration of 5 x 10^7 CFU/ml, failed to cause abscesses in the soft tissue infection model. However, implants of the same inoculum size of B. fragilis combined with 50% sterile cecal contents resulted

Table 5. Results of Implanting Various Inocula into Rats Through a Skin Incision

Inoculum	Mortality	Abscess	Positive Blood Culture
Cecal contents + $BaSO_4$	0/10[a]	10/10[b]	1/10 (E. coli)
Cecal contents	0/10	10/10	0/10
Broth cultures of:			
B. fragilis	0/10	0/10	0/10
B. melaninogenicus	0/10	0/10	0/10
E. coli	0/5	0/5	0/5

[a] No. died/no. tested
[b] No. with abscess/no. tested

in abscess formation in all 15 recipients (Table 6). Interestingly, animals immunized with the capsular polysaccharide from the homologous strain of B. fragilis prior to implantation (12) also developed abscesses. These data suggest that circulating antibody has little ability to prevent abscess formation or to eliminate B. fragilis from the abscess during wound infection. Implants of other closely related Bacteroides spp. combined with 50% sterile cecal contents showed abscess formation in 6 of 15 animals (Table 6).

Additional studies have been performed using inocula composed of 50% sterile cecal contents combined with B. asaccharolyticus (382,536). This organism was of particular interest in view of recent studies showing the presence of a capsular polysaccharide (15). All fifteen animals implanted with this inoculum developed abscesses. Additionally, 10 animals implanted with B. melaninogenicus subsp. intermedius (10946, BVA 1-21), a phenotypically similar species, also developed abscesses. These data indicate that a number of Bacteroides species have the ability to potentiate subcutaneous abscess in this model.

DISCUSSION

The rat model for intraabdominal sepsis has been used in a number of studies to explore the role of anaerobes in the infectious process and to test the virulence of selected bacterial species. In the course of these studies certain unanticipated observations led to further experimentation in an effort to better understand certain in vivo results. The discrepancy between in vitro susceptibility of the major microbial components of experimentally produced abscesses

Table 6. Results of Implanting Various Bacteroides Species into Rats Through a Skin Incision

Inoculum[a]	Mortality	Abscess	(mm)[b]
B. fragilis	0/15	15/15	(6.0)
B. fragilis after immunization	0/5	5/5	(6.0)
B. distasonis	0/5	0/5	
B. thetaiotaomicron	0/5	3/5	(3.2)
B. vulgatus	0/5	3/5	(4.0)
B. asaccharolyticus	0/15	15/15	
B. melaninogenicus subsp. intermedius	0/10	10/10	

[a] All cultures contain 5 x 10^7 CFU and 50% sterile cecal contents.
[b] No. positive/no. tested (mean abscess diameter).

to chloramphenicol and the observed in vivo lack of efficacy of this antimicrobial is one such example. It was found that chloramphenicol did not prevent abscess formation in infected animals despite the in vitro sensitivity of the dominant bacterial species to this antimicrobial. Further research revealed that, in the presence of anaerobes, chloramphenicol rapidly lost biological activity. Acetylation is a major mechanism of resistance for facultative species (2), but has not been described for anaerobes. Therefore, other mechanisms of inactivation were explored and these studies showed both B. fragilis and C. perfringens reduce chloramphenicol to an aminophenyl compound which is biologically inactive. Previous investigations had reported such activity in clostridia (9) but little was known about the role of this nitroreductase activity in Gram-negative anaerobes. The possible importance of this reduction in vivo was suggested by the high incidence of abscesses present in chloramphenicol treated animals. It should be noted that there are relatively few clinical studies of chloramphenicol efficacy in bacteriologically confirmed anaerobic infections. Therapeutic failures have been reported (21), but controlled trials are necessary to place these observations in a proper perspective.

Metronidazole also showed unanticipated results in the animal model since this drug reduced mortality rates despite the lack of in vitro activity against coliforms. This observation suggested that either anaerobes contributed substantially to early lethality in the model or that metronidazole had an in vivo effect on coliforms not anticipated from routine susceptibility tests. Subsequent experiments suggested that B. fragilis reduced metronidazole to the biologically active form (13) which, in turn, was active against E. coli. This effect was not due simply to the death of the anaerobic component, since similar studies using clindamycin in the animal model and in the chemostat had no apparent effect on E. coli. The inhibitory effect of metronidazole on coliforms during mixed infections of facultative and anaerobic bacteria has been reported in human infections as well (24).

More recent studies have dealt with the development of a wound abscess model simulating post-operative wound infections. This model was of interest because of the possibility that the host defenses during soft tissue infection are considerably different from those found in the peritoneum. It was found that cecal contents with or without the inclusion of barium sulfate caused abscess when implanted subcutaneously in Wistar rats. In contrast to the intraperitoneal infection with the same inoculum, no mortality was noted and bacteremia was rarely detected. Additionally, the adjuvant effect of barium sulfate was not required for abscess formation. These results indicate that the host response to the same inoculum was dependent to some extent on the site of the infection. These observations are also supported by the finding that animals immunized with the capsular polysaccharide of B. fragilis developed subcutaneous abscesses when challenged with the homologous strain of this organism. Previous research has shown this immunization protects against abscess formation when animals are challenged with B. fragilis introduced intraperitoneally. Additionally, a comparison of the ability of B. fragilis and related species to cause abscess showed that unencapsulated strains of organisms previously classified as B. fragilis caused abscesses in some animals challenged subcutaneously, but not intraperitoneally. Subcutaneous challenge of another encapsulated Bacteroides spp., B. asaccharolyticus, also resulted in abscess formation. Interestingly, a closely related species, B. melaninogenicus subsp. intermedius also produced abscesses; the presence of a capsular polysaccharide for this organism is undetermined. These results suggest that one criterion for virulence among the Bacteroides appears to be a capsular polysaccharide although the unique composition of the LPS of other organisms may play a significant role in their pathogenicity.

The information provided in the present report points out several important features of animal models. The most essential feature of any animal model is the similarity of animal infection to human disease. Previous researchers (1,6,7,16) have reported the ability of obligate anaerobes alone and in conjunction with other facultative bacterial species to cause disease in animals. These investigations suggested a significant pathogenic role for anaerobes, but clinical utility of the data was limited by the failure of the models to simulate human disease. An attractive feature of the model described here is that it simulates intraabdominal sepsis as it is encountered clinically by both pathologic and bacteriological parameters.

Another important consideration in evaluating animal models for human infections are bacterial-bacterial interactions. These interactions are important not only to the infectious process itself, but also may alter the outcome of antimicrobial therapy of the infection. Examples of these bacterial-bacterial interactions in experimental models are provided by the synergy between facultative and anaerobic species during intraabdominal abscess formation, and by the inactivation of chloramphenicol or the effect of metronidazole on coliforms during the same experimental disease. These bacterial-bacterial interactions may not be predicted by in vitro studies since these are generally performed using various bacteria in pure cultures.

A final consideration essential to evaluation of animal models for human infection is the host response to bacterial challenge. The ability of an animal host to respond in a particular manner to infectious insult is governed in large part by the animals' own immune response. The similarity of animal and human humoral and cell mediated immunity are necessary important considerations. Additionally, the host response to challenge may vary depending on the site of the infectious focus. This point has been demonstrated experimentally by comparing host response to intraperitoneal and subcutaneous challenge with an identical inoculum in the Wistar rat. The finding that mortality and relative virulence of certain species was different suggests that a single animal model cannot be used to draw conclusions about bacteriologically similar lesions in different tissues and demonstrates the organotropism of certain pathogenic species. Intraabdominal abscesses and subcutaneous abscesses both harbored a microflora which was identical, yet the development of the lesions, the role of specific species in the infection, and the role of circulating antibody were different. These data suggest that in order to apply the lessons learned from animal models to human disease, the site of infection must be similar.

Despite the wealth of empirical and experimental information available on bacterial infections of humans, animal models remain an important tool in elucidating the etiology of certain infections and in identifying the pathogenic factors associated with the infecting microflora. The judicious use of animal models continues to increase our understanding of the infectious process and often provides data not readily available through the study of human subjects.

ACKNOWLEDGEMENT

This research was supported by grants from the Veterans Administration, the Upjohn Company and by contract N. DAMD-17-74C-4056 from United States Army Medical Research and Development Command.

LITERATURE CITED

1. Altemeier, W.A. 1942. The pathogenicity of the bacteria of appendicitis. Surgery. 11: 374-384.

2. Benvenisk, R. and J. Davies. 1973. Mechanism of antibiotic resistance. Ann. Rev. Biochem. 42: 495-497.

3. Blair, J.E. 1970. E.H. Lennette and J.P. Truant (ed.). Manual of clinical microbiology. American Society for Microbiology, Bethesda, Maryland.

4. Cato, E.P., and J.L. Johnson. 1976. Reinstatement of species rank for Bacteroides fragilis, B. ovatus, B. distasonis, B. thetaiotaomicron and B. vulgatus: designation of neotype strains for Bacteroides fragilis (Veillon and Zuber) Castellani and Chalmers and Bacteroides thetaiotaomicron (Distaso) Castellani and Chalmers. Int. J. Syst. Bacteriol. 26: 230-237.

5. Gorbach, S.L., and J.G. Bartlett. 1974. Anaerobic infections. N. Engl. J. Med. 290: 1177-1184, 1237-1245, 1289-1294.

6. Hill, G.B., S. Osterhout, and C. Pratt. 1974. Liver abscess production by non-sporeforming anaerobic bacteria in a mouse model. Infect. Immun. 9: 559-603.

7. Hite, K.E., M. Locke, and H.C. Hesseltine. 1949. Synergism in experimental infections with nonsporulating anaerobic bacteria. J. Infect. Dis. 84: 1-9.

8. Holdeman, L.V., E.P. Cato, and W.E.C. Moore (ed.). 1977. Anaerobe laboratory manual, 4th ed. Virginia Polytechnic Institute and State University, Blacksburg.

9. Kanazawa, Y., T. Kuramats, and S. Miyamurci. 1969. Inactivation of chemotherapeutic agents by clostridia. Jpn. J. Bacteriol. 24: 281-289.

10. Kasper, D.L., and M.W. Seiler. 1975. Immunochemical characterization of the outer membrane complex of Bacteroides fragilis subspecies fragilis. J. Infect. Dis. 132: 440-450.

11. Kasper, D.L., M.E. Hayes, B.G. Reinap, F.O. Craft, A.B. Onderdonk, and B.F. Polk. 1977. Isolation and identification of encapsulated strains of Bacteroides fragilis. J. Infect. Dis. 136: 75-81.

12. Kasper, D.L., A.B. Onderdonk, and J.G. Bartlett. 1977. Quantitative determination of the antibody response to the capsular polysaccharide of Bacteroides fragilis in an animal model of intra-abdominal abscess formation. J. Infect. Dis. 136: 789-795.

13. Lindmark, D.G., and M. Muller. 1976. Antitrichomonad action mutagenicity and reduction of metronidazole and other nitroimidazoles. Antimicrob. Agents Chemother. 10: 476-482.

14. Louie, T.J., F.P. Tally, J.G. Bartlett, and S.L. Gorbach. 1976. Rapid microbiologic assay for chloramphenicol and tetracyclines. Antimicrob. Agents Chemother. 9: 874-878.

15. Mansheim, B.J., A.B. Onderdonk, and D.L. Kasper. 1978. Immunochemical and biologic studies of the lipopolysaccharide of Bacteroides melaninogenicus subspecies asaccharolyticus. J. Immunol. 120: 72-78.

16. Meleney, F.L. 1931. Bacterial synergy in disease process. Ann. Surg. 44: 961-981.

17. Onderdonk, A.B., W.M. Weinstein, N.M. Sullivan, J.G. Bartlett, and S.L. Gorbach. 1974. Experimental intraabdominal abscess in rats: Quantitative bacteriology of infected animals. Infect. and Immun. 10: 1256-1259.

18. Onderdonk, A.B., J.G. Bartlett, T.J. Louie, N. Sullivan-Sigler, and S.L. Gorbach. 1976. Microbial synergy in experimental intraabdominal abscess. Infect. and Immun. 13: 22-26.

19. Onderdonk, A.B., J. Johnston, J.W. Mayhew, and S.L. Gorbach. 1976. Effect of dissolved oxygen and Eh on the growth of Bacteroides fragilis during continuous culture. Appl. Environ. Microbiol. 31: 168-172.

20. Onderdonk, A.B., D.L. Kasper, R.L. Cisneros, and J.G. Bartlett. 1977. The capsular polysaccharide of B. fragilis as a virulence factor: Comparison of the pathogenic potential of encapsulated and unencapsulated strains. J. Infect. Dis. 136: 82-89.

21. Thadepalli, H., S.L. Gorbach, and J.G. Bartlett. Apparent failure of chloramphenicol in anaerobic infections. Curr. Ther. Res. (in press).

22. Weinstein, W.M., A.B. Onderdonk, J.G. Bartlett, and S.L. Gorbach. 1974. Experimental intraabdominal abscesses in rats: Development of an animal model. Infect. and Immun. 10: 1250-1259.

23. Weinstein, W.M., A.B. Onderdonk, J.G. Bartlett and S.L. Gorbach. 1975. Treatment of experimental intraabdominal sepsis in rats. J. Infect. Dis. 132: 282-286.

24. Willis, A.T., C.L. Bullen, I.R. Ferguson, P.H. Jones, K.D. Phillips, P.V. Tearle, K. Williams, S.E.J. Young, G.C. Brentnall, G.H. Bancroft-Livingstone, S.A. Seligman, J. Abrahams, A. Collyer, C. Lush, and D. Wilkenson. 1974. Metronidazole in the prevention and treatment of Bacteroides infections in gynecological patients. Lancet 2: 1540-1545.

25. Varel, W.H., and M.P. Bryant. 1974. Nutritional features of Bacteroides fragilis subspecies fragilis. Appl. Microbiol. 28: 251-257.

SEROLOGY OF BACTEROIDACEAE

Dwight W. Lambe, Jr.

Department of Microbiology, College of Medicine
East Tennessee State University
Johnson City, Tennessee 37601

INTRODUCTION

The anaerobic, Gram-negative non-sporing rods that comprise a large and important group of pathogenic bacteria in man include the Bacteroidaceae which is composed of Bacteroides, Fusobacterium, and Leptotrichia. The Bacteroides are found as indigenous flora of the mouth, the upper respiratory tract, and the intestinal and genital tracts. Bacteroides and Fusobacterium are found frequently in human disease whereas the other Gram-negative anaerobic genera are found less frequently if at all as a cause of human disease. The serology discussed here will be limited to the Bacteroides.

BLACK PIGMENTING ANAEROBES

Pathogenicity

The black pigmenting anaerobes include: Bacteroides asaccharolyticus, Bacteroides melaninogenicus subsp. intermedius, Bacteroides melaninogenicus subsp. melaninogenicus, and Bacteroides melaninogenicus subsp. levii. These organisms can cause a wide variety of human diseases including orafacial infections, gingival infections, liver and lung abscesses, infected surgical wounds, and other less frequent infections such as septicemia. Gibbons et al. (8) reported B. melaninogenicus as a key agent in certain mixed anaerobic infections. It rarely occurs in pure culture from clinical infections. Several virulence factors appear to be important in disease. Gibbons and McDonald (7) demonstrated a collagenase; Hausman and Kaufman (9) reported that collagenase was bound to the particulate fraction of the cell. An endotoxic lipopolysaccharide (11,12,13,15,24,32) is produced that is capable of producing a local Schwartzman reaction as well as lethality in mice. Fibrinolysin (35), deoxyribonuclease and ribonuclease (22) have also been reported.

Pigment Production and Colony Description

An important characteristic of these anaerobes is the pigment produced on laked blood agar; this pigment is rarely if ever produced on whole blood agar. Pigment production is important in recognition and classification. The incubation period required for pigment production varies with the subspecies, the strain, the medium, and the number of times the strain has been transferred on artificial medium. Fresh clinical isolates usually require from four to 21 days to produce pigment, although strains transferred over a period of time may initiate pigmentation within two or three days after subculture. B. asaccharolyticus does not produce a black pigment on whole blood agar even after 14 days incubation although a black pigment is produced within five days on laked blood agar.

B. asaccharolyticus colonies are 1.5 to 2.0 mm in diameter, moist, and produce a reddish-black pigment which may become black with age. This organism is common in clinical specimens.

B. melaninogenicus subsp. melaninogenicus colonies are usually small (0.5-2.0 mm in diameter), dry, and produce a dark brown to brown-black pigment. This organism is not commonly found in clinical specimens. However, it may grow under, or at the edge of, colonies of B. melaninogenicus subsp. intermedius and is, therefore, easily missed. It is a fastidious organism and grows much better, or only, in the presence of other anaerobes or aerobes such as Propionibacterium acnes or Staphylococcus aureus.

B. melaninogenicus subsp. intermedius colonies are 0.5 mm in diameter, dry and may have a black center with a brown edge that becomes black after a few days.

Both B. asaccharolyticus and B. melaninogenicus subsp. intermedius are much easier to grow in pure culture than B. melaninogenicus subsp. melaninogenicus and occur more commonly in clinical specimens than B. melaninogenicus subsp. melaninogenicus.

B. melaninogenicus subsp. levii produces a greenish-black to black pigment and is rarely found in clinical specimens. A number of greenish-black colonies have appeared in clinical specimens in my laboratory that die before we can identify them. I suspect that these may be B. melaninogenicus subsp. levii.

Serology

Shevky (30), Pulverer (28), Courant and Gibbons (3), and Werner and Sebald (36) used the agglutination test to study B. melaninogenicus. Some of these workers reported heterogenicity of B. melaninogenicus.

From 1973 until the present (18,19), we have developed fluorescent antibody (FA) reagents, called fluorescein isothiocyanate (FITC) labeled conjugates, which we have used for the direct fluorescent-antibody technique. Ninety-six percent of more than 300 strains tested by the direct FA were classified into one of five serogroups. Three of these serogroups are shown in Table 1. Ten strains were B. melaninogenicus subsp. melaninogenicus serogroup A; 68 strains were B. melaninogenicus subsp. intermedius serogroup C; and nine strains were serogroup C-1. Each serogroup was specific, and no cross reaction occurred.

The remaining two of the five serogroups are shown in Table 2. One hundred fifty-three strains of B. asaccharolyticus were in sero-

Table 1. Direct FA Staining Method with Selected Bacteroides Conjugates

	Conjugate		
	B. melaninogenicus subsp. melaninogenicus	B. melaninogenicus subsp. intermedius	
Organism[a]	Serogroup A (138-71)[b]	Serogroup C (275-70A)	Serogroup C-1 (532-70A)
B. melaninogenicus subsp. melaninogenicus (10 strains)	+	-	-
B. melaninogenicus subsp. intermedius (68 strains)	-	+	-
B. melaninogenicus subsp. intermedius (9 strains)	-	-	+

[a] All strains negative with conjugates to: B. asaccharolyticus serogroup 1 and B. melaninogenicus subsp. levii serogroup 1.

[b] Immunizing strain.

Table 2. Direct FA Staining Method with Selected Bacteroides Conjugates

Organism[a]	Conjugate: B. asaccharolyticus Serogroup 1 (207-72C)[b]	Conjugate: B. melaninogenicus subsp. levii Serogroup 1 (189-75)
B. asaccharolyticus		
(153 strains)	+	-
(10 strains)	-	-
B. melaninogenicus subsp. levii		
(3 strains)	-	+

[a] All strains negative to conjugates: B. melaninogenicus subsp. melaninogenicus serogroup A; B. melaninogenicus subsp. intermedius serogroups C and C-1.

[b] Immunizing strain.

group 1. This serogroup used to be designated serogroup B when this organism was classified as B. melaninogenicus subsp. asaccharolyticus. I am making this change in serogroup of B. asaccharolyticus because of the change in status from subspecies to species. Ten strains of B. asaccharolyticus failed to stain with serogroup 1 conjugate as well as with all other conjugates; therefore, they will represent one or more new serogroups of B. asaccharolyticus. Three strains of B. melaninogenicus subsp. levii comprise serogroup 1 of this organism.

A polyvalent conjugate which contains serogroup A of B. melaninogenicus subsp. melaninogenicus and serogroups C and C-1 of B. melaninogenicus subsp. intermedius, and B. melaninogenicus subsp. levii is now recommended. B. asaccharolyticus which now has species status is no longer appropriate in a B. melaninogenicus conjugate.

Twenty-eight species of anaerobes other than B. melaninogenicus and B. asaccharolyticus, as well as aerobes, failed to react with all of the conjugates listed above.

The FA conjugates also permit detection of mixtures of B. melaninogenicus subsp. melaninogenicus and B. melaninogenicus subsp. intermedius within what appear to be a pure culture. That is, some bacterial cells stain with the serogroup A, and other cells stain with the serogroup C conjugate. Biochemical reactions do not discern the mixture of these two subspecies. Serogroup C can be subcultured from a mixture in pure culture easily. However, serogroup A (B. melaninogenicus subsp. melaninogenicus) was successfully separated in pure culture from only one of eight mixtures; the other isolates grew only in the presence of B. melaninogenicus subsp. intermedius. This phenomenon suggests a possible symbiotic relationship between certain strains of B. melaninogenicus subsp. melaninogenicus and B. melaninogenicus subsp. intermedius. Apparently B. melaninogenicus subsp. intermedius is producing a factor necessary for the growth of B. melaninogenicus subsp. melaninogenicus. B. asaccharolyticus is independent of B. melaninogenicus subsp. intermedius and of B. melaninogenicus subsp. melaninogenicus for growth.

Johnson (personal communication) has performed DNA homology studies on some of the B. melaninogenicus strains described above. Our immunizing strain of B. melaninogenicus subsp. melaninogenicus (strain 138-71), my serogroup A, is in Johnson's DNA homology group A. The type strain for this DNA homology group is VPI #2381. The immunizing strain of B. asaccharolyticus, my serogroup 1, is in Johnson's DNA homology group A of this organism. The type strain for this DNA homology group is VPI #4198. The immunizing strain of B. melaninogenicus subsp. intermedius (strain 275-70A), my serogroup C, is in Johnson's DNA homology group A. The type strain for this DNA homology group is VPI #4197. The immunizing strain of B. melaninogenicus subsp. intermedius (strain 532-70A), my serogroup C-1, is the reference strain (VPI #9342) for Johnson's DNA homology group C. Some of my strains which are nonreactors also fail to fall into any of Johnson's well defined DNA homology groups. These strains may represent new species of B. melaninogenicus.

My immunofluorescence work using specific conjugates has several important applications in clinical and research laboratories: (i) rapid identification of B. melaninogenicus from an agar medium even before pigmentation develops; (ii) FA can be used for delineation of the specific serogroups; (iii) FA is an aid in distinguishing B. melaninogenicus and B. asaccharolyticus from certain organisms which are biochemically similar to the two species; and (iv) FA aids in the separation of specific serogroups in a culture with more than one serogroup and, therefore, the separation of two subspecies of B. melaninogenicus.

On initial isolation from clinical specimens, several species of Bacteroides which produce tan to brown pigment at 48-96 h can be confused with B. melaninogenicus or B. asaccharolyticus; these include Bacteroides oralis and Bacteroides putredinis. In addition, we have also seen strains of Bacteroides ruminicola that produce tan colonies. B. oralis is biochemically similar to B. melaninogenicus subsp. melaninogenicus, and B. putredinis is biochemically similar to B. asaccharolyticus. However, B. oralis and B. putredinis do not react with the B. melaninogenicus or the B. asaccharolyticus conjugates.

BACTEROIDES FRAGILIS

Pathogenicity

In 1976, we reported that Bacteroides fragilis was the most frequent anaerobic Gram-negative non-sporing bacillus found in clinical specimens. Since then others have confirmed these findings. B. fragilis causes a variety of human infections such as septicemia, endocarditis, abdominal wound infections, joint infections, and other multiple infections. The virulence and potential virulence factors of B. fragilis include: lipopolysaccharide (LPS) O antigen (14,16, 23,33), neuraminidase (25,26), fibrinolysin (38), and deoxyribonuclease (37). The role of neuraminidase, fibrinolysin, and deoxyribonuclease in pathogenicity is unclear and needs to be investigated experimentally. The capsule reported by Kasper (17) and later studied by Onderdonk et al. (27) is important in virulence.

Agglutination

The early agglutination work of other investigators (2,4,10, 29, 31,34) on B. fragilis showed that multiple serotypes existed. We began our agglutination study on B. fragilis in 1973, and later, we developed a classification scheme for B. fragilis by agglutination (20). We used a formalin treated antigen for preparation of antisera so that antibodies produced in rabbits were to proteins as well as to other compounds such as the lipopolysaccharides. Our serological classification scheme was similar to the method Pulverer and Ko (28) used to serogroup P. acnes.

We used absorbed antisera which were monospecific with respect to the immunizing antigen. This serological scheme was composed of 21 serogroups. Some serogroups had subserogroups so that there are a total of 45 serological patterns. We classified 98 strains of B. fragilis from clinical specimens and normal human feces according to this scheme. The first seven serogroups were monospecific (Table 3). Thirty-three percent of 98 strains of B. fragilis occurred in one of these seven serogroups. The other 67 strains occurred in the remaining 14 serogroups.

An example of another serogroup is shown in Table 4. There are six major antigens, more than one of which may appear in some strains. For example, all strains in Serogroup VIII have group components 1 and 3 in common, and in addition, have subserogroup components 4,5, 6, or 7 alone or in combination.

Each of the seven reference antisera used for the serogrouping scheme failed to react with 11 other Bacteroides species tested. Therefore, using our antisera, there were no cross reactions between B. fragilis antisera and Bacteroides thetaiotaomicron, Bacteroides distasonis, Bacteroides vulgatus, or Bacteroides ovatus.

Table 3. Agglutination Scheme of Bacteroides fragilis Using Seven Absorbed B. fragilis Antisera

	Absorbed Antisera (Strain No.)						
	1	2	3	4	5	6	7
Serogroup	(289)	(322)	(586)	(531)	(988)	(270)	(898)
I	+	–	–	–	–	–	–
II	–	+	–	–	–	–	–
III	–	–	+	–	–	–	–
IV	–	–	–	+	–	–	–
V	–	–	–	–	+	–	–
VI	–	–	–	–	–	+	–
VII	–	–	–	–	–	–	+

Distribution of Serogroups

Once we established a serological classification by agglutination, we examined the distribution of serogroups of 89 strains of B. fragilis isolated from clinical specimens from different patients, as well as the distribution of serogroups of 16 strains of B. fragilis isolated from the same patient. All of these B. fragilis isolates were serogrouped by our agglutination method employing the seven reference antisera.

Strains from a particular source were classified into one or more serogroups (Table 5), for example, blood isolates occurred in 14 different serogroups. The four fecal isolates occurred in four different serogroups. Eight different serogroups were represented among the abdominal wound isolates. Thus, there was no apparent relationship between the clinical source of the strains and the

Table 4. Agglutination Scheme of Bacteroides fragilis Using Seven Absorbed B. fragilis Antisera

Serogroup	Subserogroup	Group Component	Subserogroup Component
VIII	a	1,3	4
	b	1,3	5
	c	1,3	5,6
	d	1,3	6,7
	e	1,3	4,6,7

Table 5. Distribution of *B. fragilis* Serogroups From Clinical Sources

Source	Serogroup
Blood isolates (27 strains):	I, II, III, VII, VIII, IX, XI, XII, XIV, XVII, XVIII, XIX, XX, and XXI
Fecal isolates (4 strains):	II, X, XV, XVI
Abdominal wound (11 strains):	I, III, VII, VIII, X, XIV, XVIII, XIX

serogroups into which the strains were placed. However, 46% of the strains, isolated from a variety of clinical sources, were placed into five serogroups. Seventy-five percent of the strains were placed into one of 11 serogroups.

We also examined 16 strains of *B. fragilis* isolated from one patient (Table 6). Three venipuncture blood specimens were cultured into pre-reduced anaerobically sterilized (PRAS) blood broth. When the broth showed growth, the specimen was subcultured to blood agar plates which were incubated anaerobically. When growth appeared, five colonies of *B. fragilis* were selected at random from one plate

Table 6. Distribution of 16 Strains of *B. fragilis* from One Patient

B. fragilis Strain	Source	Serogroup	
1A;B	1st Venipuncture	XVIII	c
C;D		XXI	d
E		VIII	e
2A;B;C; D;E	2nd Venipuncture	XXI	d
3A;B;C	3rd Venipuncture	XXI	d
D		VIII	d
E		VIII	f
4A	Abdominal mesentery	XXI	d

of each of the three venipuncture specimens. These 15 colonies were then serogrouped. The five colonies from the first venipuncture were of three different serogroups. All five colonies from the second venipuncture were serogroup XXI d. Two serogroups were found in the five colonies from the third venipuncture.

One colony from the abdominal mesentery was serogroup XXI d which was the serogroup found in all three blood specimens. Unfortunately, due to spreading growth on the original plate of the abdominal mesentery culture, it was not possible to study several colonies from this specimen. To summarize this patient, only three serogroups occurred among the 16 isolates of B. fragilis and most isolates were of serogroup XXI d.

In 1977, Elhag et al. (5) reported an agglutination scheme for B. fragilis. Elhag used a heat-killed antigen for immunization whereas we used a formalin killed antigen. Therefore, our agglutination scheme and Elhag's agglutination scheme are not comparable. Twenty antisera were prepared by Elhag and absorbed to remove cross-reactions. There were multiple serotypes of B. fragilis, B. thetaiotaomicron, B. vulgatus, B. distasonis, and B. ovatus, and there were some cross reactions between these species. Unlike our findings, there was no correlation between the antigenic and biochemical characteristics of these organisms.

In 1978, Elhag and Tabaqchali (6) reported distribution of B. fragilis serotypes by their agglutination scheme among various clinical specimens. They tested 322 strains of B. fragilis from infected patients at three different hospitals with the 20 type specific antisera. Forty-one and three tenths percent were assigned to a single O-serotype, an additional 20.5% were agglutinated by several antisera and could not be classified, and the remaining strains showed no reactions. As was true with our findings, Elhag found no correlation between serotypes and the origin of infection.

Direct Immunofluorescent Antibody (FA) Test

From 1974 to the present, I developed and tested a fluorescent antibody conjugate for B. fragilis (21). This polyvalent conjugate contained conjugates prepared against three strains of B. fragilis. The polyvalent conjugate stained 93% of the 111 B. fragilis strains isolated from clinical specimens (Table 7). The other eight strains stained at certain times but not others. This conjugate is specific for B. fragilis, since 91 strains of anaerobes other than B. fragilis failed to give a positive fluorescence. The advantage of this conjugate is a faster and less expensive identification of B. fragilis than the use of the PRAS biochemical media and gas chromatography. The direct FA test provides a rapid, presumptive identification which can be supported by biochemical testing if desired.

Table 7. Direct FA Staining Method with a Polyvalent B. fragilis Conjugate

Organism	B. fragilis Polyvalent Conjugate (anti-289-71, 586-71, 814-72A)
B. fragilis	
(111 strains)	+[a]
(8 strains)	+ or -[b]

[a] 3+ to 4+ fluorescence.

[b] 0 to 1+ fluorescence.

Abshire et al. (1) have also reported a polyvalent conjugate for B. fragilis. Their work with agglutination and FA agrees with our findings that multiple serotypes of B. fragilis exist.

SUMMARY

We have developed specific FITC conjugates for the identification of various Bacteroides species. These conjugates are specific and may be used for rapid identification. Agglutination, crossed-immunoelectrophoresis, and co-agglutination also provide useful information regarding the antigenic structure of these Bacteroides species.

LITERATURE CITED

1. Abshire, R.L., G.L. Lombard, and V.R. Dowell, Jr. 1977. Fluorescent-antibody studies on selected strains of Bacteroides fragilis subspecies fragilis. J. Clin. Microbiol. 6: 425-432.

2. Beerens, H., P. Wattre, T. Shinjo, and C. Romond. 1971. Premiers résultats d'un essai de classification sérologique de 131 souches de Bactéroides du groupe fragilis (Eggerthella). Ann. Inst. Pasteur (Paris) 121: 187-198.

3. Courant, P.R., and R.J. Gibbons. 1967. Biochemical and immunological heterogeneity of Bacteroides melaninogenicus. Archs. Oral Biol. 12: 1605-1613.

4. Eggerth, A.H., and B.H. Gagnon. 1933. The bacteroides of human feces. J. Bacteriol. 25: 389-413.

5. Elhag, K.M., K.A. Bettelheim, and S. Tabaqchali. 1977. Serological studies of Bacteroides fragilis. J. Hyg. Camb. 79: 233-241.

6. Elhag, K.M., and S. Tabaqchali. 1978. The distribution of Bacteroides fragilis serotypes amongst clinical strains. J. Hyg. 81(1): 89-97.

7. Gibbons, R.J., and J.B. MacDonald. 1961. Degradation of collagenous substrates by Bacteroides melaninogenicus. J. Bacteriol. 81: 614-621.

8. Gibbons, R.J., S.S. Socransky, S. Sawyer, B. Kapsimalis, and J.B. MacDonald. 1963. The microbiota of the gingival crevice area of man. II. The predominant cultivable organisms. Arch. Oral Biol. 8: 281-289.

9. Hausman, E., and E. Kaufman. 1969. Collagenase activity in a particulate fraction from Bacteroides melaninogenicus. Biochem. Biophys. Acta. 194: 612-615.

10. Henthorne, J.C., L. Thompson, and D. Beaver. 1936. Gram-negative bacilli of the genus Bacteroides. J. Bacteriol. 31: 255-274.

11. Hofstad, T. 1968. Chemical characteristics of Bacteroides melaninogenicus endotoxin. Arch. Oral Biol. 13: 1149-1155.

12. Hofstad, T. 1969. Serological properties of lipopolysaccharide from oral strains of Bacteroides melaninogenicus. J. Bacteriol. 97: 1078-1082.

13. Hofstad, T. 1970. Biological activities of endotoxins from Bacteroides melaninogenicus. Arch. Oral Biol. 15: 343-348.

14. Hofstad, T., and T. Kristoffersen. 1970. Chemical characteristics of endotoxin from Bacteroides fragilis NCTC 9343. J. Gen. Microbiol. 61: 15-19.

15. Hofstad, T., and T. Kristoffersen. 1971. Lipopolysaccharide from Bacteroides melaninogenicus isolated from the supernatant fluid after ultracentrifugation of the water phase following phenol-water extraction. Acta. Path. Microbiol. Scand. 79: 12-18.

16. Hofstad, T., T. Kristoffersen, and K.A. Selvig. 1972. Electron microscopy of endotoxic lipopolysaccharide from Bacteroides, Fusobacterium, and Sphaerophorus. Acta. Path. Microbiol. Scand. 80: 413-419.

17. Kasper, D.L., and M.W. Seiler. 1975. Immunochemical characterization of the outer membrane complex of Bacteroides fragilis subsp. fragilis. J. Infect. Dis. 132: 440-450.

18. Lambe, D.W., Jr. 1974. Determination of Bacteroides melaninogenicus serogroups by fluorescent antibody staining. Appl. Microbiol. 28: 561-567.

19. Lambe, D.W., Jr., and R.C. Jerris. 1976. Description of a polyvalent conjugate and new serogroup of Bacteroides melaninogenicus by fluorescent antibody staining. J. Clin. Microbiol. 3: 506-512.

20. Lambe, D.W., Jr., and D.M. Moroz. 1976. Serogrouping of Bacteroides fragilis subsp. fragilis by the agglutination test. J. Clin. Microbiol. 3: 586-592.

21. Lambe, D.W., Jr. 1979. Characterization of a polyvalent conjugate of Bacteroides fragilis by fluorescent antibody staining. Am. J. Clin. Pathol. 71: 97-101.

22. MacDonald, J.B., and R.J. Gibbons. 1962. The relationship of indigenous bacteria to peridontal disease. J. Dent. Res. 41: 320-326.

23. Meisel-Mikolajczyk, F., and A. Dworczynski. 1973. Chemical composition of endotoxins of Eggerthella convexa (Bacteroides fragilis) strain. Bull. Acad. Polonaise Sci. Ser. Sci. Biol. 6: 193-197.

24. Mergenhagen, S.E., E.G. Hampp, and H.W. Scherp. 1961. Preparation and biological activities of endotoxins from oral bacteria. J. Infect. Dis. 108: 304-310.

25. Müller, H.E., and H. Werner. 1970a. Die Neuraminidase als pathogenetischer Fator bei eivem durch Bacteroides fragilis bedingten Abscess. Z. Med. Mikerobiol. U. Immunol. 156: 98-106.

26. Müller, H.E., and H. Werner. 1970b. In vitro Untersuchungen uber das Vorkommen von Neuraminidase bei Bacteroides arten. Path. Microbiol. 36: 135-152.

27. Onderdonk, A.B., D.L. Kasper, R.L. Cisneros, and J.G. Bartlett. 1977. The capsular polysaccharide of Bacteroides fragilis as a virulence factor: comparison of the pathogenic potential of encapsulated and unencapsulated strains. J. Infect. Dis. 136: 82-89.

28. Pulverer, G. 1958. Zur morphologie, biochemie, und serologie des Bacteroides melaninogenicus. Z. Hyg. Infektionskr. Med. Mikrobiol. Immunol. Virol. 145: 293-303.

29. Romond, C., H. Beerens, and P. Wattre. 1972. Identification sérologique des Bactéroides en relation avec leur pouvoir pathogene. Arch. Roumaines Pathol. Exp. Microbiol. 31: 351-355.

30. Shevky, M., C. Kohl, and M.S. Marshall. 1934. Bacterium melaninogenicum. J. Lab. Clin. Med. 19: 689-694.

31. Shinjo, T., H. Beerens, and C.H. Romond. 1971. Classification sérologique de 131 souches de Bactéroides du groupe fragilis (Eggerthella). Ann. Inst. Past. - Lille XXII: 85-100.

32. Sonnenwirth, A.C., E.T. Yin, E.M. Sarmiento, and S. Wessler. 1972. Bacteroidaceae endotoxin detection by Limulus assay. Am. J. Clin. Nutr. 25: 1452-1454.

33. Ushijima, T., K. Ueno, S. Suzuki, and U. Kurimoto. 1971. Morphology and chemistry of the bacterial cell wall. II. Sugar composition and location of O-antigen in the cell wall of Bacteroides convexus. J. Electron Microscopy 20: 32-39.

34. Weiss, J.E., and L.F. Rettger. 1937. The gram-negative bacteroides of the intestine. J. Bacteriol. 33: 423-434.

35. Weiss, C. 1943. The pathogenicity of Bacteroides melaninogenicus and its importance in surgical infections. Surgery 13: 683-691.

36. Werner, H., and M. Sebald. 1968. Etude sérologique d'anaerobies Gram-négatif asporulés, et particulièrement de Bacteroides convexus et Bacteroides melaninogenicus. Ann. Inst. Pasteur (Paris) 115: 350-366.

37. Werner, H., and G. Rintelen. 1968. Untersuchungen über die Konstanz der Kohlenhydratspaltung bei intestinal Bacteroides (Eggerthella) - Arten. Zen. Bakt. Orig. 208: 521-528.

38. Werner, H., and H.E. Müller. 1971. Immunelektrophoretishe Untersuchungen über die Einwirkung von Bacteroides -, Fusobacterium -, Leptotrichia -, and Sphaerophorus - Atten auf menschliche Plasmaproteine. Zbl. Bakt. I. Abt. Orig. 216: 96-113.

DEMONSTRATION OF HEAT STABLE AND HEAT LABILE ANTIGENS OF BACTEROIDES FRAGILIS WITH THE USE OF CO-AGGLUTINATION AND IMMUNOELECTROPHORESIS TECHNIQUES

Dan Danielsson+, Dwight W. Lambe, Jr.[1] and Kaethe P. Ferguson[1]

[1]Department of Microbiology, College of Medicine
East Tennessee State University
Johnson City, Tennessee 37601

+Department of Clinical Microbiology and Immunology
Central County Hospital
S-701 85 Örebro, Sweden

INTRODUCTION

Bacteroides constitute an important group of the anaerobic non-sporulating Gram-negative rods isolated from clinical specimens; Bacteroides fragilis (4) has been of particular clinical interest since it is the causative agent of various types of human infections (6,7,12,13,14,18). Several studies have shown that B. fragilis is the most frequent anaerobic Gram-negative bacillus in clinical specimens (19,28). Serious infections with this penicillin resistant organism have been reported (11,20,27).

Early serological work on Bacteroides (9,24) gave little evidence of the existence of distinct serological groups that could form the basis of a serological classification. Recently, others have indicated that different serogroups of B. fragilis exist (3,10,19,23, 25,26). Kasper and Seiler (15) described an antigen associated with the outer membrane complex which formed subspecies specific immunoprecipitins when tested with serum from hyperimmunized rabbits. Studies of the immune response in humans to B. fragilis infections have also indicated the existence of more than one serotype as well as serologically related strains (6,7,18,22).

Recently, Lambe and Moroz (19) described a serological classification scheme for B. fragilis with the tube agglutination test. As a continuation of these studies, we used co-agglutination (COA) and one- and two-dimensional immunoelectrophoresis (IE) to demonstrate heat stable and heat labile antigens of B. fragilis strains.

MATERIALS AND METHODS

Strains

B. fragilis (24 strains) used in the present study were lyophilized stock strains in our laboratory which had been isolated predominantly from clinical specimens. B. fragilis strains 289-71, 322-72A, 586-71, 531-71A, 988-72B, 270-72A and 898-72 were used as reference strains; these seven strains represented the seven serogroups described by Lambe and Moroz (19) with the agglutination test. The seven B. fragilis strains were encapsulated (21). Other B. fragilis strains studied were: 913-70, 2-72, 168-72, 357-72, 513-72, 814-72A, 1344-72, 1280-73A, 141-74, 371-74, 565-74, 897-74A, 1270-74, 1586-74, 274-75 and 288-75. Other Bacteroides species included two strains of Bacteroides thetaiotaomicron (70-71C, 123-71D), three strains of Bacteroides vulgatus (335-73B, 934-70, 1041-70B), two strains of Bacteroides distasonis (356-71D, 842-73C), and three strains of Bacteroides ovatus (201-74B, 720-74, 721-74).

Culture and Identification

Anaerobic strains were cultured on freshly prepared supplemented blood agar plates (SBAP) composed of brain heart infusion agar (Difco) supplemented with 5% sheep blood (vol/vol), 0.5% yeast extract, 0.0005% hemin and 0.00005% Vitamin K_1 (wt/vol) (19). Identification of anaerobic bacteria was performed as previously described (19) with prereduced, anaerobically sterilized media (Carr-Scarborough Microbiologicals Inc., Stone Mountain, Ga.).

Antigens

Bacteroides strains were grown anaerobically on SBAP for 42-48 h at 35-36 C, harvested in 0.15 M saline (membrane filtered and sterilized), and centrifuged at 4,000 x g for 20 min. The wet weight of sedimented organisms was estimated and antigenic preparation of the organisms prepared in one of the three following ways: (i) Whole cells were suspended in 0.15 M saline at a concentration of 1% (wt/vol) and used in COA tests either untreated, treated with formalin (19), or treated with heat at 56 C, 63 C, 73 C, 80 C, or 100 C for 30 min. (ii) Sonic treated cells. Organisms were suspended in 0.15 M saline at a concentration of 200 or 300 mg/ml, placed in an ice water bath and sonicated with a Bronson ultrasonic apparatus operated at 6-7 D.C. amperes for periodic intervals of 60 s for a total of 360 s. The sonic treated organisms were centrifuged at 7,700 x g for 30 min. The supernatant was collected and used in IE and COA tests either untreated or after treatment with heat. (iii) Boiled saline extracts. Organisms were suspended in 0.15 M saline at a concentration of 200 or 300 mg/ml (wt/vol), heated at 100 C for 30 min and then centrifuged at 7,700 x g for 30 min. The supernatant was collected and used in COA and IE tests.

Antisera

Antisera against the seven reference strains of B. fragilis were obtained from rabbits immunized with formalin treated whole cells as previously described (19) and stored at -80 C. After thawing, merthiolate (1:10,000 wt/vol) was added to the serum which was stored at 4 C and used within four months. Absorptions of antisera were performed with formalin treated or heat treated organisms. One volume of antiserum was mixed with one volume of packed organisms, incubated in a water bath at 37 C for 2-3 h, and stored at 4 C overnight. Absorbed antiserum was recovered by centrifugation at 4,000 x g for 20 min. In some experiments, antisera were absorbed with heat treated organisms and then absorbed with formalin treated bacilli or antisera were absorbed with formalin treated organisms followed by absorption with heat treated organisms. This additional absorption was performed at 37 C for 4 h followed by centrifugation as described above. Absorbed antisera not used the same day were stored at -80 C until used.

Coagglutination

The production and stabilization of protein A-containing staphylococci for COA reagents were performed by the procedures of Kronvall (17). Staphylococci were coated with antibodies by adding 1.0 ml of a 10% suspension of staphylococci (vol/vol) to 0.1 ml of undiluted absorbed or unabsorbed rabbit B. fragilis antiserum. The staphylococci and antiserum were mixed, allowed to stand for 5 min at room temperature, centrifuged at 4,000 x g for 15 min and washed once with 0.01 M phosphate buffered saline, pH 7.2 (PBS). The coated staphylococci were suspended to a concentration of 1% (vol/vol) in PBS containing 0.1% (wt/vol) sodium azide. Control reagent consisted of staphylococci, uncoated or coated with IgG from preimmune rabbit serum. Prepared reagents were stable for at least three months when stored at 4 C.

COA tests were performed with untreated, formalin treated, or heated organisms. The supernatant of sonicated organisms or saline extracts of boiled cells were used as antigens. One drop of a 1% (vol/vol) suspension of the organisms was thoroughly mixed with one drop of reagent staphylococci on a glass slide. The slide was then tilted approximately once per second for 30-45 s and left for 1-2 min after which the reaction was read in oblique light under a magnifying glass (Luxo magnifier, Luxo Lamp Corp., Port Chester, N.Y.). A negative reaction was defined as a turbid suspension of reagent staphylococci and test organisms with no agglutination. A positive COA reaction was agglutination of staphylococci in a clear fluid. Weak positive reactions were +, moderate positive reactions were ++, and strong COA reactions +++. Some untreated and formalin treated B. fragilis strains formed a pseudo-positive reaction (psr). These reactions appeared as small granules which were graded as (+) or (++); in contrast to a true COA reaction the suspension remained milky. Another type of psr appeared as heavy floccules, usually forming within 10-15 tilts of the slide. The suspension of the reagents cleared less than a true COA reaction. These psr's were graded (+++). Negative and positive COA reactions as well as pseudopositive reactions are illustrated in Fig. 1. Wells A1 and C3 were +++; well B2 was ++. These COA reactions represented typical positive reactions seen with homologous strains and antisera. Wells B1 and C1 demonstrated (++) and (+++) psr's respectively; wells A2, A3, B3, and C2 were negative reactions.

Immunoelectrophoresis

One- and two-dimensional IE with an antigen-containing intermediate agar gel were performed as described by Axelsen et al. (2) and referred to as rocket line IE (R-LIE) and crossed line IE (C-LIE) respectively by these authors. The micromodification with 5 x 5 cm

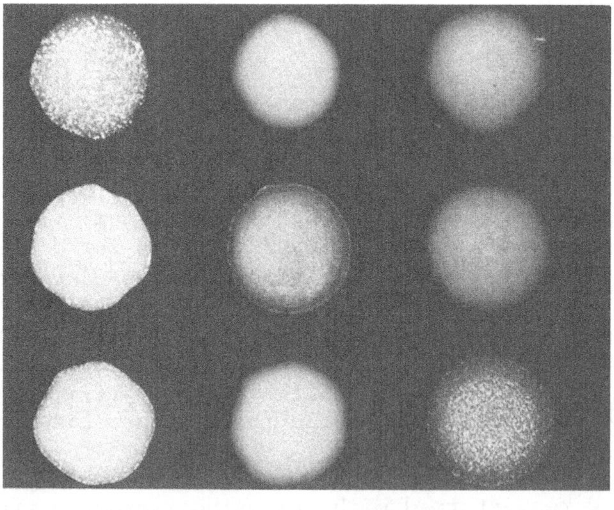

Fig. 1. Co-agglutination patterns obtained with reagent staphylococci coated with specific antibodies against different B. fragilis strains, and formalin treated or heat treated B. fragilis organisms. Anti-B. fragilis 586-71 absorbed with heated organisms of 586-71 in horizontal row A; anti-289-71 absorbed with 531-71A and 988-72B in row B; anti-988-72B absorbed with 531-71A in row C; formalin treated organisms of 586-71 in the wells A1 and B1; formalin treated cells of 289-71 in C1; heated organisms of 289-71 in vertical row 2; and heated organisms of 988-72B in vertical row 3.

glass plates was used. Agarose type I (Sigma) low electroendosmosis (lot 48C-0011) was used throughout this study and was melted at 1% (wt/vol) in sodium barbital-barbital buffer, pH 8.6, 0.02 M, with sodium azide as preservative (2). Figs. 2,3, and 4 show antigen wells (area A), the intermediate agar gel containing the reference antigen (area B), and reference anti-B. fragilis agar gel (area C) for the R-LIE and C-LIE tests. The area containing the antigen wells was 7.5 cm^2; the area of the intermediate agar gel was 5.0 cm^2; the gel containing the B. fragilis antiserum was 12.5 cm^2; the thickness of the agar gel in each of these three areas was 1.5 mm. A 0.12 ml sample of the heated saline extract or the supernatant of the sonicated organisms was included in the intermediate gel, and 200 ul of antiserum was incorporated in the reference antibody gel. The antigen wells, 4 mm in diameter, were filled with 12.5 ul of the untreated or heated supernatant of sonicated organisms or with the saline extracts of organisms heated at 100 C. Reference antigens were tested in concentrations from 50 - 300 mg/ml (wt/vol) as related to the wet weight of sedimented organisms. Optimal results were obtained with 200 mg/ml in C-LIE tests, and with 100 mg/ml in R-LIE tests. The tests were run in an LKB electrophoresis apparatus, with an LKB 3371E D.C. power supply or a Pharmacia power supply CEPS 2000/300. The barbital buffer (pH 8.6, 0.067 M) in the electrophoresis vessels was mixed after each run and changed after five runs. R-LIE was run overnight with a potential gradient of 1.5 - 2.0 V/cm. The first dimension of C-LIE was electrophoresed at 6.0 V/cm for 45 min and the second dimension was electrophoresed at 1.5 - 2.0 V/cm overnight. After electrophoresis the plates were washed in saline and distilled water, pressed under moist filter paper and soft blotting paper, dried and stained with Coomassie blue (2) after which the preciptin reactions were recorded.

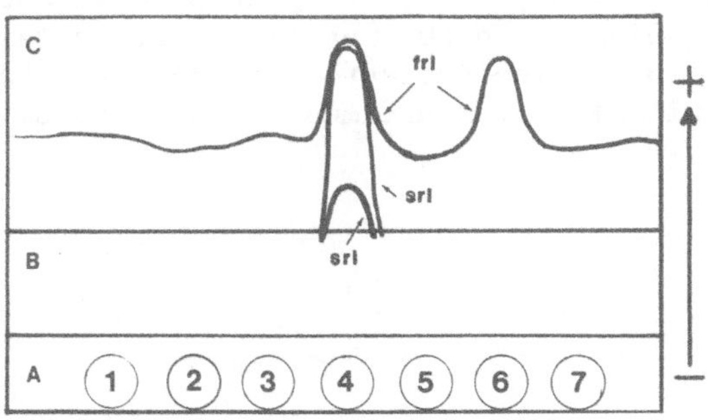

Fig. 2. Schematic drawing of rocket-line immunoelectrophoresis with intermediate agar gel. The rectangular area B contained agarose with saline extract of heated organisms of B. fragilis 898-72, and area C contained agarose with anti-B. fragilis 270-72B. Before the electrophoretic run in the vertical direction, wells 1-7 were filled with saline extracts of B. fragilis strains: (1) 289-71, (2) 322-72A, (3) 586-71, (4) 270-72B, (5) 531-71A, (6) 898-72 and (7) 988-72B.

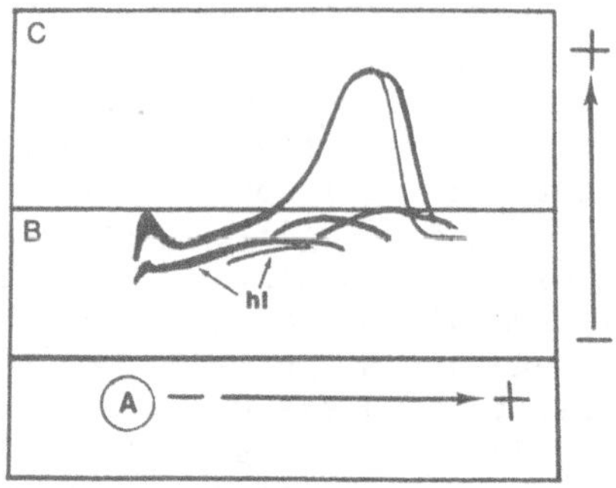

Fig. 3. Schematic drawing of crossed-line immunoelectrophoresis with intermediate agar gel. Before the first electrophoretic run in the horizontal direction, well A was filled with supernatant of sonicated cells of B. fragilis 586-71. Before the second electrophoretic run in the vertical direction, rectangular area B was filled with agarose containing supernatant of sonicated cells of B. fragilis 270-72B, and area C was filled with anti-B. fragilis 586-71.

RESULTS

Heat Stable Antigens

Reagent staphylococci coated with unabsorbed antibodies gave strong or very strong COA reactions with the heated (100 C) homologous B. fragilis organisms, and some gave strong COA reactions with heterologous organisms (Table 1). The same results were obtained with the saline extracts. Absorption of the antibodies with cross-reacting organisms made the antibody-coated reagent staphylococci specific for the homologous organisms. No COA reactions were obtained between heated whole cells or saline extracts with reagent staphylococci uncoated or coated with IgG from preimmune rabbit serum.

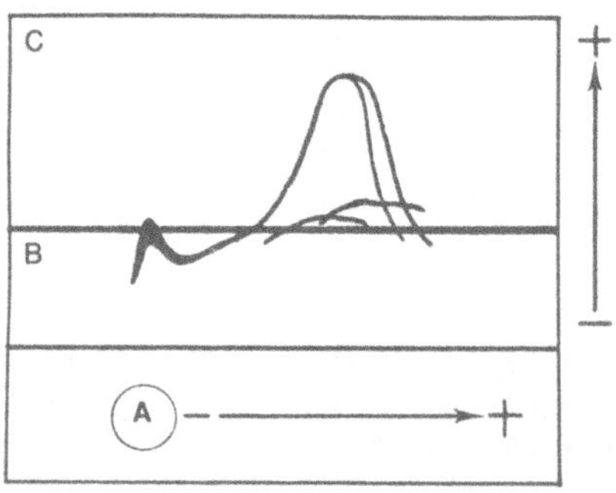

Fig. 4. The same arrangement as in Fig. 3 but with the boiled saline extract of B. fragilis 270-72B included in the intermediate agar gel.

Table 1. Demonstration of Heat Stable Antigens of Whole Cells and Saline Extracts of Heated (100 C) Bacteroides fragilis Organisms with the Use of Co-agglutination

B. fragilis Antiserum for Coating Reagent Staphylococci	B. fragilis Strains Used for Absorption	Co-agglutination Results with Whole Cells and Saline Extracts of Heated (100 C) B. fragilis Organisms						
		289-71	322-72A	586-71	531-71A	988-72B	270-72A	898-72
Anti-289-71	None	+++	[a]		++	+		
	988-72B	+++			+			
	531-71A	+++				+		
	531-71A & 988-72B	+++						
Anti-322-72A	None		+++					
Anti-586-71	None			+++			++	
	270-72A			+++				
Anti-531-71B	None				+++			
Anti-988-72B	None					+++		
Anti-270-72A	None			+++			+++	++
	898-72						++	
Anti-898-72	None			++			+++	+++
	586-71						+++	++
	270-72A							++

[a] Empty space = negative reaction.

Because the saline extracts of the heated B. fragilis organisms gave the same results as the heated whole cells in COA tests, these extracts were used as antigens in R-LIE tests. Saline extracts of boiled organisms or the supernatant of sonicated cells of heterologous strains were included in the intermediate agar gel to absorb in situ cross-reacting antibodies when necessary. Under these conditions the homologous antigen-antibody combinations formed specific rocket precipitin lines as will antigen-antibody combinations with any antigenically related organisms (2). Antigens in the intermediate agar gel cross reacting with the antibodies in the reference antiserum agar gel formed a fused horizontal precipitin line(s) and the corresponding antigen in the antigen well formed a rocket line fusing with the horizontal one (2). The arrangement of the R-LIE tests and the appearance of both specific and fused rocket precipitin lines (srl and frl respectively) are illustrated in Fig. 2. B. fragilis 270-72A in well 4 formed two srl with homologous antiserum. Antigens of strains 270-72A and 898-72 formed a frl with the horizontal line formed by 898-72 in the intermediate agar gel, indicating that strains 270-72A and 898-72 shared a common antigen.

The results of the R-LIE tests with saline extracts of the heated organisms of the seven reference strains are summarized in Table 2. One, two or three rocket lines were formed with the homologous antigen-antibody combinations which indicated that the corresponding B. fragilis strains contained at least one, two or three heat stable antigens. By comparing the results presented in Table 2 with those in Table 1 it will be seen that there was a good agreement between the results of COA and R-LIE. Common heat stable antigens of strains 289-71, 531-71A and 988-72B and of strains 270-72A and 898-72 demonstrated in the COA tests were also demonstrated in R-LIE tests. Common heat stable antigens were demonstrated by COA for strains 586-71 and 898-72, although these common antigens were not shown by R-LIE.

Heat Labile Antigens

The seven B. fragilis reference strains were further investigated with R-LIE and C-LIE and with COA tests for heat labile antigens. To avoid interference with the heat stable antigens, saline extracts of heated (100 C) homologous organisms were included in the intermediate agar gels in the IE tests to absorb corresponding antibodies against heat stable antigens. The antibodies for coating reagent staphylococci were absorbed with homologous cells heated at 100 C.

The sonicated cells of six B. fragilis reference strains demonstrated common antigens in the R-LIE test. However, strain 322-72A shared no common antigens with the other six B. fragilis strains. The supernatant of the sonicated strains 586-71 and 270-72A formed

Table 2. Demonstration of Heat Stable Antigens of Bacteroides fragilis with the Use of Rocket-Line Immunoelectrophoresis with Intermediate Agar Gel Containing Antigen

Anti-B. fragilis Antiserum Used in R-LIE	B. fragilis Antigen in Intermediate Agar Gel	Number of Rocket Lines Formed with Saline Extracts of Heated (100 C) B. fragilis Organisms						
		289-71	322-72A	586-71	531-71A	988-72B	270-72A	898-72
Anti-289-71	988-72B	3			1	1[a]		
Anti-322-72A	None		2					
Anti-586-71	None			3				
Anti-531-71A	None				3			
Anti-988-72B	None					1		
Anti-270-72A	898-72			1			3	1[a]
Anti-898-72	586-71						2	3

[a] Rocket line fusing with horizontal line formed between antigen in intermediate agar gel and reference antibody.

three rocket lines with both of their corresponding antisera. Reactions of identity were shown for all three lines by arranging the antigen wells close to each other. Strains 531-71A and 898-72 shared two antigens with 586-71 and 270-72A. Strains 289-71 and 988-72B shared one antigen with 586-71 and 270-72A. All three antigens were stable at 63 C; two antigens were inactivated at 80 C and the third antigen was inactivated at 100 C. Both heat stable and heat labile antigens of B. fragilis strain 586-71 were demonstrated using two dimensional IE tests with an antigen containing intermediate agar gel. Precipitin lines representing heat stable antigens only were obtained by incorporating strain 270-72A sonicate in the intermediate gel (Fig. 3). This procedure absorbed the antibodies to only heat labile antigens since strains 586-71 and 270-72A shared common heat labile antigens but did not share heat stable antigens (Table 3).

R-LIE and C-LIE tests using the untreated supernatant of sonicated organisms and preimmune rabbit serum gave no precipitin lines. Heat stable and heat labile antigens of strain 586-71 are shown in Fig. 4. Common heat labile antigens of strain 270-72A were destroyed by boiling. When this boiled extract was incorporated into the intermediate agar gel (Fig. 4), absorption of antibodies to heat labile antigens did not occur and precipitin lines representing both heat stable and labile antigens were demonstrated.

The results of COA tests are summarized in Table 4. Formalin treated or untreated organisms of all the B. fragilis strains except strain 322-72A gave moderate or strong COA reactions with reagent staphylococci coated with homologous antibodies. This was due to a heat labile antigen since tests with heated organisms were all negative. However, the same six strains also gave (+), (++) or (+++) psr's with all the reagent staphylococci coated with B. fragilis antibodies as well as with those coated with IgG of preimmune rabbit serum. These psr's were not observed with uncoated staphylococci, nor with organisms heated at 100 C. They were not eliminated by absorbing the antisera or preimmune rabbit sera with formalin treated organisms of strains 289-71 or 531-71A. The weak and moderately strong psr's were almost eliminated after absorption of the antisera with formalin treated organisms of 586-71 and 270-72A; however, this absorption also eliminated the true COA reactions with these strains. Strain 289-71 still gave a moderate psr after absorption. All psr's were eliminated by heating the organisms at 73 C for 30 min. However, the true COA reactions for the heat labile antigens were also eliminated. COA tests were also performed with the supernatant of the sonicated organisms to ascertain that the same antigens were being examined in both COA and R-LIE tests. The same reactivity pattern shown in Table 4 was obtained although the reactions in these tests were more like true COA reactions.

Table 3. Demonstration of Heat Labile Antigens of Bacteroides fragilis with the Use of Rocket-Line Immunoelectrophoresis (R-LIE) with Intermediate Agar Gel Containing Antigen

Anti-B. fragilis Antiserum Used in R-LIE	B. fragilis Antigen in Intermediate Agar Gel[a]	Number of Rocket Lines Formed with Untreated Supernatant of Sonicated B. fragilis Strains						
		289-71	322-72A	586-71	531-71A	988-72B	270-72A	898-72
Anti-289-71	289-71	1	0	1	1	1	1	1
Anti-322-72A	322-72A	0	0	0	0	0	0	0
Anti-586-71	586-71	1	0	3	2	1	3	2
Anti-531-71A	531-71A	1	0	1	1	1	1	1
Anti-988-72A	988-72B	1	0	1	1	1	1	1
Anti-270-72A	270-72A	1	0	3	2	1	3	2
Anti-898-72	898-72	1	0	2	1	1	2	2

[a] Saline extracts of organisms heated at 100 C for 30 min.

Table 4. Demonstration of Heat Labile Antigens of Whole Cells of Bacteroides fragilis with the Use of Co-agglutination and the Occurrence of Pseudo-positive Reactions

Immunoglobulin (IgG) for Coating Reagent Staphylococci (B. fragilis Antiserum)	B. fragilis Strains Used for Absorption	Co-agglutinations and Pseudo-positive Reactions Obtained with Formalin Treated and Untreated Whole Cells of B. fragilis						
		289-71	322-72A	586-71	531-71A	988-72B	270-72A	898-72
289-71	289-71[a]	+++	-	(++)[b]	(+)	(+)	(++)	(++)
322-72A	322-72A[a]	(+++)	-	(++)	(+)	(+)	(++)	(++)
586-71	586-71[a]	(+++)	-	+++	(+)	(+)	+++	(++)
531-71A	531-71A[a]	(+++)	-	(++)	++	(+)	(++)	(++)
988-72B	988-72B[a]	(+++)	-	(++)	(+)	+++	(++)	(++)
270-72A	270-72A[a]	(+++)	-	+++	(+)	(+)	+++	(++)
898-72	898-72[a]	(+++)	-	(++)	(+)	(+)	(++)	++
898-72	289-71[c]	(+++)	-	(++)	(+)	(+)	(++)	++
586-71	586-71[c]	(++)	-	-	-	-	-	-
Preimmune rabbit	None	(+++)	-	(++)	(+)	(+)	(++)	(++)
None	-	-	-	-	-	-	-	-

[a] Absorption with whole cells treated by heat at 100 C.

[b] Reactions within parenthesis indicate pseudo-positive reaction.

[c] Absorption with formalin treated organisms.

COA Tests with B. fragilis and Bacteroides Species

Formalin treated and heat treated organisms of 17 B. fragilis strains and ten strains of other Bacteroides species were subjected to COA with reagent staphylococci coated with B. fragilis antibodies specific for heat stable antigens of the seven reference strains (Table 1). The 27 Bacteroides strains were also tested with COA reagents for heat labile antigens. In addition, reagent staphylococci coated with rabbit preimmune IgG were included in these tests. Thirteen of the 17 B. fragilis strains gave psr's with reagent staphylococci coated with anti- B. fragilis IgG or with rabbit preimmune IgG (Table 5). Six of these strains shared a heat stable antigen with one of the seven reference strains. One strain shared two heat stable antigens. Three of four strains that gave no psr reacted with the COA reagents; two strains reacted with two reagents each; and the third strain reacted with one reagent. None of these four strains reacted with COA reagents for heat labile antigens. The COA reactions for heat labile antigens of the other 13 strains were difficult to interpret because of the moderate, strong or very strong psr's. The ten non-B. fragilis Bacteroides species were negative in the COA tests, and no psr's were demonstrated for any of these strains (Table 5).

DISCUSSION

A serological classification scheme based on the agglutination test was described by Lambe and Moroz (19). This classification was composed of seven serogroups that contained only one group component, and 14 other serogroups that contained group and subgroup components. Forty-five serological patterns were described. The antigenic components of the seven B. fragilis strains were heat resistant. In the present study, the same seven reference strains of B. fragilis were studied by COA and one- and two-dimensional IE techniques.

The seven serogroups of Lambe and Moroz were confirmed by COA. Minor cross reactions were demonstrated in these groups by COA and R-LIE; these minor cross reactions were not observed in the tube agglutination tests. Therefore, COA and R-LIE were sensitive in detecting minor antigens.

Heat stable antigens of the seven B. fragilis reference strains were either strain specific or shared by more than one strain. These heat stable antigens were demonstrated by COA, R-LIE, and C-LIE. One or more of these antigens were also shown in ten additional strains of B. fragilis. Such antigens might form the basis of the serological classification of B. fragilis into serogroups and subserogroups described by Lambe and Moroz (19), or the serotypes described by Elhag et al. (10).

Pseudo-positive reactions occurred when reagent staphylococci coated with B. fragilis antibodies, or with preimmune rabbit serum,

Table 5. Results of Co-agglutination Tests of Formalin Treated and Heat Treated (100 C) Cells of 17 B. fragilis and 10 Strains of Bacteroides Species with Reagent Staphylococci Coated with Specific Rabbit Anti-B. fragilis IgG, or with Rabbit Preimmune IgG

Bacteroides Strains	Number of Strains	Number of Strains[a] Reacting with Reagent Staphylococci Coated with Specific B. fragilis Antibodies for: 289-71	322-72A	586-71	531-71A	988-72B	270-72A	898-72	Number of Strains Pseudo-positive Reactions[b]
B. fragilis	7[c]	1	1	2	2	2	0	1	7
B. fragilis	6[d]	0	0	0	0	0	0	0	6
B. fragilis	3[e]	0	1	0	1	3	0	1	0
B. fragilis	1[f]	0	0	0	0	0	0	0	0
B. thetaio-taomicron	2	0	0	0	0	0	0	0	0
B. vulgatus	3	0	0	0	0	0	0	0	0
B. distasonis	2	0	0	0	0	0	0	0	0
B. ovatus	3	0	0	0	0	0	0	0	0

[a] Tests performed with formalin fixed and heated organisms.

[b] Pseudo-positive reactions obtained in tests between formalin treated cells and reagent staphylococci coated with anti-B. fragilis IgG or with rabbit preimmune IgG.

[c] B. fragilis strains 274-75, 288-75, 371-74, 814-72A, 897-74A, 1344-72 and 1586-74.

[d] B. fragilis strains 2-72, 141-74, 168-72, 513-72 and 913-70.

[e] B. fragilis strains 565-74, 357-72 and 1280-73A.

[f] [illegible]

were mixed with most formalin treated B. fragilis strains. These psr's were not demonstrated with uncoated staphylococci which indicated that IgG was involved. The psr's were not formed when reagent staphylococci were mixed with heat treated B. fragilis organisms showing that the antigens responsible for the psr's were heat labile. Since psr's occurred with preimmune rabbit serum, only heat treated B. fragilis organisms should be used in COA tests.

Heat labile antigens were demonstrated in six of the seven B. fragilis reference strains by R-LIE; these six strains also showed psr's in COA. Heat labile antigens were not observed when preimmune rabbit serum was used in R-LIE, although psr's resulted between B. fragilis and preimmune serum in some COA tests. Therefore, psr's may be caused by one or more heat labile components of B. fragilis strains. These components may or may not be associated with the heat labile antigens observed in R-LIE. Kasper (16) also reported reactivity between rabbit preimmune serum and a protein-polysaccharide complex isolated from the outer membrane complex of B. fragilis. Whether the same antigen or antigen complex demonstrated by Kasper was responsible for the psr's in the COA method was not investigated in this study.

There were no cross reactions between the antigens of B. distasonis, B. ovatus, B. thetaiotaomicron, or B. vulgatus and reagent coated staphylococci; these four Bacteroides species did not form psr's with COA reagents.

The COA method is a rapid, sensitive, and simple test for identification of other pathogenic bacteria (5,8,17). Testing of more B. fragilis strains is needed to evaluate the COA method as a potential diagnostic test for B. fragilis.

LITERATURE CITED

1. Abshire, R.L., G.L. Lombard, and V.R. Dowell, Jr. 1977. Fluorescent-antibody studies on selected strains of Bacteroides fragilis subspecies fragilis. J. Clin. Microbiol. 6:425-432.

2. Axelsen, N.H., J. Kroll, and B. Weeke. 1973. A manual of quantitative immunoelectrophoresis. Methods and applications. Scand. J. Immunol. (Suppl. 1).

3. Beerens, H., P. Wattre, T. Shinjo, and C. Romond. 1971. Premiers résultats d'un essai de classification sérologique de 113 soches de Bactéroides du groupe fragilis (Eggerthella). Ann. Inst. Pasteur (Paris) 121:187-198.

4. Cato, E.P., and J.L. Johnson. 1976. Reinstatement of species rank for Bacteroides fragilis, B. ovatus, B. distasonis, B. thetaiotaomicron and B. vulgatus: designation of neotype strains for Bacteroides fragilis (Veillon and Zuber) Castellani and Chalmers and Bacteroides thetaiotaomicron (Distso) Castellani and Chalmers. Int. J. System. Bacteriol. 26:230-237.

5. Christensen, P., G. Kahlmeter, S. Jonsson, and G. Kronvall. 1973. New methods for the serological grouping of streptococci with specific antibodies absorbed to protein A-containing staphylococci. Infect. Immun. 7:881-885.

6. Danielsson, D., D.W. Lambe, Jr., and S. Persson. 1972. The immune response in a patient to an infection with Bacteroides fragilis ss. fragilis and Clostridium difficile. Acta Pathol. Microbiol. Scand. Sect. B, 80:709-712.

7. Danielsson, D., D.W. Lambe, Jr., and S. Persson. 1974. Immune response to anaerobic infections, p. 173-191. In A. Balows, R.M. DeHaan, V.R. Dowell, and L.B. Guze (ed.), Anaerobic bacteria: role in disease. International Conference on Anaerobic Bacteria, Center for Disease Control, 1972. Charles C. Thomas, Springfield, Ill.

8. Danielsson, D., and G. Kronvall. 1974. Slide agglutination method for the serological identification of Neisseria gonorrhoeae with antigonococcal antibodies absorbed to protein A-containing staphylococci. Appl. Microbiol. 27:368-374.

9. Eggerth, A.H., and B.H. Gagnon. 1933. The Bacteroides of human feces. J. Bacteriol. 25:389-413.

10. Elhag, K.M., K.A. Bettelheim, and S. Tabaqchali. 1977. Serological studies of Bacteroides fragilis. J. Hyg. (Camb.). 79:233-241.

11. Felner, J.M., and V.R. Dowell, Jr. 1970. Anaerobic bacterial endocarditis. N. Engl. J. Med. 283:1188-1192.

12. Finegold, S.M. 1977. Anaerobic bacteria in human disease, p. 71, Academic Press, Inc., New York.

13. Gorbach, S.L., H. Thadepalli, and J. Norsen. 1974. Anaerobic microorganisms in intraabdominal infections, p. 370-384. In A. Balows, R.M. DeHaan, V.R. Dowell, and L.C. Guze (ed.), Anaerobic bacteria: role in disease. International Conference on Anaerobic Bacteria, Center for Disease Control, 1972. Charles C. Thomas, Springfield, Ill.

14. Gorbach, S.L., and J.G. Bartlett. 1974. Anaerobic infections (Second of three parts). N. Engl. J. Med. 290:1237-1245.

15. Kasper, D.L., and M.W. Seiler. 1975. Immunochemical characterization of the outer membrane complex of Bacteroides fragilis subspecies fragilis. J. Infect. Dis. 132:440-450.

16. Kasper, D.L. 1976. The polysaccharide capsule of Bacteroides fragilis subspecies fragilis: Immunochemical and morphologic definition. J. Infect. Dis. 133:79-87.

17. Kronvall, G. 1973. A rapid slide agglutination method for typing pneumococci by means of specific antibody absorbed to protein A-containing staphylococci. J. Med. Microbiol. 6:187-190.

18. Lambe, D.W., Jr., D. Danielsson, D.H. Vroon, and R.K. Carver. 1975. Immune response in eight patients infected with Bacteroides fragilis. J. Infect. Dis. 131:499-508.

19. Lambe, D.W., Jr., and D.A. Moroz. 1976. Serogrouping of Bacteroides fragilis ss. fragilis by the agglutination test. J. Clin. Microbiol. 3:586-592.

20. Leigh, D.A. 1975. Wound infections due to Bacteroides fragilis following intestinal surgery. Br. J. Surg. 62:375-382.

21. Moller, O. 1951. A new method for staining bacterial capsules. Acta Path. Microbiol. Scand. 28:127-131.

22. Rissing, J.P., J.G. Crowder, J.W. Smith, and A. White. 1974. Detection of Bacteroides fragilis infection by precipitin antibody. J. Infect. Dis. 130:70-71.

23. Sonnenwirth, A.C. 1960. A study of certain Gram-negative non-sporulating anaerobic bacteria indigenous to man, with special reference to their classification by serological means. Thesis, Washington University (Ann Arbor, Michigan), Dissertation Abstracts 21: 1336.

24. Weiss, J.F., and L.F. Rettger. 1937. The gram-negative Bacteroides of the intestine. J. Bacteriol. 33:423-434.

25. Werner, H., and M. Sebald. 1968. Etude sérologique d'anaerobies gram-négatifs asporulés, et particulièrement de Bacteroides convexus et. Bacteroides melaninogenicus. Ann Inst. Pasteur (Paris) 115:350-366.

26. Werner, H. 1969. Das serologische Verhalten von Stammen der Species Bacteroides convexus, B. thetaiotaomicron, B. vulgatus and B. distasonis. Zbl. Bakt. Orig. 210:192-201.

27. Wilson, W.R., W.J. Martin, C.J. Wilkowske, and J.A. Washington II. 1972. Anaerobic bacteremia. Mayo Clin. Proc. 47:639-646.

28. Zabransky, R.J. 1970. Isolation of anaerobic bacteria from clinical specimens. Mayo Clin. Proc. 45:256-264.

SURFACE ANTIGENS AS VIRULENCE FACTORS IN INFECTION WITH BACTEROIDES FRAGILIS

Dennis L. Kasper,* Andrew B. Onderdonk, B. Frank Polk, and John G. Bartlett

Channing Laboratory, Department of Medicine, Harvard Medical School, and Peter Bent Brigham Hospital, Division of Affiliated Hospitals Center, Inc., and Infectious Diseases Research Laboratory, Veterans Administration Hospital, Boston, Department of Medicine, Tufts University School of Medicine, Boston, Massachusetts 02115

INTRODUCTION

The virulence properties of bacteria have been attributed to a number of substances that appear to help the organism invade tissues. Although many bacteria elaborate virulence-enhancing substances, such as enzymes and toxins, in others the pathogenic properties are structurally integrated into the cell wall. For example, the virulence of bacteria that behave as extracellular parasites is often caused, at least in part, by antiphagocytic polysaccharide capsules that form a gel-like matrix around the cell. When the Streptococcus pneumoniae was studied in mice, it was found that unencapsulated strains were virtually avirulent because they are readily phagocytosed, but encapsulated strains were highly virulent because of their resistance to phagocytosis (17). Similarly, the virulence of Gram-negative bacteria is thought to be caused, in part, by the presence of endotoxins in the outer membrane. Endotoxins are complex lipopolysaccharides (LPS), whose toxicity resides in the lipid A portion of the molecule, and these lipids have numerous direct biologic effects. In animals LPS cause fever, transient leukopenia followed by leukocytosis, hyperglycemia, purpura, and the Schwartzman phenomenon. In addition, large intravenous doses result in irreversible shock. Our studies are concerned with the capsular polysaccharide

* Recipient of U.S.P.H.S. Research Career Development Award 1K04AI00126.

and LPS components of anaerobic bacteria and the role of these substances in the development of infection.

CLINICAL AND MICROBIOLOGIC ASPECTS OF BACTEROIDES

Among the diseases commonly caused by anaerobes are brain abscess, chronic sinusitis, dental infections, aspiration pneumonitis, lung abscess, empyema, liver abscess, intraabdominal sepsis, and infections of the female genital tract (6). When optimal bacteriologic techniques are used, anaerobic bacteria can be isolated from 70%-95% of patients with these diseases. A common denominator in this seemingly diverse array of septic processes is that the source of the bacteria responsible is the patient's own microflora. Thus, the anaerobic bacteria that are isolated from infected sites are normal inhabitants of the oral cavity, gastrointestinal tract, lower female genital tract, or skin. The pathogenic mechanism is usually a disruption of anatomic barriers and of other host-defense mechanisms that allows the bacteria that colonize mucocutaneous surfaces to gain access to normally sterile sites.

The bacteriology of these infections might be expected to reflect the flora of the source of the inoculum. Yet, although 400 bacterial species reside in the colon and 200 are thought to colonize healthy oral cavities, the average number of bacterial species in infections associated with colonic perforation is five (25), the average in dental infections is six (2), and for aspiration pneumonia the average is three (1). The anaerobic bacteria that dominate in these types of diseases include Bacteroides fragilis, Bacteroides melaninogenicus, Fusobacterium nucleatum, Clostridium perfringens, Peptostreptococcus anaerobius, and Peptococcus asaccharolyticus - six species that probably account for the great majority of anaerobic isolates in clinical laboratories (5). Thus, from a seemingly endless array of anaerobic bacteria in the normal flora, only a few are common in septic processes; it is likely that virulence is an important factor in their selection.

Of all the anaerobes, B. fragilis is the most frequently encountered in intraabdominal sepsis or bacteremia. Members of the genus Bacteroides were second only to Escherichia coli as a cause of Gram-negative septicemia in patients at the Mayo Clinic (Rochester, Minn.), and 78% of these Bacteroides were B. fragilis (27). Studies of intraabdominal sepsis and infection of the female genital tract indicated that B. fragilis is the most common cause of bacteremia in these clinical settings (25,26). Much of our work is focused on this common anaerobe.

Organisms classified as B. fragilis were formerly subdivided into six subspecies: fragilis, distasonis, vulgatus, thetaiotaomicron, ovatus, and an unspecified group, subspecies "other." These subspecies share many phenotypic characteristics, including resistance to penicillins, and their separation was based on minor variations in biochemical reactions. Although they have been reclassified into distinct species on the basis of studies of DNA homology (3), the older, more familiar classification is used.

The distribution of the B. fragilis subspecies is markedly different in normal flora and infected sites. In the colon, the usual source of B. fragilis in septic processes, the numerically dominant subspecies are distasonis, vulgatus, and thetaiotaomicron; subspecies fragilis accounts for only about 0.5% of the colonic microflora (20). In clinical specimens, however, B. fragilis subsp. fragilis is most often encountered. During a two-year period we observed 338 strains of B. fragilis in blood cultures or exudates from clinical infections. Of these organisms, 260 (78%) were subspecies fragilis. Thus, when compared to the numerical concentrations in normal flora, B. fragilis subsp. fragilis is present in a disproportionately large number of clinical isolates (10,24); its predominance in exudate and blood strongly suggests that this subspecies has unique virulence properties.

THE OUTER MEMBRANE OF B. FRAGILIS

We conducted several studies to determine whether any unique bacterial components of B. fragilis subsp. fragilis could account for its enhanced virulence. We began with immunochemical analysis of the outer membrane structure, and this investigation provided some insight into the virulence of the components of the membrane.

In B. fragilis and other Gram-negative bacteria, the cell wall consists of an outer membrane, an inner, or cytoplasmic membrane, and a rigid peptidoglycan layer, which separates the two trilaminar membranes (Fig. 1). The cytoplasmic membrane is generally the site of membrane synthesis and thus contains most of the biosynthetic enzymes. The outer membrane contains the antigens that are encountered by the host, in other words, the surface components of the bacteria.

The outer membranes were loosened from intact B. fragilis by heating of organisms that were suspended in a buffer that contained 10 mM EDTA. This procedure was followed by gentle shearing through a 25-gauge needle and purification by differential ultracentrifugation (11). The purity of the membrane fraction was assessed by isopycnic ultracentrifugation on a 30%-65% sucrose density gradient. A single peak was identified (Fig. 2); its density was 1.23 g/ml, a value similar to that reported for other bacterial outer membranes (9).

The outer membrane in Gram-negative bacteria contains protein,

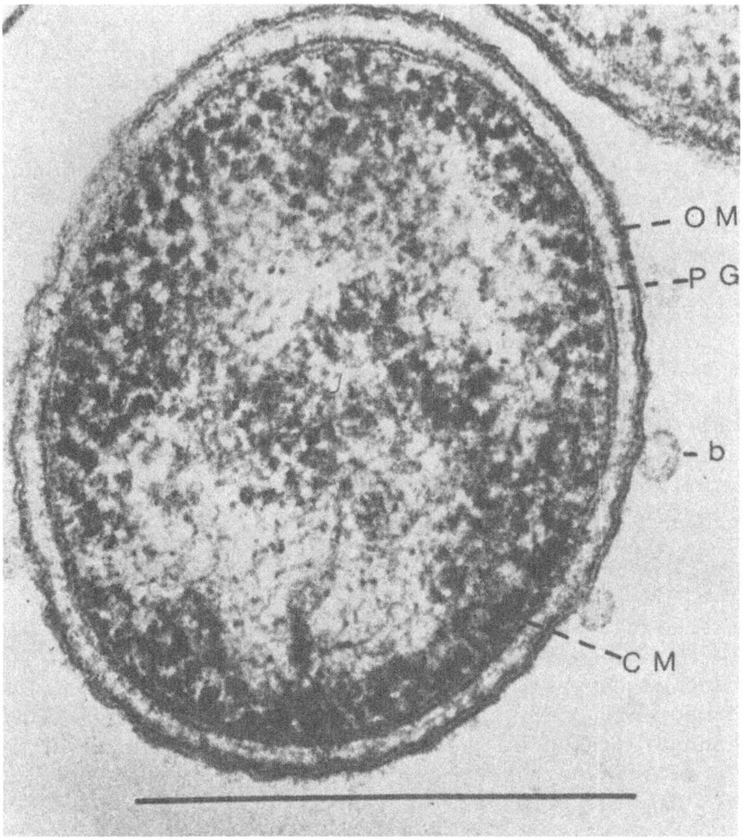

Fig. 1. Electron micrograph of Bacteroides fragilis subsp. fragilis stained by standard techniques (x 120,000). OM = outer membrane; PG = peptidoglycan; b = bleb of outer membrane that is extruded into the growth medium; CM = cytoplasmic membrane. The scale marker denotes 1 um.

LPS, and loosely bound lipids. Capsular polysaccharide is also present in some bacteria, including B. fragilis (12). When we studied the protein component of the outer membranes of strains of B. fragilis by means of electrophoresis in sodium dodecyl sulfate-polyacrylamide gels, the representative strains from each subspecies had distinct peptide-band patterns (Fig. 3a). This finding was not surprising since the outer membrane proteins in other bacteria are biochemically and genetically heterogeneous. Of greater interest was the observation that strains of B. fragilis subsp. fragilis had nearly identical peptide-band patterns (Fig. 3b), a similarity that is unusual within a biochemical group.

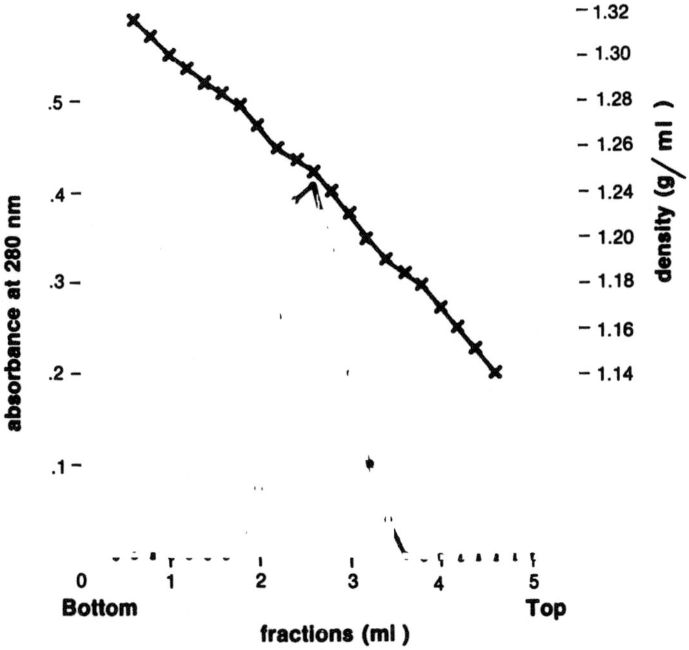

Fig. 2. Absorption at 280 nm of fractions collected from a 30%-65% discontinuous sucrose density gradient centrifugation of the outer membrane fraction of Bacteroides fragilis subsp. fragilis (strain ATCC 23745, American Type Culture Collection, Rockville, Md.). Density (X X) was determined with a refractometer.

As stated above, the LPS component is regarded as a major virulence factor of Gram-negative bacteria. However, the LPS of B. fragilis is biologically distinct from that of aerobic Gram-negative bacteria (13). Although, chemically, it is a lipopolysaccharide, it does not function as an endotoxin. The LPS of aerobic Gram-negative bacteria contains a lipid (lipid A) portion (Fig. 4), which consists primarily of a disaccharide backbone highly substituted with long-chain fatty acids (8). This portion is linked to a carbohydrate core, which contains two unusual sugars (2-keto-3-deoxyoctonate and a heptose), as well as glucose, galactose, and glucosamine. The core is linked to the repeating carbohydrates of the O side chain. Most aerobic Gram-negative bacteria have biologically similar lipopolysaccharide cores, and antibodies to these cores are cross-reactive between bacterial species. However, the O side chain differs markedly between strains even of the same species and thus is the basis of serologic typing schemes for the Enterobacteriaceae (8). The core of the major pathogenic Bacteroides species (fragilis and melaninogenicus) is quite distinct from the

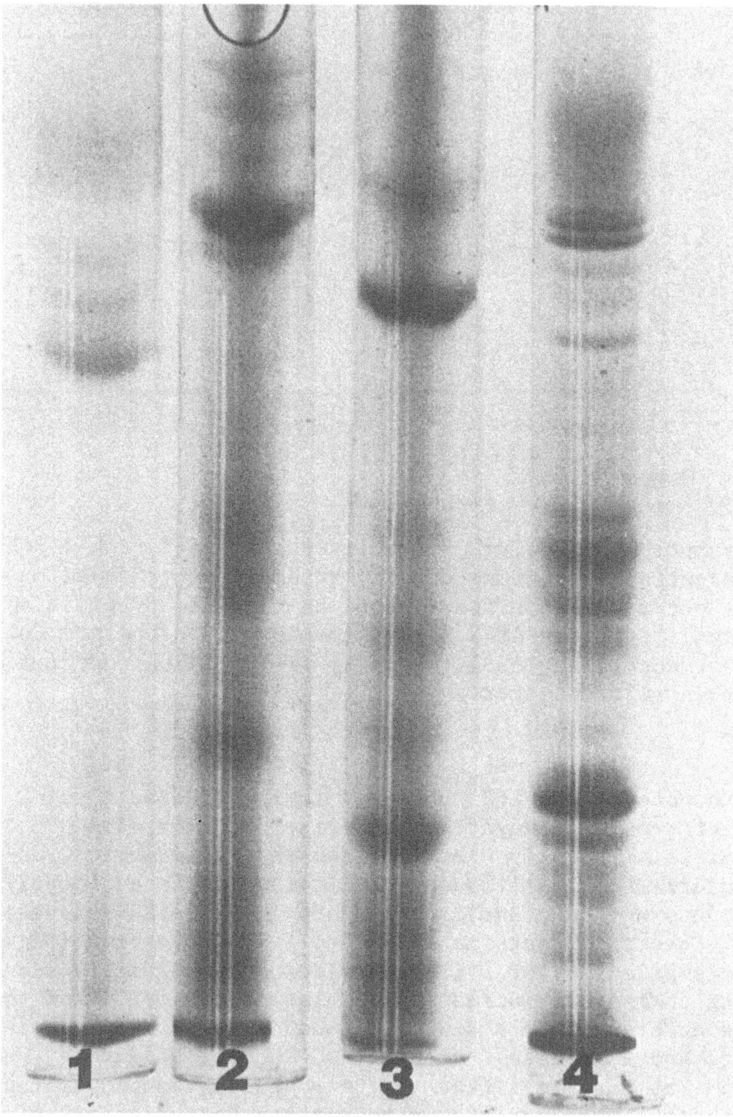

Fig. 3a. (See p. 179)

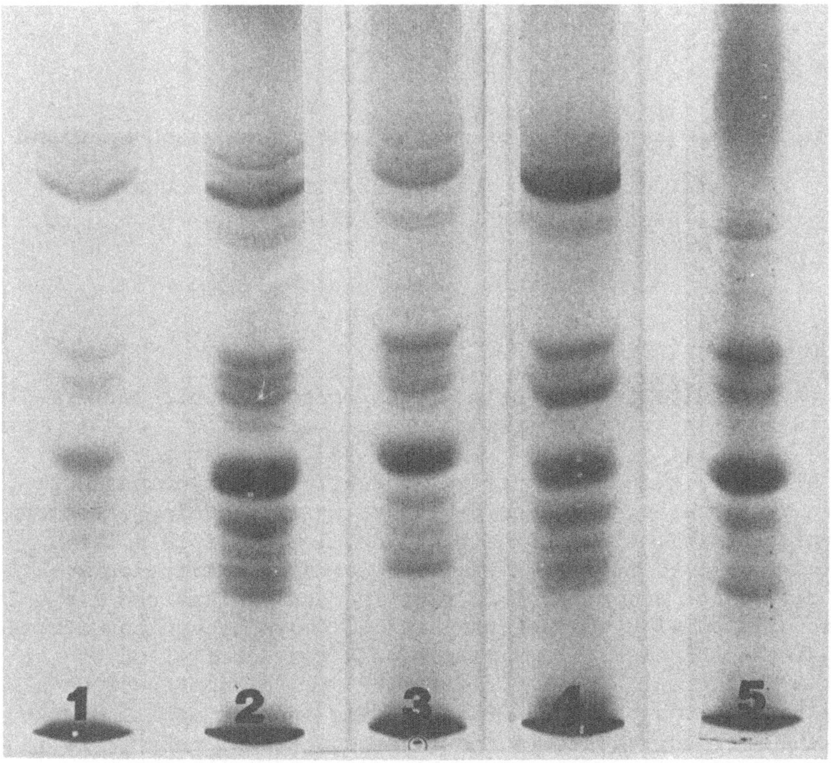

Fig. 3b. Electrophoretic studies of structural proteins in outer membranes of cells that represent four subspecies of Bacteroides fragilis (Fig. 3a.) and of cells that represent five strains of _B._ fragilis subsp. fragilis (Fig. 3b.). Electrophoresis was performed in sodium dodecyl sulfate-polyacrylamide gels. The subspecies shown in Fig. 3a. are distasonis (strain 8503), vulgatus (strain 8482), thetaiotaomicron (strain 12290), and fragilis (strain 23745). The strains of subspecies fragilis shown in the Fig. 3b. are 2429 (Los Angeles, Calif.), ATCC 23745 (American Type Culture Collection, Rockville, Md.), 1262 (Philadelphia, Pa.), 2244 (Los Angeles, Calif.), and 26747 (Boston, Mass.). These strains have nearly identical peptide-band patterns.

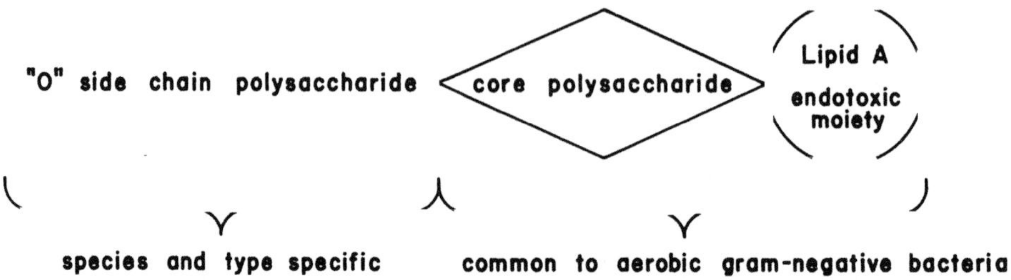

Fig. 4. Schematic diagram of the typical lipopolysaccharide or endotoxin of Gram-negative bacteria.

core of other facultative and of at least some anaerobic bacteria (7,13,18,19).

The LPS of B. fragilis contains no 2-keto-3-deoxyoctonate or heptose in the inner core and no B-hydroxy myristic acid, a common constituent of aerobic lipopolysaccharides, in the lipid moiety. Over 98% of the lipid moiety is easily removed by extraction with chloroform-methanol and ethanol, a fact indicating that the lipid is loosely associated with the polysaccharide. Physicochemical studies showed that the LPS of B. fragilis has some characteristics of the LPS of other bacteria. The B. fragilis LPS can disaggregate to a monomeric unit in the presence of detergents such as sodium deoxycholate, and it reaggregates in the absence of these detergents (13). In biologic studies, it causes gelation of the limulus lysate only at a much higher concentration than that of the endotoxin of Salmonella typhi. Furthermore, the LPS of B. fragilis is not lethal in 10-day-old chick embryos at doses 100 times higher than the lethal dose of S. typhi. Whereas the S. typhi LPS induces the local Schwartzman reaction at a dose of 3 ug per rabbit; the B. fragilis LPS fails to provoke this reaction at a dose of 1 mg per rabbit; furthermore, intact, oxygen-killed B. fragilis is ineffective at a dose of 2.5 mg. These findings indicate that the LPS of B. fragilis is different from that of most Gram-negative bacteria. Although it has some of the chemical and physical properties of an endotoxin, it lacks the biologic properties of a true endotoxin.

An understanding of the LPS component of the Bacteroides may have important clinical implications. Patients with bacteremia due to Bacteroides rarely have either disseminated intravascular coagulation or purpural skin lesions, disorders that are clearly attributable to endotoxins, and the absence of these disorders probably reflects the biologic impotence of these LPS.

BACTERIAL CAPSULES

Another possible virulence factor, the bacterial capsule, is exemplified by the polysaccharide of S. pneumoniae. Some strains of B. fragilis possess a capsular polysaccharide of large molecular size. Immunochemical purification can be achieved by gentle separation of the polysaccharide from the outer membrane (12). Capsules can be demonstrated by several techniques, and a possible explanation for the higher rates of recovery associated with subspecies fragilis as compared with other subspecies found in clinical specimens may be apparent from these studies.

Thirty strains of B. fragilis, characteristic of the various subspecies, were studied with the electron microscope and stained with ruthenium red. Fifteen strains of subspecies fragilis were examined, and a distinct capsule could be seen on the external surface of the outer membrane of 14 of the 15 strains. Capsules were absent from most strains from the other subspecies; however, with one strain of subspecies vulgatus, a dense capsular material was present in 20% of the organisms in the microscopic field. Also, a distinct capsule could be seen in one strain of subspecies thetaiotaomicron. In several strains of subspecies other than fragilis, a less dense material giving a "hairy" surface appearance to the outer membrane was seen, but it was easily differentiated from the electron-dense capsules of the strains of subspecies fragilis. Fig. 5 shows eight strains of various subspecies of B. fragilis.

Quellung reactions with antiserum specific for the polysaccharide of subspecies fragilis demonstrated capsular swelling in 10 strains of this subspecies. Five strains from each of the other subspecies failed to swell with this antiserum or with antisera to isolates of homologous subspecies. An indirect immunofluorescence assay was developed for identification of clinical isolates; capsular material immunologically similar to that in a reference strain of subspecies fragilis was used. In this assay all 132 strains from the other subspecies were negative (14). The fluorescence-positive strain of other subspecies of B. fragilis was of the subspecies B. thetaiotaomicron.

The Role of Encapsulation as a Virulence Factor in an Animal Model of Intraabdominal Sepsis

Initial experiments for development of an animal model were designed to simulate the septic consequence of colonic perforation in human beings (21,28). Gelatin capsules containing an inoculum that included anaerobes (Eubacterium, Clostridium, Bacteroides, Peptococcus, and Fusobacterium) and aerobes (E. coli, enterococcus) in a ratio of 100:1 (anaerobes:aerobes) were implanted in the peritoneal cavity of Wistar rats. The natural course of infection was

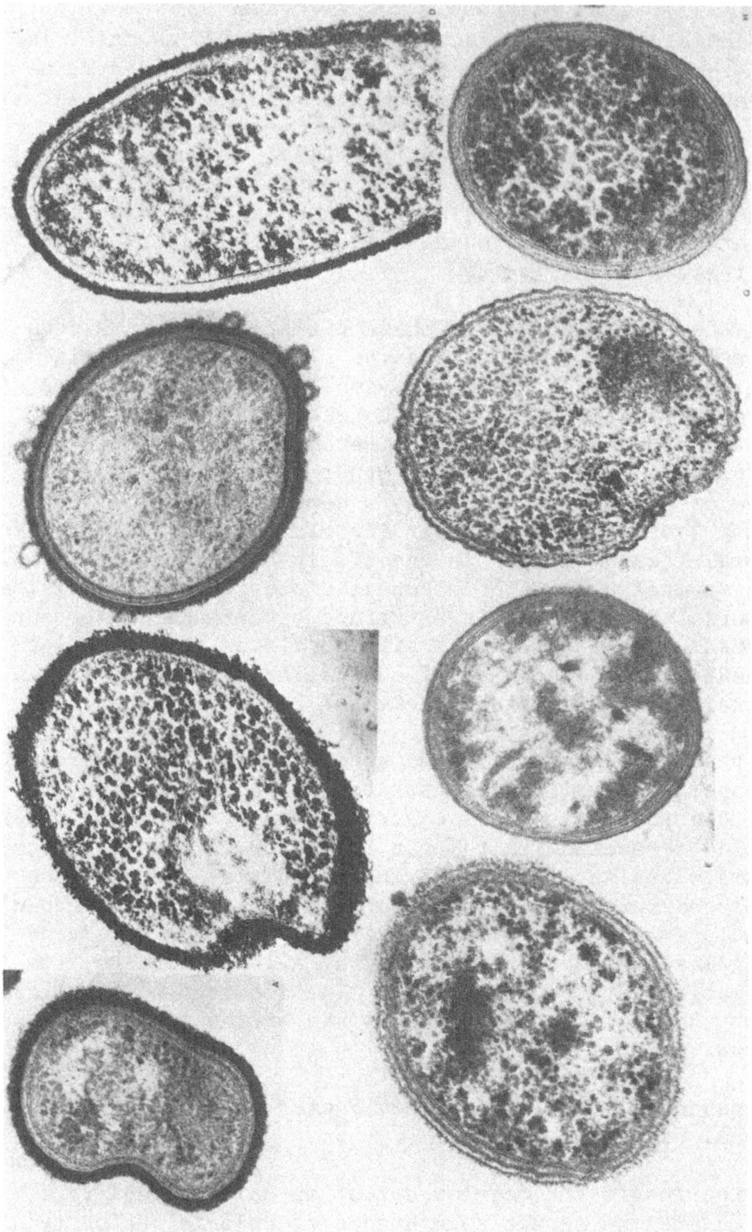

Fig. 5. Electron micrographs of cells of four strains of *Bacteroides fragilis* subsp. *fragilis* (top row) and of four strains of the other subspecies of *B. fragilis* (bottom row) stained with ruthenium red for the detection of capsules (CAP) (x 53,800).

biphasic. The early phase (less than five days) was characterized by acute peritonitis with free-flowing exudate; the mortality was 43%. In the second phase all animals that survived for seven days after challenge had intraabdominal abscesses. Quantitative bacteriologic studies of both phases of illness showed an average of 6.2 bacterial species per specimen. The four most prevalent organisms were E. coli, enterococci, Bacteroides, and Fusobacterium. The two aerobes outnumbered the anaerobes in the peritoneal exudates, whereas anaerobes predominated in the abscess contents. Blood cultures were predictably positive for E. coli during the early (peritonitis) phase and were seldom positive for this microbe in cultures obtained after the third postoperative day. The use of antimicrobial probes further clarified the role of various organisms in the disease process (29). Treatment with gentamicin, which is inactive against the anaerobes, reduced the early mortality to 4% but failed to prevent abscesses. In contrast, clindamycin, which is inactive against E. coli, failed to reduce early mortality but nearly eliminated formation of abscesses among survivors. A combination of the two antibiotics showed the salutory effects of each in that there was a reduction of both early mortality and the second-phase abscess formation noted in untreated animals. Thus, it appeared that the coliforms were responsible for early death, whereas the anaerobes appeared to cause abscess formation.

In another series of experiments, the animals were challenged with various bacterial species instead of with the complex fecal inoculum. These studies showed that E. coli was required to produce mortality, whereas abscesses occurred only when an anaerobe and an aerobe were combined (22). However, the strain of B. fragilis used in this experiment was subsequently shown to be unencapsulated, and further studies showed that the aerobe was unnecessary as an adjunct for abscess development when encapsulated B. fragilis was used as the anaerobe for infection of animals (23). Subsequently, it was shown that heat-killed B. fragilis produced abscesses indistinguishable from those resulting from infection with viable organisms. Finally, when purified capsular material from B. fragilis was implanted, abscesses again resulted. Control studies, including the implantation of capsular polysaccharide of E. coli and heat-killed type III S. pneumoniae, failed to produce detectable disease.

This group of experiments has provided an approach to the study of pathogenesis of anaerobic infection by analysis of specific virulence factors in a model that simulates infection in humans.

Antibody Response to the B. fragilis Capsule in the Rat Peritonitis Model

The humoral antibody response to the capsular polysaccharide of B. fragilis was quantitated in animals with intraabdominal abscesses by means of a sensitive, radioactive antigen-binding assay (16). The antibody detected by this technique correlated highly with that measured by quantitative precipitin analysis (r=0.943). Animals infected with encapsulated B. fragilis had high levels of circulating serum antibody to the capsular polysaccharide (Fig. 6). This antibody could be induced by implantation of live organisms, heat-killed organisms, heterologous strains of B. fragilis, or various outer-membrane components that contained the capsular antigen, and the immunogenicity of the capsular polysaccharide could be enhanced by complexing to the outer membrane or to outer-membrane proteins.

Antibody Response of Women with Pelvic Inflammatory Disease to the Capsular Polysaccharide of B. fragilis

By the use of the radioactive antigen-binding assay, the antibody response to the B. fragilis capsule was quantitated in women with acute pelvic inflammatory disease (15). Table 1 lists the antibody levels in paired sera from 33 patients, the interval (in days) between collection of the two samples of serum, and the change in antibody concentration during the interval. Patients were categorized according to the results of cultures of fluid from their cul-de-sac and cervical swabs; those yielding B. fragilis subsp. fragilis alone or in mixed culture from the cul-de-sac are listed first (group 1), followed by those yielding strains of B. fragilis that were not subspeciated (group 2), and those with no evidence (on the basis of culdocentesis cultures) of infection with B. fragilis (group 3). The mean difference in concentrations of serum antibody between acute- and convalescent-phase specimens for women with B. fragilis subsp. fragilis was 10.47 ug/ml (group 1). For those with cervical cultures negative for Neisseria gonorrhoeae, the mean change was 2.58 ug/ml (group 2). The mean change in antibody concentration in the first group was significantly higher than for each of the other groups or for a group of healthy female volunteers ($P < 0.01$, one-way analysis of variance). Changes in antibody levels in group 2 were not significantly different from those of volunteer laboratory workers. These results demonstrate much greater changes in levels of serum antibody to the capsule of B. fragilis subsp. fragilis in patients from whom this organism was isolated by culdocentesis or laparoscopy as compared with changes in antibody levels of other patients.

The data support the bacteriologic evidence (4) that B. fragilis subsp. fragilis is a more important etiologic agent in acute nongonococcal than in gonococcal pelvic inflammatory disease; however, these rises in titer of antibody cannot be interpreted as absolute proof of causality of the infection. This argument could be misleading; one needs only to be reminded of the frequent finding of Neisseria meningitidis in the nasopharynx of military recruits with pharyngitis due to adenovirus disease. These recruits simultaneously develop antibodies to N. meningitidis and to adenovirus; yet N. meningitidis is

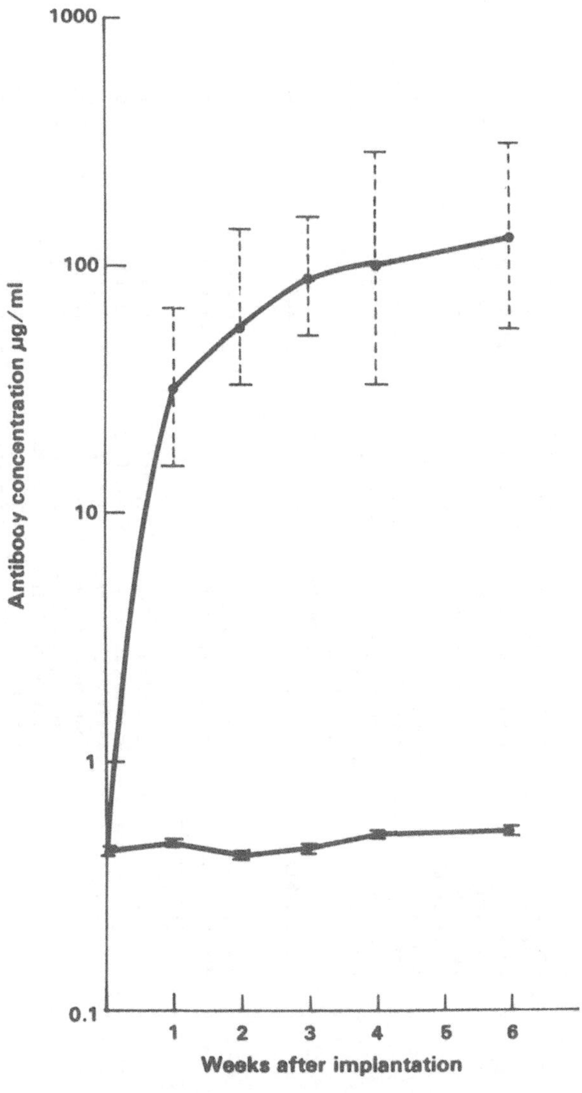

Fig. 6. Quantitative antibody response to the capsular polysaccharide of Bacteroides fragilis for groups of 10 rats implanted with encapsulated B. fragilis (line with dashed brackets) and unencapsulated B. fragilis (line with solid brackets). Means ± SD are plotted for each weekly sampling of blood after implantation (week zero). Implants for both groups included 5 x 10^7 viable enterococci, sterile cecal contents, $BaSO_4$, and either the encapsulated B. fragilis or the unencapsulated strain of Bacteroides.

Table 1. Results of Culture and Concentrations of Serum Antibody to the Capsule of Bacteroides fragilis Subsp. fragilis in 33 Selected Cases of Pelvic Inflammatory Disease (PID)

Group, Patient No.	PID Episode[a]	Neisseria gonorrhoeae Isolated from Cervix	Cul-de-sac Isolate(s): B. fragilis Subspecies	Cul-de-sac Isolate(s): Other Organism	Antibody Concentration in ug/ml (Interval in Days): Acute-Phase Serum	Antibody Concentration in ug/ml (Interval in Days): Convalescent-Phase Serum	Change in Antibody Concentration (ug/ml)[b]
Group 1							
201	I	-	fragilis, thetaiotaomicron	Aerobes	9.86(2)[c]	14.26(7)[d]	4.40
219	I	-	fragilis	Aerobes, anaerobes	31.79(7)	19.08(30)	12.71
247	R	-	fragilis	Anaerobes, aerobes	16.75(1)	9.87(14)	6.88
263	I	+	fragilis, distasonis	Anaerobes, aerobes	12.89(1)	11.45(34)	1.44
264	I	-	fragilis	Aerobes	30.55(1)	59.69(5)	29.14
282	I	-	fragilis	Aerobe	24.26(2)	10.66(14)	13.60
300	I	-	fragilis	Anaerobes, aerobe	12.78(6)	17.89(20)	5.11
259	R	-	Unavailable	Bacteroides capillosus, anaerobes, aerobe	16.39(14)	25.21(23)	8.82
069	R	-	Unavailable	...	14.74(I)	22.64(7)	7.90
Group 2							
233	I	-	distasonis	Anaerobes, aerobes	23.13(10)	21.65(46)	1.48
245	I	-	distasonis, vulgatis, thetaio-taomicron	Anaerobes, aerobe	15.15(14)	13.33(21)	1.82
268	I	-	...	Anaerobes	12.03(7)	13.16(21)	1.13
301	I	-	...	Anaerobes	13.66(15)	11.65(10)	2.01
248	R	-	...	Anaerobe, aerobes	45.55(1)	43.05(10)	2.50
258	R	-	...	Anaerobe, aerobe	20.78(7)	17.10(28)	3.68
262	I	-	...	Aerobes, Mycobacterium hominis	9.44(4)	15.49(14)	6.05
202	R	-	...	Aerobe	15.14(1)	12.73(34)	2.41
209	I	-	...	Aerobe	12.37(1)	13.65(180)	1.28
229	I	-	...	Aerobes	17.36(1)	18.77(33)	1.41
243	I	-	...	Aerobe	8.01(1)	8.51(34)	0.50
269	I	-	...	Aerobe	8.63(5)	8.73(21)	0.10
272	I	-	...	Aerobe	14.24(4)	24.60(18)	10.36
290	R	-	...	Aerobe	9.88(4)	8.57(14)	1.31

Table 1. (Continued)

Group, Patient No.	PID Episode[a]	Neisseria gonorrhoeae Isolated from Cervix	Cul-de-sac Isolate(s): *B. fragilis* Subspecies	Cul-de-sac Isolate(s): Other Organism	Antibody Concentration in ug/ml (Interval in Days): Acute-Phase Serum	Antibody Concentration in ug/ml (Interval in Days): Convalescent-Phase Serum	Change in Antibody Concentration (ug/ml)[b]
Group 3							
206	I	+	distasonis	Aerobes	8.18(2)	9.69(20)	1.51
212	R	+	...	*N.* gonorrhoeae, *B.* capillosus, aerobe	13.51(2)	13.45(30)	0.06
235	I	+	...	*N.* gonorrhoeae, aerobe	19.47(10)	19.84(64)	0.37
276	I	+	...	*N.* gonorrhoeae	22.21(14)	11.21(14)	10.99
284	I	+	...	*N.* gonorrhoeae	22.59(2)	20.38(20)	2.21
295	I	+	...	*N.* gonorrhoeae, aerobe	14.28(1)	14.84(34)	0.56
307	I	+	...	*N.* gonorrhoeae	28.88(1)	26.67(6)	2.21
308	R	+	...	*N.* gonorrhoeae	26.49(3)	17.70(9)	8.79
227	I	+	No growth		15.02(2)	12.87(60)	2.15
236	I	+	No growth		11.66(3)	10.40(18)	1.26

NOTE. Tables with total identification of all isolates are available upon request from the authors.

[a] I = initial, R = recurrent.

[b] The mean changes for groups 1,2, and 3 were 10.00, 2.58, and 3.01, respectively.

[c] Interval from onset of abdominal pain until sample was obtained. I = indeterminate.

[d] Interval between samples.

not the primary pathogen. The clinical setting of pelvic inflammatory disease and B. fragilis is not completely analogous, however. B. fragilis is a part of the normal colonic flora of humans. Therefore, the isolation of this organism from an infected site with a concomitant rise in titer of antibody, although not fulfilling Koch's postulates, does provide supportive evidence for the causation of disease.

Antibody Response of Women with Abscesses after Hysterectomy to the Capsular Polysaccharide

To determine the possible role of B. fragilis in the development of infectious complications of hysterectomy, we measured serum antibody to the capsular polysaccharide in 53 women before and several days after elective surgery.

Specimens of serum were collected from potential participants before surgery. At the time of discharge, a second specimen of serum was collected from five categories of patients: (i) those with an uncomplicated postoperative course; (ii) those with febrile illness (oral temperature of ≥100.4 F on at least two days after surgery, excluding the first 24 h); (iii) those with abdominal or wound infection; (iv) those with pelvic cellulitis; and (v) those with abscess (cuff abscess or pelvic abscess).

The base-line concentrations of antibody of these individual subjects varied widely (2.0–17.7 ug/ml), as did the final concentrations (Table 2).

Table 2. Results of Determinations of Concentration of Serum Antibody to the Capsule of Bacteroides fragilis subsp. fragilis in Women Undergoing Hysterectomy

Group (n)	Median Antibody Concentration in ug/ml (Range) Before Surgery	After Surgery[a]
No complications (21)	5.2 (2.0–11.3)	6.6 (2.5–10.6)
Wound infection (4)	4.1 (3.1– 4.8)	5.5 (3.6– 8.7)
Pelvic cellulitis (4)	4.3 (3.7–10.3)	5.5 (3.6–10.4)
Abscess (9)	5.6 (3.1–17.7)	13.0 (4.0–17.9)
Fever (15)	5.6 (3.0–13.3)	7.8 (3.2–13.0)

[a] Antibody concentration was measured in samples of sera obtained at the time of discharge from the hospital.

The changes in antibody concentrations for each of the five groups are listed by diagnosis in Table 2. Analysis of variance demonstrated that the five groups differed significantly in their mean changes in concentration of antibody between the pre- and post-operative specimens ($F_{4,48}=6.54$; $p < 0.05$). Further analysis revealed that the mean rise in concentration of antibody (4.91 ug/ml), in the group with abscesses was significantly greater than the mean rise among patients with no complications (0.62 ug/ml), wound infection (1.90 ug/ml), pelvic cellulitis (0.63 ug/ml), and febrile illness (0.95 ug/ml) ($t = 4.52$, $p < 0.05$). The mean changes in antibody concentrations among the latter four groups of patients were not significantly different from each other ($t=1.35$; $0.20 < p < 0.10$). Two of the five patients without abscess who had an increase in antibody concentration of 3.0 ug/ml had pathologic findings of pelvic inflammatory disease. Another of these five patients had a wound infection from which were cultured two types of anaerobic Gram-negative bacilli that were not identified further.

The data presented here suggest that the majority of abscesses following hysterectomy, either cuff or pelvic abscesses, are associated with an increase in antibody to the capsular polysaccharide of B. fragilis. The data presented here suggest that the majority of abscesses are associated with an increase in antibody to the capsular polysaccharide of B. fragilis. The data further suggest that, with the possible exception of wound infections, the other infectious or presumably infectious complications of this procedure are uncommonly associated with such changes in antibody concentrations.

CONCLUSION

One traditional school of thought has promulgated the belief that anaerobes are merely commensals and that they play no important part in clinical infection. Current thinking, based largely on clinical evidence, has begun to refute this notion, and the experimental data reviewed herein also indicate that anaerobes have a role in the septic process. The bacterial species in patients with clinically important infections do not reflect the normal bowel flora. In addition, the prevalence of certain anaerobic bacteria may, in part, be explained by the immunochemical properties of the cell wall. The most prevalent anaerobe in clinical infections, B. fragilis, has an LPS with no endotoxic activity and a capsular polysaccharide that induces intraabdominal abscess in an animal model and antibody in infected hosts. These features may account for the types of disease caused by this species of bacteria.

ACKNOWLEDGMENTS

This work was supported by contract numbers DAMD-17-78C-8019 and DAMD-17-74C-4056 from the U.S. Army Medical Research and Development Command.

LITERATURE CITED

1. Bartlett, J.G., S.L. Gorbach, and S.M. Finegold. 1974. Bacteriology of aspiration pneumonia. Am. J. Med. 56:202-207.

2. Bartlett, J.G., and S.L. Gorbach. 1976. Anaerobic infections of the head and neck. Otolaryngol. Clin. North Am. 9:655-678.

3. Cato, E.P., and J.L. Johnson. 1976. Reinstatement of species rank for Bacteroides fragilis, B. ovatus, B. distasonis, B. thetaiotaomicron, and B. vulgatus: designation of neotype strains for Bacteroides fragilis (Veillin and Zuber) Castellani and Chalmers and Bacteroides thetaiotaomicron (Distaso) Castellani and Chalmers. Int. J. Syst. Bacteriol. 26:230-237.

4. Eschenbach, D.A., T.M. Buchanan, H.M. Pollock, P.S. Forsyth, E.R. Alexander, J.S. Lin, S.P. Wang, B.B. Wentworth, W.M. McCormack, and K.K. Holmes. 1975. Polymicrobial etiology of acute-pelvic inflammatory disease. N. Engl. J. Med. 293:166-171.

5. Finegold, S.M., W.E. Shepard, and E.H. Spaulding. 1977. Practical anaerobic bacteriology, p. 1-14. CUMITECH no. 5, American Society for Microbiology, Washington, D.C.

6. Gorbach, S.L., and J.G. Bartlett. 1974. Medical progress: anaerobic infections. N. Engl. J. Med. 290: 1177-1184; 1237-1245; 1289-1294.

7. Hofstad, T. 1974. The distribution of heptose and 2-keto-3-deoxyoctonate in Bacteroidaceae. J. Gen. Microbiol. 85: 314-320.

8. Jann, K., and O. Westphal. 1975. Microbial polysaccharides, p. 1-125. In M. Sela (ed.), The antigens. Vol. 3. Academic Press, New York.

9. Johnston, K.H., and E.C. Gotschlich. 1974. Isolation and characterization of the outer membrane of Neisseria gonorrhoeae. J. Bacteriol. 119: 250-257.

10. Jones, R.N., and P.C. Fuchs. 1976. Identification and antimicrobial susceptibility of 250 Bacteroides fragilis subspecies by broth dilution methods. Antimicrob. Agents Chemother. 9: 719-721.

11. Kasper, D.L., and M.W. Seiler. 1975. Immunochemical characterization of the outer membrane complex of Bacteroides fragilis subspecies fragilis. J. Infect. Dis. 132: 440-450.

12. Kasper, D.L. 1976. The polysaccharide capsule of Bacteroides fragilis subspecies fragilis: immunochemical and morphologic definition. J. Infect. Dis. 133: 79-87.

13. Kasper, D.L. 1976. Chemical and biological characterization of the lipopolysaccharide of Bacteroides fragilis subspecies fragilis. J. Infect. Dis. 134: 59-66.

14. Kasper, D.L., M.E. Hayes, B.G. Reinap, F.O. Craft, A.B. Onderdonk, and B.F. Polk. 1977. Isolation and identification of encapsulated strains of Bacteroides fragilis. J. Infect. Dis. 136: 75-81.

15. Kasper, D.L., D.A. Eschenbach, M.E. Hayes, and K.K. Holmes. 1978. Quantitative determination of the serum antibody response to the capsular polysaccharide of Bacteroides fragilis ss fragilis in women with pelvic inflammatory disease. J. Infect. Dis. 138: 74-80.

16. Kasper, D.L., A.B. Onderdonk, and J.G. Bartlett. 1978. Quantitative determination of the antibody response to the capsular polysaccharide of Bacteroides fragilis in an animal model of intraabdominal abscess formation. J. Infect. Dis. 136: 789-795.

17. MacLeod, C.M., and M.R. Kraus. 1950. Relation of virulence of pneumococcal strains for mice to the quantity of capsular polysaccharide formed in vitro. J. Exp. Med. 92: 1-9.

18. Mansheim, B.J., and D.L. Kasper. 1977. Purification and immunochemical characterization of the outer membrane complex of Bacteroides melaninogenicus subspecies asaccharolyticus. J. Infect. Dis. 135: 787-799.

19. Mansheim, B.J., A.B. Onderdonk, and D.L. Kasper. 1978. Immunochemical and biologic studies of the lipopolysaccharide from Bacteroides melaninogenicus subspecies asaccharolyticus. J. Immunol. 120: 72-78.

20. Moore, W.E.C. 1977. Anaerobes as normal flora: gastrointestinal tract, p. 222-228. In S.M. Finegold (ed.), Proceedings of the International Metronidazole Conference, Montreal, Quebec, Canada. Excerpta Medica, Princeton, N.J.

21. Onderdonk, A.B., W.M. Weinstein, N.M. Sullivan, J.G. Bartlett, and S.L. Gorbach. 1974. Experimental intraabdominal abscesses in rats. II. Quantitative bacteriology of infected animals. Infect. Immun. 10: 1256-1259.

22. Onderdonk, A.B., J.G. Bartlett, T.J. Louie, N. Sullivan-Siegler, and S.L. Gorbach. 1976. Microbial synergy in experimental intraabdominal abscess. Infect. Immun. 13: 22-26.

23. Onderdonk, A.B., D.L. Kasper, R.L. Cisneros, and J.G. Bartlett. 1977. The capsular polysaccharide of B. fragilis as a virulence factor: comparison of the pathogenic potential of encapsulated and unencapsulated strains. J. Infect. Dis. 136: 82-89.

24. Polk, B.F., and D.L. Kasper. 1977. Bacteroides fragilis subspecies in clinical isolates. Ann. Intern. Med. 86: 569-571.

25. Thadepalli, H., S.L. Gorbach, and P.N. Broido. 1973. Abdominal trauma: anaerobes and antibiotics. Surg. Gynecol. Obstet. 137: 270-276.

26. Thadepalli, H., S.L. Gorbach, and L. Keith. 1973. Anaerobic infection of the female genital tract: bacteriologic and therapeutic aspects. Am. J. Obstet. Gynecol. 117: 1034-1040.

27. Washington, J.A., II. 1971. Comparison of two commercially available media for detection of bacteremia. Appl. Microbiol. 22: 604-607.

28. Weinstein, W.M., A.B. Onderdonk, J.G. Bartlett, and S.L. Gorbach. 1974. Experimental intraabdominal abscesses in rats. I. Development of an experimental model. Infect. Immun. 10: 1250-1255.

29. Weinstein, W.M., A.B. Onderdonk, J.G. Bartlett, and S.L. Gorbach. 1975. Antimicrobial therapy of experimental intra-abdominal sepsis. J. Infect. Dis. 132: 282-286.

ANTIGENIC ANALYSIS OF ACTINOMYCES SPECIES

George E. Kenny and Betsy L. Williams

Department of Pathobiology SC-38
School of Public Health and Community Medicine and
Department of Periodontics SM-44, School of Dentistry
University of Washington, Seattle, WA 98195

INTRODUCTION

Patients with chronic periodontal inflammation frequently have a predominance of Actinomyces species in their lesions. For example, of the first four patients in a study by Williams et al. (8), three patients had a predominance of Actinomyces species at the subgingival sites. When the patients, all with six to eight mm pockets, were compared with age matched controls, the Actinomyces viscosus-naeslundii group of organisms were statistically more prominent than in the controls. Although we now realize that the current activity of periodontal destruction of tissues in these patients was not well characterized and that six to eight mm pockets do not necessarily mean active periodontal disease, nevertheless, Actinomyces were possible agents of inflammatory periodontal disease. In addition, Loesche (6) has shown that cessation of oral hygiene measures promptly results in gingivitis associated with an increase in numbers of Actinomyces in dental plaque.

In characterizing Actinomyces, it became evident that we were observing a large number of organisms in the A. viscosus-naeslundii group. Their biochemical reactions, particularly carbohydrate fermentation, varied; and the differences in carbohydrate fermentation might be associated with differences in colonial morphology and surface antigens. In a 1976 report (8), one patient had antibodies to a smooth strain of A. viscosus isolated from another patient, but only the rough strain was recovered from the former patient in fairly high numbers. Since Actinomyces and the other organisms are constantly bathed by antibodies in the cervicular fluid which flows from the underlying connective tissues towards the gingival margin, they may be subjected to continuous selective pressures by antibody. Actinomycotic lesions commonly occur in the head, neck, thorax and abdomen; the mouth is the most probable reservoir for such infection. Fig. 1 shows an actinomycotic lesion following the extraction of a tooth. The ability of Actinomyces to infect is not surprising: from their niche on the root surface where they are the prominent organism in root caries, they could easily penetrate into deeper tissues or gain access to the bloodstream. Emphasis has been placed on the taxonomy of these organisms because of the growing recognition of their importance.

The purpose of the present study was to investigate the taxonomic relationships in the Actinomycetes by quantitative immunoelectrophoretic methods. We then compared the relationships shown by numerical taxonomy and DNA homology with the serological characteristics. In addition we also attempted to identify and characterize antigens important in taxonomy and in disease. Such antigens include surface antigens, cell wall antigens and other components common to the Actinomycetes.

MATERIALS AND METHODS

Organisms were grown in defined medium (Socransky, personal communication), centrifuged, and suspended in buffered 0.15 M NaCl at a concentration 200 times that of the original culture. Concentrated organisms were disrupted by shaking with glass beads (Bronwill cell disintegrator). For most experiments, excluding the charge-shift experiments, 2% Triton X-100 and 0.25% sodium deoxycholate were added and the antigen was sonicated. Two-dimensional immunoelectrophoresis was carried out using methods developed in this laboratory

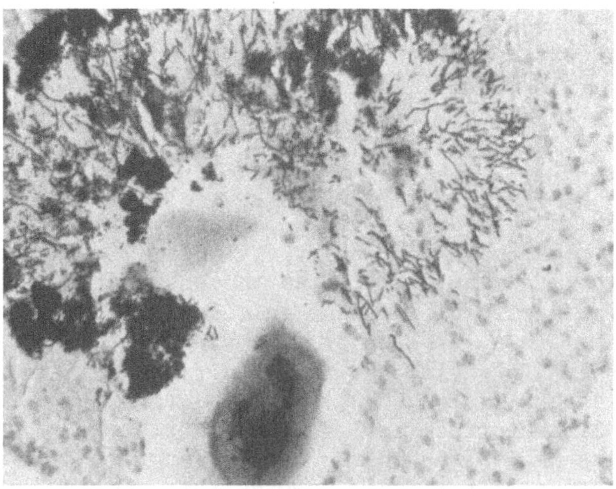

Fig. 1. An actinomycotic lesion at the site of a tooth extraction.

(1,2,7). Glass slides (4.2 x 4.2 cm) were coated with 2.0 ml of 0.5% agarose suspended in veronal buffer (pH 8.6, 0.05 M) containing 0.5% Triton X-100 and 0.05% sodium deoxycholate except where indicated. The running buffer was the same buffer at 0.1 M. First phase electrophoresis (Fig. 2) with bovine albumin as the marker for electrophoretic mobility was run at 3 to 4 V/cm for 90 min, which was sufficient to move the albumin marker 3/4 of the length of the slide. The agarose on the upper half of the slide was removed and replaced with agarose containing antiserum to the organism and sufficient antibody to the bovine albumin to provide a visible rocket. Second phase electrophoresis was carried out at 1 V/cm for 18 h. Slides were observed, washed with 0.15 M NaCl for 24 h, washed in distilled water for 24 h and stained with Coomassie brilliant blue.

Antisera were prepared in rabbits using whole live organisms cultivated and concentrated as above. The immunization scheme was the one described previously (5). Rabbits were injected intramuscularly with 2 ml of immunogen mixed with 2 ml of incomplete Freund's adjuvant. After three weeks, rabbits were injected intravenously with increasing dosages (0.1, 0.2, 0.3, and 0.4 ml) of fluid immunogen twice weekly for a total of four injections. Blood was collected from rabbits one week later (six weeks after the primary immunization).

RESULTS

Solubilization of the antigens and quantitation of the amount of material used in the immunoelectrophoresis tests were difficult. Dis-

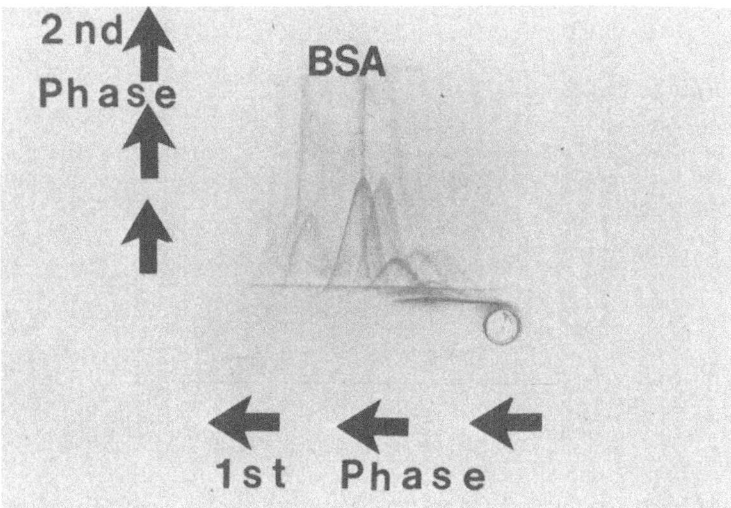

Fig. 2. Illustration of two-dimensional immunoelectrophoresis. *A. viscosus* strain 28 run against homologous antiserum.

integration of the organisms with glass beads provided excellent solubilization for most of the antigens detectable on the profiles (Fig. 2); however, the low lying precipitin line seen near the origin could not be increased in height by increasing the amount of antigen tested on the slide. Solubilization of the cell wall antigens by autoclaving eliminated most of the electrophoretically fast peaks and two antigens could be detected in the autoclaved preparation for A. viscosus strain 28 (Fig. 3). The picture was more clear-cut for Actinomyces israelii where the antiserum gave considerably better resolution of the profile. Six antigens remained after autoclaving, two of which could be identified in the profile of the control antigen (Fig. 4). Quantitation of the amount of antigen actually used on the slides was difficult because optimum solubilization required: disintegration with glass beads, filtration to remove the glass beads, and sonication of the resulting suspension of disrupted organisms in the presence of both Triton X-100 and deoxycholate were performed. A large amount of material remained insoluble and did not migrate from the antigen well.

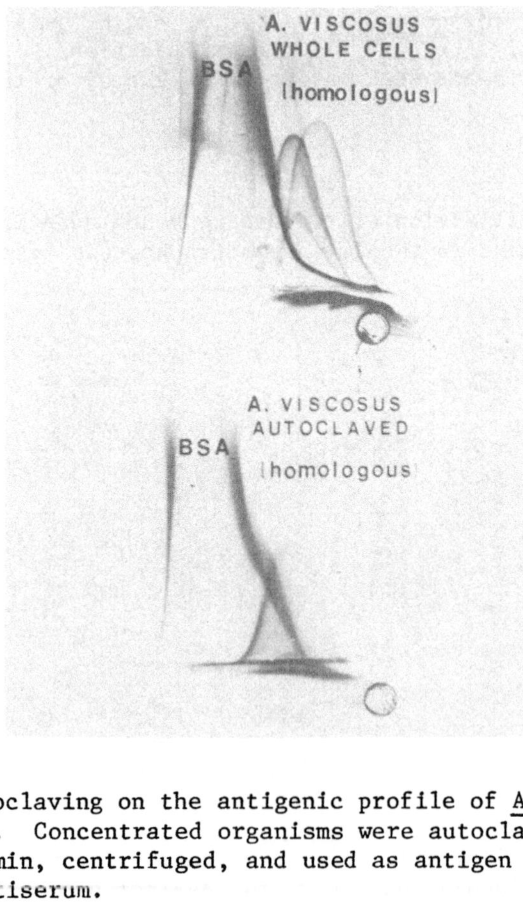

Fig. 3. Effect of autoclaving on the antigenic profile of A. viscosus strain 28. Concentrated organisms were autoclaved at 121 C for 30 min, centrifuged, and used as antigen against homologous antiserum.

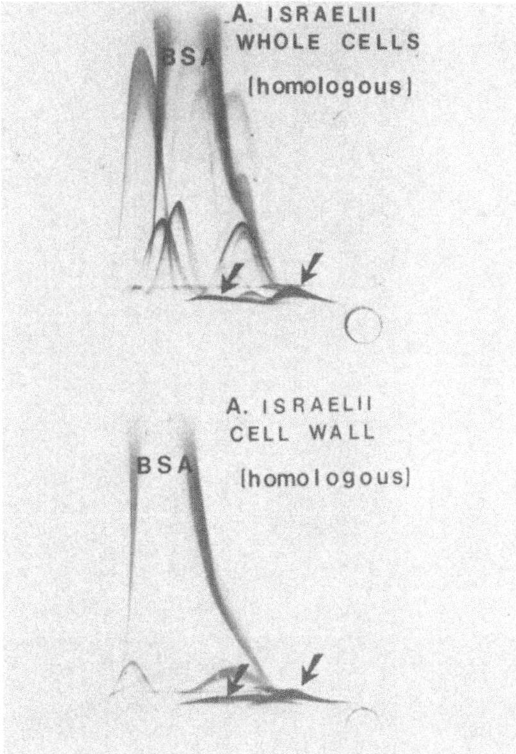

Fig. 4. Effect of autoclaving on the antigenic profile of A. israelii ATCC 12103. Concentrated organisms were autoclaved at 121 C for 30 min, centrifuged, and used as antigen against homologous antiserum.

Centrifugation of the antigen improved profiles because it removed the trailing seen from the antigen well with uncentrifuged antigens. Thus, the amount of material actually run on the immunoelectrophoresis slide is not known. The results were reproducible in that peak heights for identical or closely related antigens were similar from one organism to another.

In an effort to improve solubility and resolution of profiles, a technique devised in our laboratory for studies with mycoplasmata termed charge-shift immunoelectrophoresis (2) was used. The addition of a negatively charge detergent such as deoxycholate increased the negative charge on amphiphilic but not on hydrophilic antigens. The amphiphilic antigens were increased in mobility and gave larger peaks (Fig. 5). The mobilities of the antigens indicated by the arrows, which were undistinguished blurs at the origin showed better profiles

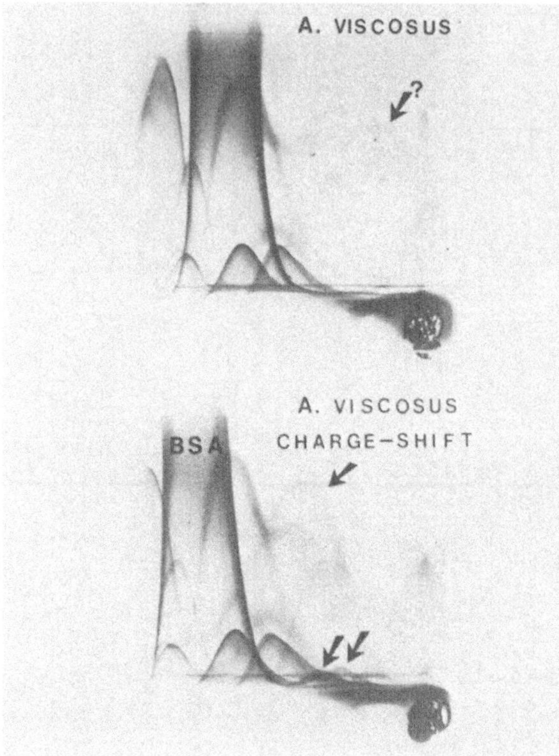

Fig. 5. Effect of deoxycholate on antigenic profile of solubilized whole cells of A. viscosus strain 28 tested against homologous antiserum. The concentration of deoxycholate was 0.05% in both first and second phase electrophoresis for the slide labeled "charge-shift" whereas deoxycholate was omitted for the upper frame of the figure. Triton X-100 was included at 0.5% in both slides.

and were more clearly separated. In the mycoplasmic model cytoplasmic antigens were not increased in mobility and could be distinguished from the membrane antigens (1). Resolution of the profiles was improved by addition of deoxycholate, and was added to all subsequent two-dimensional immunoelectrophoresis runs. This was important since some of the surface antigens required charge-shift conditions for demonstration.

The initial comparison of Actinomyces species by two-dimensional immunoelectrophoresis showed that the organisms classified as A. viscosus and A. naeslundii were closely related (Table 1) and shared six of the nine to 12 precipitin lines shown in the homologous system.

Table 1. Comparison of Four Species in Actinomycetales by Two-Dimensional Immunoelectrophoresis Using Disrupted Cells as Antigen

Antigen	Antiserum 1	2	3	4
1. A. viscosus (ATCC 19246)	12[a]	6	2	2
2. A. naeslundii (WVU 820)	6	9	2	2
3. A. israelii (ATCC 12103)	1	1	12	1
4. R. dentocariosa (ATCC 17931)	0	0	0	20

[a] Number of precipitin lines; homologous reactions underlined.

In contrast, Rothia dentocariosa and A. israelii were clearly distinct from each other and from A. viscosus. When the antigens were autoclaved for 30 min at 121 C to solubilize cell wall components and to eliminate heat labile soluble protein antigens, the same relationships were seen (Table 2). A. viscosus and A. naeslundii shared at least one putative cell wall antigen. Neither of these organisms shared components with R. dentocariosa or A. israelii both of which differed from each other.

The technique of two-dimensional immunoelectrophoresis is advantageous for the demonstration of surface antigens (1). The area of

Table 2. Comparison of Autoclaved Antigens of Four Species in Actinomycetales by Two-Dimensional Immunoelectrophoresis

Antigen	Antiserum 1	2	3	4
1. A. viscosus (ATCC 19246)	4[a]	2	0	0
2. A. naeslundii (WVU 820)	1	2	0	0
3. A. israelii (ATCC 12103)	0	0	5	0
4. R. dentocariosa (ATCC 17931)	0	0	1?	7

[a] Number of precipitin lines; homologous reactions are underlined.

the peak is directly proportional to the amount of antigen and inversely proportional to the amount of antibody. Therefore, absorption of the serum with whole organisms removes antibody to surface components only (1). The resolving power of the assay system removes 50% of the antibody which can be detected by an increase in peak height or area of the affected antigen. Absorption of antibody to cells of strain 28 caused the elimination of one peak indicated by the arrow on the control slide (Fig. 6), and an increase in the height of another peak indicated by the arrow on the absorbed slide. When this absorbed antiserum was tested with autoclaved antigen containing only putative cell wall antigens (Fig. 7), two peaks disappeared, indicated by arrows on the control slide; this suggested that the cell wall components were on the surface of this strain.

A comparison of solubilized whole organisms of A. viscosus strains with a similar A. israelii antigen by two-dimensional immunoelectrophoresis showed that the five A. viscosus strains were closely related; there were six to 13 lines in the homologous systems and in the heterologous cross-reactions (Table 3). In contrast, A. israelii antiserum showed only two components with the A. viscosus antigens whereas 13 components were recognized in the homologous reactions. The A. israelii antiserum showed two fast components, which had an electrophoretic mobility greater than that of bovine albumin, in each

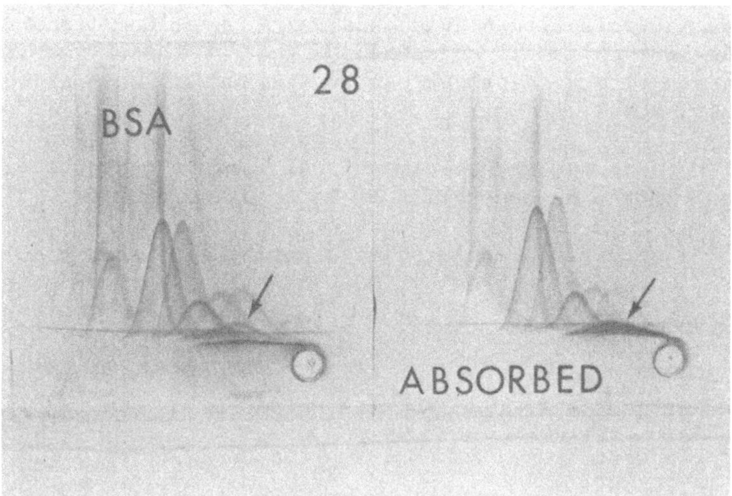

Fig. 6. Demonstration of surface antigens of A. viscosus strain 28 by absorption of antiserum with concentrated live organisms. Pelleted organisms were added to antiserum at approximately 10% by volume. Serum was incubated for 1 h at 4 C and organisms were removed by centrifugation. Antiserum was tested against solubilized whole cell antigen.

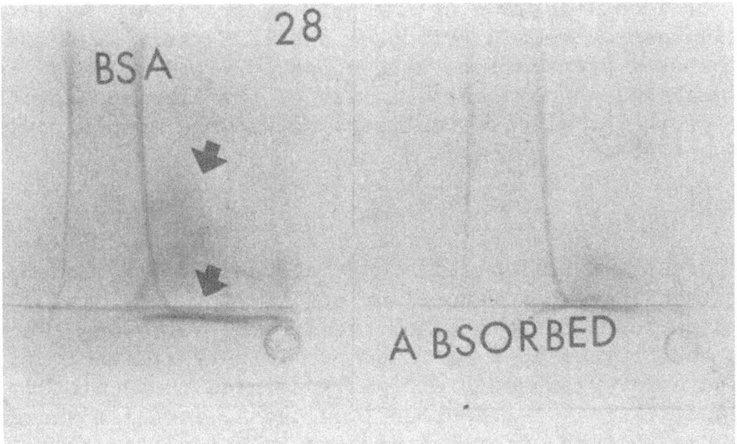

Fig. 7. Demonstration of surface antigens of A. viscosus. Antiserum was absorbed as described in Fig. 6 and tested against autoclaved cells as antigen.

A. viscosus strain. These components were heat labile and did not shift in charge, which suggested that they are cytoplasmic components. In addition, both components were detected by any method of disruption which suggests that they readily spill from the cytoplasm of the organism. If we are able to produce monospecific antiserum to one or both components, such antisera might have considerable taxonomic

Table 3. Comparison of Solubilized Whole Cell Antigens of Five Strains of Actinomyces viscosus with Actinomyces israelii by Two-Dimensional Immunoelectrophoresis

	Antiserum					
	A. viscosus strains					A. israelii
Antigen	T14	28	A30A	A32B1	19246	12103
T14	<u>6</u>[a]	13	7	6	8	3
28	8	<u>12</u>	5	7	8	2
A30A	8	14	<u>8</u>	8	8	2
A32B1	9	13	8	<u>9</u>	10	2
ATCC 19246	6	13	4	6	<u>9</u>	3
ATCC 12103	0	5	2	1	2	<u>15</u>

[a] Number of precipitin lines; homologous reactions are underlined. Organisms solubilized by glass beads and run under charge-shift conditions.

utility for identification of Actinomyces species. The antigenic distinctiveness between A. viscosus and A. israelii was more evident when autoclaved preparations were compared (Table 4). A. israelii antiserum showed no components in any of the A. viscosus strains and only two of the A. viscosus antisera showed one component in the A. israelii antigen.

DISCUSSION

The present results indicated that quantitative immunoelectrophoretic techniques have excellent utility for determining the antigenic structure of the Actinomycetes. The following general conclusions can be reached from these preliminary studies: (i) Strains classified as A. viscosus are closely related to each other and to A. naeslundii. (ii) R. dentocariosa and A. israelii showed little relationship to each other and distant relationships to the A. viscosus-naeslundii complex. (iii) For A. viscosus, the surface antigens appeared to be cell wall components. (iv) Cell wall components appeared to be more species-specific than cytoplasmic components since A. viscosus shared at least two specific cytoplasmic antigens with A. israelii. The resolving power of our antisera is comparable to those of Holmbert et al. who detected up to 10 antigens in two-dimensional immunoelectrophoretic studies (3,4). They showed, as we verified in the present study, that the number of antigens detected depends on the method of solubilization.

Table 4. Comparison of Autoclaved Extracts of Five Strains of Actinomyces viscosus with Actinomyces israelii by Two-Dimensional Immunoelectrophoresis

	Antiserum					
	A. viscosus strains					A. israelii
Antigen	T14	28	A30A	A32B1	19246	12103
T14	1[a]	3	1	3	1	0
28	2	3	1	2	1	0
A30A	2	3	1	4	1	0
A32B1	2	2	2	3	1	0
ATCC 19246	3	3	3	3	3	0
ATCC 12103	0	1	0	1?	0	5

[a] Number of precipitin lines; homologous reactions are underlined. Organisms solubilized by glass beads, autoclaved, and run under charge-shift condition.

ACKNOWLEDGMENTS

This study was supported in part by grant DE 02600 from the National Institute of Dental Research and by RR-0571407 from the General Research Support Branch, Division of Research Resources, National Institutes of Health. We are grateful to S. Jenkins for skilled assistance.

LITERATURE CITED

1. Alexander, A.G., and G.E. Kenny. 1977. Characterization of membrane and cytoplasmic antigens of Mycoplasma arginini by two-dimensional (crossed) immunoelectrophoresis. Infect. Immun. 15:313-321.

2. Alexander, A.G., and G.E. Kenny. 1978. Application of charge-shift electrophoresis to antigenic analysis of mycoplasmic membranes by two-dimensional (crossed) immunoelectrophoresis. Infect. Immun. 20:861-863.

3. Holmberg, K., C.E. Nord, and T. Wadström. 1975. Serological studies of Actinomyces israelii by crossed immunoelectrophoresis: standard antigen-antibody system for A. israelii. Infect. Immun. 12:387-397.

4. Holmberg, K., C.E. Nord, and T. Wadström. 1975. Serological studies of Actinomyces israelii by crossed immunoelectrophoresis: taxonomic and diagnostic applications. Infect. Immun. 12: 398-403.

5. Kenny, G.E. 1971. Immunogenicity of Mycoplasma pneumoniae. Infect. Immun. 3:510-515.

6. Loesche, W.J. 1975. Bacterial succession in dental plaque: role in periodontal disease, p. 132-136. In D. Schlessinger (ed.), Microbiology. American Society of Microbiology, Washington, D.C.

7. Thirkill, C.E., and G.E. Kenny. 1974. Serological comparison of five arginine-utilizing Mycoplasma species by two-dimensional immunoelectrophoresis. Infect. Immun. 10:624-632.

8. Williams, B.L., R.M. Pantalone, and J.C. Sherris. 1976. Subgingival microflora and periodontitis. J. Periodont. 11:1-18.

SEROLOGY OF PROPIONIBACTERIA

Cecil S. Cummins

Anaerobe Laboratory
Virginia Polytechnic Institute and State University
Blacksburg, Virginia 24061

INTRODUCTION

The propionibacteria are Gram-positive, non-sporing, anaerobic to aerotolerant, irregular rods, which produce propionic and acetic acids as the major end-products of fermentation.

In the eighth edition of Bergey's Manual of Determinative Bacteriology (3), two groups of strains, of generally different origins, are classified in the genus Propionibacterium. The first group is what might be called the "classical" propionibacteria - that is a group of strains isolated from cheese and dairy products, including such species as P. freudenreichii, P. jensenii, P. thoenii and P. acidipropionici. These organisms are very important in cheesemaking and thereby do much good for the human race. However they do not cause disease in man, and I do not propose therefore to consider them further.

The other group of strains classified in Propionibacterium are the anaerobic (or micro-aerophilic) diphtheroids from skin, the cutaneous propionibacteria. This group was, until recently, generally classified in Corynebacterium, the commonest species being, of course, called C. acnes. One may refer to them colloquially perhaps as the "acne group" or the "anaerobic diphtheroids". As pointed out by Douglas and Gunter (8) and Moore and Cato (15) the principal end-products of carbohydrate metabolism in the acne group of organisms are acetic and propionic acids, and these organisms differ in a number of major ways from the classical corynebacteria as exemplified by C. diphtheriae. For example, cell walls of the acne group do not contain the arabino-galactan characteristic of the classical corynebacteria, and the diamino-acid of the peptidoglycan is (with very few exceptions) the L-isomer of diamino-pimelic acid (DAP) and not the meso-isomer. Also, they do not synthesise mycolic acids, and their cell lipids are characterized by a high proportion of branched-chain C_{15} fatty acids, as are found in the lipids of propionibacteria from cheese and dairy products.

For all of these reasons, these anaerobic diphtheroids seem to fit much better with Propionibacterium than with the classical corynebacteria such as _C_. diphtheriae, _C_. xerosis, _C_. pseudodiphtheriticum, etc. This is summarized in Table 1.

SEROLOGY AND CLASSIFICATION OF ANAEROBIC DIPHTHEROIDS

Serological investigations in this, as in other groups, have been intimately connected with classification, and so I propose to discuss the classification first and then relate the serological results to it.

Views on the classification of the group have varied from regarding all strains as belonging to one species, _C_. acnes, to having 12 named species whose separation depended on fermentation tests with various sugars, the production of indole, the liquefaction of gelatin and other biochemical parameters.

Table 1. Comparison of Anaerobic Coryneforms with Classical Corynebacteria

Characteristic	Anaerobic Coryneforms	Classical Corynebacteria
Relation to oxygen	Microaerophilic to anaerobic	aerobic
Presence of mycolic acids	-	+++
DAP isomer in cell walls	LL- (occ. DL-)	DL-
Presence of arabino-galactan	-	+++
Characteristic fatty acids in cell lipids	C15 branched	C14, C16, C18

The names of the 12 species (Table 2) will be found in the literature. However, it would not be easy to allocate strains to any of these species on the basis of published descriptions, and we believe, that the group has been over-speciated.

Classification of the group originated in a collaborative study by Johnson and Cummins (12) into homology relationships and cell wall composition in a group of strains which included many from Prévot's collection at the Institut Pasteur in Paris. Cell wall composition in these studies included an analysis of polysaccharide antigens extracted with trichloroacetic acid as well as the determination of cell wall sugar patterns.

As a result of these studies we were able to define three principal homology groups and five serological types (Table 3). It also became evident that strains in each homology group could be recognized by the application of a small number of physiological tests (Table 4). These facts seemed to support the idea of three species, Propionibacterium acnes, Propionibacterium avidum and Propionibacterium granulosum, with two serological types in P. acnes and two in P. avidum. I have already given the reason we considered Propionibacterium, rather than Corynebacterium, a suitable genus for these organisms. The separation of strains classified as acnes and granulosum had in fact already been suggested by Brzin (2) and Voss (20) who noted that indole negative strains were generally able to ferment disaccharides. The status of P. avidum strains was not so obvious, until the homology results were obtained. Recognition of P. avidum strains may have been delayed because, unlike the other two groups, they often grow quite well under aerobic conditions, and therefore may not have been considered as belonging to the acne group. In

Table 2. Named Species of Anaerobic Coryneforms

Corynebacterium anaerobium
Corynebacterium granulosum
Corynebacterium liquefaciens
Corynebacterium pyogenes
Corynebacterium lymphophilum
Corynebacterium hepatodystrophicans
Corynebacterium adamsoni
Corynebacterium parvum
Corynebacterium avidum
Corynebacterium diphtheroides
Corynebacterium renale cuniculi
Corynebacterium acnes

(from Prevot and Fredette, 1966)

Table 3. Homology Groups and Cell Wall Composition in Anaerobic Coryneforms

Organisms; Serotype		Cell Wall Components		DNA Homology % Homology to Reference Strains		
		Sugars	DAP	0389 (Acnes)	0575 (Avidum)	0507 (Granulosum)
P. acnes	type I	Galactose, glucose, mannose	LL-	97	51	16
	type II	Glucose, mannose	LL-, occ. meso-			
P. avidum	type I	Galactose, glucose, mannose	LL-	50	90	17
	type II	Glucose, mannose	LL-, occ. meso-			
P. granulosum		Galactose, mannose (occ. trace glucose)	LL	12	15	95

discussing the serology of the group, therefore, and the antigens responsible for it, I am going to assume the validity of the classification in Bergey's Manual, with three species: *P.* acnes, *P.* avidum and *P.* granulosum.

SEROLOGY OF THE ACNE GROUP

The acne bacillus was first described by Unna (19) as a rod-shaped organism in the lesions of acne vulgaris, and it was cultured a few years later by Sabouraud (18). However, not much attention was paid to the serology of the group until 1942, when Craddock (5) described two different serological types among 47 strains isolated from acne lesions. It seems likely that one of Craddock's types was *P.* avidum, since these strains formed large, yellowish colonies which were hemolytic, and the organisms fermented sucrose and maltose. However, the other type was also described as fermenting sucrose which would suggest that it was not *P.* acnes either. In any case, the two groups were very distinct serologically, since they did not cross-react by agglutination at a serum dilution of 1/10.

Table 4. Physiological Tests to Separate P. acnes, P. avidum and P. granulosum

Organism	Glucose	Sorbitol	Maltose	Sucrose	Esculin Hydrolysis	Indole Production	Gelatin Liquefaction	Nitrate Reduction
P. acnes I	+	+ or -	-	-	-	+	+	+
P. acnes II	+	-	-	-	-	+	+	+
P. avidum I	+	-	+	+	+	-	+	-
P. avidum II	+	-	+	+	+	-	+	-
P. granulosum	+	-	+	+	-	-	-	-

More detailed studies of the acne group of organisms were made by workers in France and Germany soon after World War II, probably because of the interest aroused at that time by the discovery of the reticulo-stimulatory abilities of some strains. This reticulo-stimulating power was especially associated with strains called Corynebacterium parvum, and we will return to the taxonomic position of C. parvum a little later.

Linzenmeier (13,14) published two papers on the serology of anaerobic coryneforms; most of the strains he studied were from the Institut Pasteur collection, but included other strains which were freshly isolated from clinical material. A large number of strains showed identical reactions with five sera (Table 5), and Linzenmeier concluded that "a large number of differently named strains are closely related to, if not identical with, C. acnes". It may also be noted that several strains labeled Actinomyces bovis or Actinomyces spp. fell into the same group. I will return to this point also a little later. Caille and Toucas (4) also examined a group of strains of anaerobic coryneforms, by the passive haemagglutination test. For the test they sensitized sheep RBC with antigens extracted from the bacteria by heating in a water bath at 100 C for 2 h. Like Linzenmeier, they found that strains of the various named species C. acnes, C. parvum, Corynebacterium avidum, Corynebacterium granulosum, Corynebacterium anaerobium and Corynebacterium liquefaciens cross reacted to a considerable extent. Two strains of Corynebacterium diphtheroides were quite distinct from the others, but two strains with these numbers in the Anaerobe Laboratory collection at VPI were identified as Ramibacterium (now Eubacterium) alactolyticum. One of these had been examined by Linzenmeier.

Table 5. Slide Agglutination of Various Anaerobic Diphtheroids with Unabsorbed Sera (From Linzenmeier, 1957)

Antigen From	Serum to: 595	379	714	961*	758*	889*	936B*	ATCC 6919*
Corynebacterium parvum 595	3+	-	-	-	-	-	-	-
C. diphtheroides 379	-	3+	-	-	-	-	-	-
C. diphtheroides 1035								
C. granulosum 714	-	-	3+	-	-	-	-	-
C. granulosum 10482/56	-	-	3+	-	-	-	-	-
C. avidum 735								
C. avidum 759								
C. avidum 760	-	-	-	3+	3+	3+	3+	3+
C. avidum 592								
C. anaerobium 678	-	-	-	3+	3+	3+	3+	3+
C. liquefaciens 889								
C. liquefaciens 2000	-	-	-	3+	3+	3+	3+	3+
C. liquefaciens 417								
C. parvum 936B								
C. parvum 643	-	-	-	3+	3+	3+	3+	3+
C. granulosum 583	-	-	-	3+	3+	3+	3+	3+
C. acnes Ger								
C. acnes Beck								
C. acnes 4 St.	-	-	-	3+	3+	3+	3+	3+
C. acnes P. Holm								
C. acnes 25 St.								
Corynebacterium spp. 7539								
Corynebacterium spp. 7772								
Corynebacterium spp. 562	-	-	-	3+	3+	3+	3+	3+
Corynebacterium spp. 563								
Actinomyces bovis AP1								
A. bovis 8373								
A. bovis 8374	-	-	-	3+	3+	3+	3+	3+
Actinomyces spp. A1								
Actinomyces spp. A5								

*961 = C. avidum; 758 = C. anaerobium; 889 = C. liquefaciens; 936B = C. parvum; ATCC 6919 = C. acnes.

A more recent study using agglutination is that of Hoeffler, Ko and Pulverer (9). In an earlier paper, Pulverer and Ko (17) had proposed eight biotypes divided among 11 serotypes. Hoeffler, Ko, and Pulverer (9) re-examined a group of 104 strains to correlate their previous results with the three species P. acnes, P. avidum and P. granulosum proposed in the eighth edition of Bergey's Manual. Using both tube and slide agglutination tests, they found an excellent correlation between their results and the classification of their strains according to the scheme proposed in Bergey's Manual. These results are summarized in Table 6, which is somewhat condensed from Table 2 in their paper.

The serological results described so far have all been obtained using agglutination tests with suspensions of intact bacteria, or in one case passive haemagglutination using RBC sensitized with soluble antigens liberated by boiling in saline. In our own work on the antigens of these strains we have used either cell wall agglutination tests or immunodiffusion tests with extracted antigens. The cell wall agglutination is generally in the form of large floccules which makes the test easy to read, and the cell wall fragments often give more stable suspension than whole cells, especially in this group where 5-10% of strains may be autoagglutinable. However, cell wall

Table 6. Tube Agglutination Tests with 104 Strains of Cutaneous Propionibacteria (from Hoeffler et al., 1977) Using Absorbed Antisera

Number of Strains	Titers with Antisera to:					
	P. acnes	P. granulosum		P. avidum		
	KB	D-34	95	0589(II)[a]	0575(I)[a]	31
56	320-640[b] (1 strain, 160)		(4 strains, 20)		(10 strains, 20)	
5		160-320				
6	(2 strains, 20)		320-640		(3 strains, 20)	
6		80-320	640			
11				320-640		
17					160-640	
4						320-640

[a] II and I indicate that the strains are P. avidum type II or P. avidum type I, respectively.

[b] Figures represent reciprocals of highest dilution giving agglutination.

fractions are somewhat tedious to prepare, and largely for this reason we investigated the use of immunodiffusion tests with extracted antigens.

POLYSACCHARIDE ANTIGENS OF THE ACNE GROUP

Like many other Gram-positive bacteria, the anaerobic coryneforms have cell wall polysaccharides which are antigenic, and can be extracted in various ways. We have found that 30 min extraction with 5% trichloroacetic acid at 56 C is a satisfactory procedure, although a number of other methods could be used. Soluble material from culture filtrates of the organisms has been employed, but this is probably a less desirable procedure since it represents an unknown mixture of various cell antigens, both protein and polysaccharide. The extraction procedure we have used is shown in Table 7.

When we apply this extraction method to strains representing the different serological types of P. acnes, P. avidum and P. granulosum, the results shown in Figs. 1-5 were obtained. The antisera used were prepared in rabbits as described previously (6) except that a partial disintegrate (a mixture of cell wall fragments and intact cells) was used for immunization. Most of the sera used were concentrated to some extent with Lyphogel (6). The extracts used in these preparations were prepared from purified cell wall fractions, but virtually identical results will be obtained using extracts of whole cells.

Table 7. Antigen Extraction Procedure

1. Extract cells with 5% Trichloroacetic acid at 56 C for 30 min (1-2 ml for growth from 10 ml culture).

2. Cool. Centrifuge. Add 5 vol acetone + 2 drops 5% potassium acetate to supernatant.

3. Keep at 4 C for several hours, or overnight.

4. Centrifuge; redissolve precipitate in 1 ml PBS*. Add 1 drop phenol red and adjust pH to 7.0 with diluted NaOH.

5. Centrifuge; use clear extract in immunodiffusion test.

PBS = phosphate buffered saline: 0.9% NaCl + 0.05 M phosphate buffer, pH 7.0

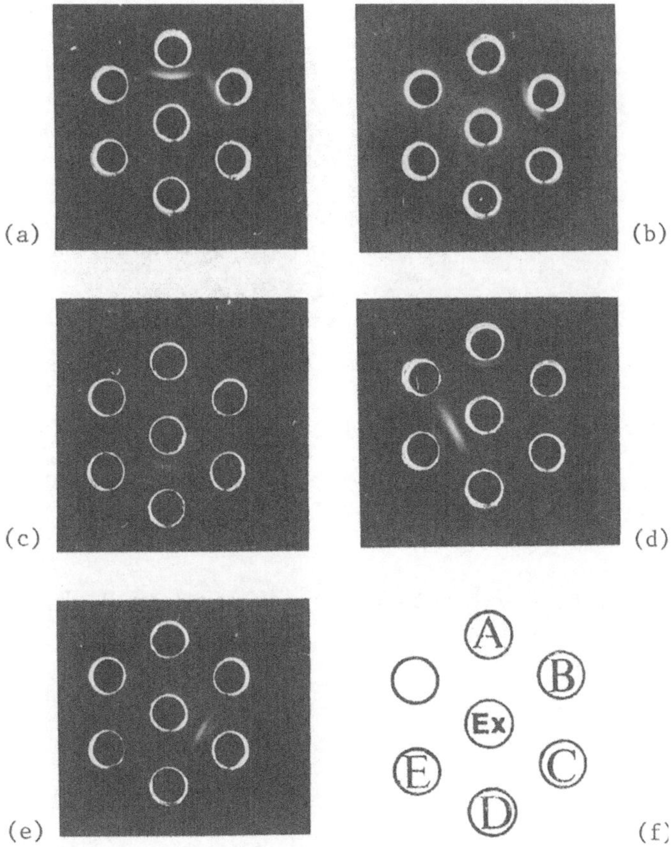

Fig. 1, a-f. Precipitin reactions of TCA extracts of P. acnes I and II, P. avidum I and II and P. granulosum with standard antisera (antigen extracts in center well, antisera in peripheral wells).

a) Extract of P. acnes type II.

b) Extract of P. acnes type I.

c) Extract of P. avidum type I.

d) Extract of P. avidum type II.

e) Extract of P. granulosum.

f) Location of sera. A = P. acnes II, B = P. acnes I, C = P. granulosum, D = P. avidum I, E = P. avidum II, Ex = Extract.

(a) 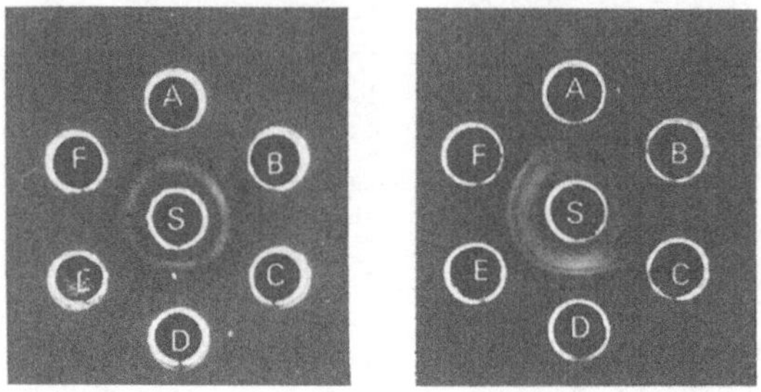 (b)

Fig. 2, a,b.

a) Extracts of P. acnes I & II strains against P. acnes I serum.

b) Extracts of P. acnes I & II strains against P. acnes II serum.

S = Serum; A, B, C extracts of type I strains; D, E, F extracts of type II strains.

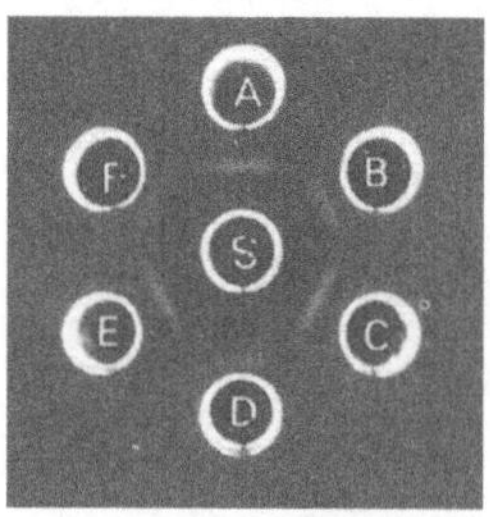

Fig. 3. Extracts of six P. avidum type I strains against P. avidum 0575 serum (type I).

S = Serum; A, B, C, D, E, F = extracts.

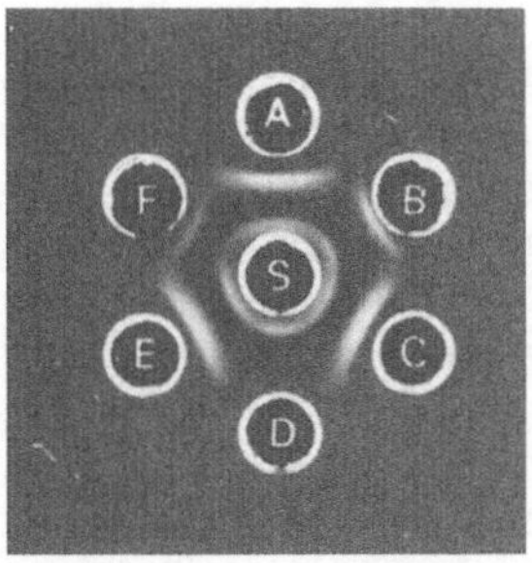

Fig. 4. Extracts of six P. avidum type II strains against P. avidum 0589 serum (type II).

S = Serum; A, B, C, D, E, F = extracts

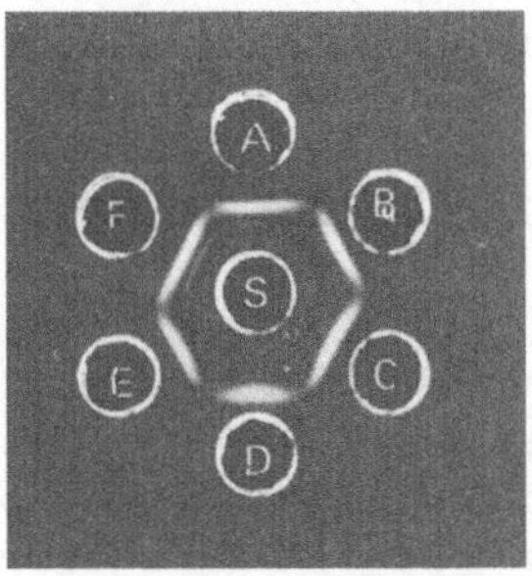

Fig. 5. Extracts of six P. granulosum strains against P. granulosum 0507 serum.

S = Serum; A, B, C, D, E, F = extracts.

One of the main points to note in these results is the marked cross-reaction between extracts of strains of P. acnes I and II and P. acnes antisera. This is more obvious with type II extracts than with type I (Fig. 1, a and b). Despite this cross-reaction, however, it is still easy to distinguish P. acnes I and P. acnes II, even with unabsorbed sera.

Cross-reaction is usually also found between extracts of P. avidum type II and P. acnes type II (Fig. 1, d). Extracts of P. avidum II strains generally show two lines against P. avidum II serum (Fig. 1, d and Fig. 4), however some strains (e.g. strain D in Fig. 4) obviously lack one of these antigens.

FLUORESCENT ANTIBODY TECHNIQUES

With suitable antisera one can get brilliant immunofluorescence of members of the acne group by either the direct or indirect techniques, and the major advantage of the method is, of course, that one can pick out individual organisms in clinical material. The method has been used successfully by Holmberg and Forsum (10). With suitable absorbed antisera they were able easily to separate P. acnes types I and II.

From a comparison of the results obtained by various techniques we may conclude that all of them essentially detect the same antigenic material, that is, the cell wall polysaccharides. Our own experience has been largely with immunodiffusion tests, and the results illustrated in Figs. 1-5 show that even with unabsorbed sera each group of strains gives a characteristic pattern of reactions. Other techniques could be used to clearly distinguish the serogroups, especially if absorbed sera were used.

In conclusion we may mention three aspects of the subject where serology has been of value.

ANAEROBIC DIPHTHEROIDS AS CULTURE CONTAMINANTS

Anaerobic coryneforms, especially P. acnes, are common contaminants of anaerobic cultures (12; Cummins, unpublished observations). This had been noted previously by Beerens (1) and Linzenmeier (13, 14). The situation becomes even more confusing when cultures of P. acnes become mixed with P. acnes of a different serological type, or with P. granulosum, and mixtures of this kind may have led to confused identifications in the past.

A further example of this problem is illustrated in Table 8, which shows what may happen to a strain over the years as it is repeatedly subcultured in different laboratories. It must be stated emphatically, of course, that this problem is in no way the fault of the American Type Culture Collection. It may be noted that Werner and Mann (21) found two different colony types in their subculture of ATCC 11829, and when the two organisms were separated they had quite different properties: from their results, one was P. granulosum (indole and gelatin $-^{ve}$; saccharose $+^{ve}$) while the other was P. acnes (indole and gelatin $+^{ve}$; saccharose $-^{ve}$). In these situations, serological tests can be very useful.

THE STATUS OF CORYNEBACTERIUM PARVUM

Strains bearing this designation have reticulo-stimulatory properties, and vaccines made from them are at present under test as immuno-stimulants in cancer therapy. We have examined many strains

Table 8. Comparison of Various Subcultures of ATCC 11829

	Cell Wall Sugars			Serological
	Galactose	Glucose	Mannose	Identification
VPI 0210	-	+	+	P. acnes II
NCTC 10387	++	±	+	P. granulosum
C. parvum A	+	+	+	P. acnes I
C. parvum B	-	+	+	P. acnes II
C. parvum C	+	trace	±	P. granulosum

Results taken from Cummins and Johnson (1974). J. Gen. Microbiol. 80: 433.

of C. parvum and have found that 90% of them are P. acnes, and the remainder, P. avidum. The name C. parvum is very firmly established in the immunological literature, and seems unlikely to be replaced for some time. It may be worth while pointing out therefore that the C. parvum vaccine commonly used in the United States and in England is made from a strain of P. acnes type I but that a similarly prepared vaccine commonly used in France is made from a strain of P. avidum type I (7). Both are referred to as "C. parvum" vaccines. Elsewhere in the literature there are references to "C. granulosum" vaccine, but these strains are also P. acnes and in fact vaccines made from strains of P. granulosum as defined earlier (12) are essentially negative as far as reticulo-stimulation is concerned.

The confusion as to which type of strain is being referred to when the designation C. parvum is used illustrates how important it is to examine these strains carefully by all available techniques.

ANTIBODIES TO P. ACNES IN MAN

It should not be forgotten that most healthy adults have a moderate to high titer of antibodies to P. acnes especially if they have acne. For example Puhvel (16) found that the average titer in acne patients was 1:320 - 1:640, while in controls the range was 1:40 - 1:80.

Antibody levels to P. acnes have become of some interest because of the use of vaccines in cancer therapy, and the results in Table 9 and Fig. 6 illustrate the range of titers that have been found in

Table 9. Antibody to C. parvum: Titration of Normal Human Sera

C. parvum Titer	No. of Sera (% of Total)	Adult Sera[a] (% of Adults)
1:8	11 (3.5)	0 (0)
1:16	30 (9.7)	1 (0.6)
1:32	33 (10.7)	8 (5.2)
1:64	56 (18.1)	17 (11.2)
1:128	58 (18.7)	24 (15.8)
1:256	37 (11.9)	21 (13.8)
1:512	41 (13.2)	38 (25.0)
1:1,024	23 (7.4)	22 (14.5)
1:2,048	14 (4.5)	14 (9.2)
1:4,096	5 (1.6)	5 (3.2)
1:8,192	2 (0.6)	2 (1.3)

[a]18 to 50 years of age.
(from Wolberg et al., 1977, Inf. Imm. 15: 1004)

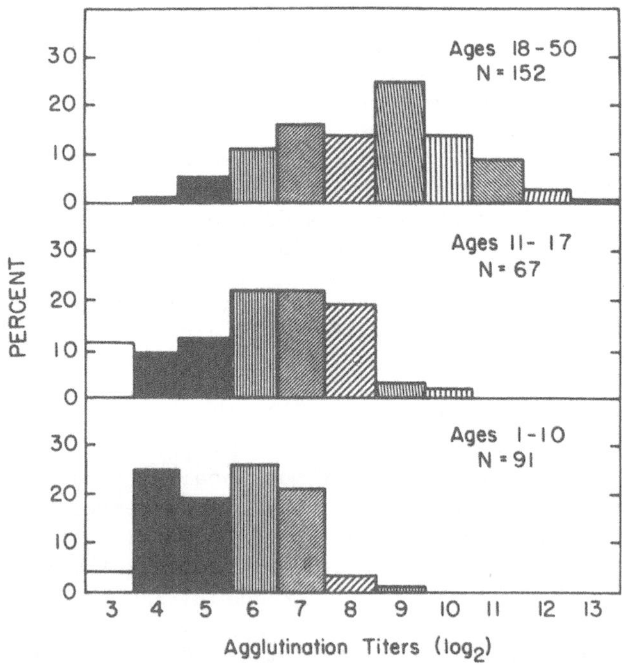

Fig. 6. Anti- C. parvum (= P. acnes I) agglutination titers of 310 normal human sera (from Wolberg et al. 1977).

normal persons of various ages in a study by Wolberg et al. (22). The C. parvum strain used to assay antibody levels is P. acnes type I according to our designation. In Fig. 1 one can see the quite marked rise in mean titer that occurs with increasing age.

Finally, Fig. 7 shows that the use of C. parvum (P. acnes) vaccines in man is associated, as one might expect, with a considerable increase in antibody levels during treatment with these vaccines. The IgG levels showed a consistent increase in these patients, but the effect on the levels of IgA, IgM and IgE was variable (11).

SUMMARY

The serology of the cutaneous propionibacteria based on cell wall polysaccharide antigens has been presented against the background of their relationships as shown by DNA homology tests. For this group of organisms, the two sets of results agree very well. It seems likely that cell wall antigens can form a satisfactory basis for classification in many Gram-positive bacteria, especially when combined with the groups which emerge from a study of DNA homology relationships.

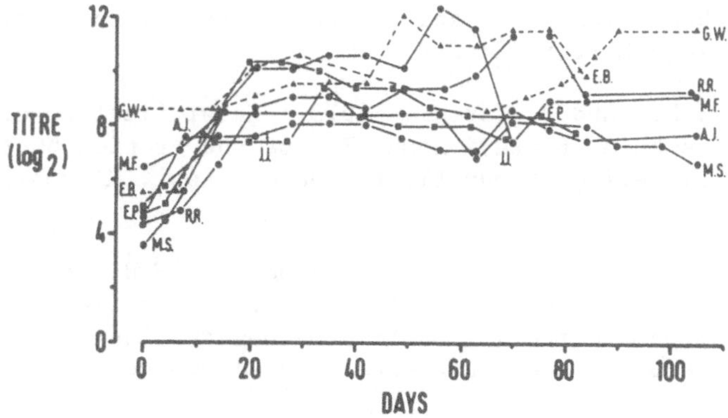

Fig. 7. Antibody response in man to multiple injections of C. parvum (= P. acnes I) (from James et al., 1975). ●-●-● Melanoma; ▲—▲ breast cancer; ■-■-■ stomach cancer.

LITERATURE CITED

1. Beerens, H. 1953. Étude comparative de six souches de bactéries anaérobies non-sporuleés. Ann. Inst. Pasteur 84: 1026-1032.

2. Brzin, B. 1964. Studies on the Corynebacterium acnes. Acta Pathologica et Microbiologica Scandanavica 60: 599-608.

3. Buchanan, R.E., and N.E. Gibbons. 1974. Bergey's Manual of Determinative Bacteriology, Eighth Edition. Williams and Wilkins, Baltimore. pp. 633-641.

4. Caille, B., and M. Toucas. 1960. Étude antigenique de Corynebacterium acnes par l'épreuve d'hemagglutination passive. Ann. Inst. Pasteur 98: 276-281.

5. Craddock, S. 1942. Use of penicillin in cultivation of the acne bacillus. Lancet i, pp. 558-559.

6. Cummins, C.S. 1975. Identification of Propionibacterium acnes and related organisms by precipitin tests with trichloroacetic acid extracts. J. Clin. Microbiol. 2: 104-110.

7. Cummins, C.S., and D.M. Linn. 1977. Reticulostimulating properties of killed vaccines of anaerobic coryneforms and other organisms. J. Natl. Cancer Inst. 59: 1697-1708.

8. Douglas, H.C., and S.E. Gunter. 1946. The taxonomic position of Corynebacterium acnes. J. Bacteriol. 52: 15-23.

9. Hoeffler, U., H.L. Ko, and G. Pulverer. 1977. Serotyping of Propionibacterium acnes and related microbial species. FEMS Microbiology Letters 2: 5-9.

10. Holmberg, K., and U. Forsum. 1973. Identification of Actinomyces, Arachnia, Bacterionema, Rothia and Propionibacterium species by defined immunofluorescence. Appl. Microbiol. 25: 834-843.

11. James, K., G.J.A. Clunie, M.F.A. Woodruff, W.H. McBride, W.H. Stimson, R. Drew, and D. Catty. 1975. The effect of Corynebacterium parvum therapy on immunoglobulin class and IgG subclass levels in cancer patients. Br. J. Cancer 32: 310-322.

12. Johnson, J.L., and C.S. Cummins. 1972. Cell wall composition and deoxyribonucleic acid similarities among the anaerobic coryneforms, classical propionibacteria and strains of Arachnia propionica. J. Bacteriol. 109: 1047-1066.

13. Linzenmeier, G. 1954. Étude serologique des corynebactéries anaérobies par la methode des agglutinins. Ann. Inst. Pasteur 87: 572.

14. Linzenmeier, G. 1957. Serologie anaerober Corynebakterien. II. Mitteilung: Serologie and pathogentische Bedeutung von Corynebacterium acnes. Zentralbl. Bakteriol. Parasitenk. Infekt. Hyg. Abt. I. Orig. 170: 85-90.

15. Moore, W.E.C., and E.P. Cato. 1963. Validity of Propionibacterium acnes (Gilchrist) Douglas and Gunter comb. nov. J. Bacteriol. 85: 870-974.

16. Puhvel, S.M., I.K. Hoffman, R.M. Reisner, and T.H. Steinberg. 1967. Dermal hypersensitivity of patients with acne vulgaris to Corynebacterium acnes. J. Invest. Dermatol. 49: 154-158.

17. Pulverer, G., and H.L. Ko. 1973. Fermentative and serological studies on Propionibacterium acnes. Appl. Microbiol. 25: 222-229.

18. Sabouraud, R. 1897. La seborhée grasse et la pelade. Ann. Inst. Pasteur 11: 134-159. Quoted by Douglas and Gunter (1946).

19. Unna, P.G. 1891. Cited in Bergey's Manual, 7th Ed.

20. Voss, J.G. 1970. Differentiation of two groups of Corynebacterium acnes. J. Bacteriol. 101: 392-397.

21. Werner, H., and S. Mann. 1968. Chemische analyse der Zellwand von Corynebacterium acnes and C. parvum. Zentralbl. Bakteriol. Parasitenk. Infektionskr. Hyg. Abt. I. Orig. 206: 286-299.

22. Wolberg, G., G.S. Duncan, C. Adlam, and J.K. Whisnant. 1977. Antibody to Corynebacterium parvum in normal human and animal sera. Infect. Immun. 15: 1004-1007.

IMMUNE RESPONSE: TO ANAEROBIC BACTERIA CAUSING SEPTICEMIA AND TO ANAEROBIC COCCI

Dwight W. Lambe, Jr. Ph.D.

Professor and Chairman
Department of Microbiology, College of Medicine
East Tennessee State University
Johnson City, Tennessee 37601

INTRODUCTION

Anaerobic bacteremia may be caused by a variety of anaerobic bacteria. The organisms which we have isolated from blood cultures over a 10 year period from 1968-1978, at Emory University Hospital in Atlanta, Georgia and at New England Deaconess Hospital in Boston, Massachusetts include: Bacteroides fragilis, Bacteroides thetaiotaomicron, Bacteroides melaninogenicus, Fusobacterium nucleatum, Fusobacterium necrophorum, Fusobacterium varium, Clostridium perfringens, Clostridium septicum, Eubacterium lentum, Eubacterium cylindroides, Eubacterium saburreum, Propionibacterium acnes, Peptococcus magnus, Peptococcus prevotii, Peptococcus asaccharolyticus, Peptostreptococcus anaerobius, Streptococcus constellatus, Streptococcus intermedius, and Streptococcus morbillorum. Other laboratories have reported some of these same species from blood cultures in addition to other species. Wilson et al. (31) reported Eubacterium alactolyticum, Bifidobacterium species, Bacteroides oralis, Bacteroides terebrans, and Clostridium paraputrificum from blood cultures.

Some blood specimens contain two or more anaerobic species. We have especially noticed the combination of B. fragilis and E. lentum in multiple blood cultures; the true significance of this combination of anaerobes, although interesting, is unknown.

In 1974, Chow and Guze (4) summarized three years experience of 112 patients with Bacteroidaceae bacteremia. Bacteroides and Fusobacterium accounted for 9.3% of all positive blood cultures in this period and these organisms were a more important cause of sepsis than had been recognized previously. Overall mortality in non-obstetrical patients was 43%. Underlying disease was the most common determinant of mortality, although age, sex, and prior history of trauma or surgery were the most significant factors in patients with non-fatal underlying disease.

In general, the most common portal of entry into the blood appears to be the gastrointestinal tract followed by the female genital tract, decubital ulcers or gangrene. The portals of entry for anaerobes which infect heart valves are the mouth (especially in cases of periodontal disease and tooth extraction), and to a lesser extent, the gastrointestinal and genitourinary tracts. The most commonly isolated organisms in endocarditis are microaerophilic and anaerobic cocci, with B. fragilis, Fusobacterium and Clostridium found less commonly.

The common clinical features of anaerobic bacteremia include: fever, leucocytosis, chills, diaphoresis and often jaundice. Other symptoms may include: thrombophlebitis, thromboembolism, shock and disseminated intravascular coagulation (4).

IMMUNE RESPONSE TO ANAEROBIC BACTEREMIA

With this background of anaerobic septicemia, let us now consider the immune response to anaerobic infection. The human immune response to a particular infectious agent is a normal host defense reaction to invading microorganisms, and the demonstration of such a response provides evidence for the clinical and pathogenic significance of anaerobic organisms in human disease. In addition, the production of antibody may be used to detect infection or to aid in the prognosis of an infectious disease.

A summary of the investigators who have published work on the human immune response to infection with the Bacteroidaceae from 1939 to 1980 is shown in Table 1. In 1970, we (6) began our work on the patient's immune response to anaerobic infection. The first patient we investigated was a patient in Sweden with Crohn's disease and a perirectal abscess. We showed a significant immune response to strains of B. fragilis and Clostridium difficile that were isolated from this patient.

Immune Response in Seven Patients with Anaerobic Septicemia

From 1970-1972, we (7) studied seven patients with anaerobic septicemia due to the following anaerobes: F. necrophorum (one patient), B. fragilis (five patients), and a combination of B. fragilis and P. asaccharolyticus (one patient). The serological results of the patient with F. necrophorum septicemia are summarized in Table 2. The antigen used in these tests was the patient's strain of F. necrophorum. The patient's first two serum specimens were negative with both passive hemagglutination (PHA) and agar gel diffusion (AGD), but the indirect immunofluorescent (IFL) test showed

Table 1. Human Immune Response to Infection With Bacteroidaceae

1939	Laporte and Brochard
1967	Courant, Gibbons
1969	Kristoffersen
1970	Kristoffersen, Hofstad
1971	Monteiro, Fossey, Shiver, Draser, Allison
1972	Quick, Goldberg, Sonnenwirth
1972	Danielsson, Lambe, Persson
1974	Danielsson, Lambe, Persson
1974	Rissing, Crowder, Smith, White
1975	Lambe, Danielsson, Vroon, Carver
1978	Schwan, Ryden
1980	Danielsson and Lambe

a four-fold increase in titer. In specimens obtained three and four weeks after symptoms appeared, both the PHA and indirect IFL titers showed four-fold, or greater, increases in titer, and one or two precipitin bands were formed in AGD. At 21 weeks, the immune response was still noted except by PHA. The patient's sera also gave positive results with a laboratory strain of F. necrophorum indicating that these two strains shared common antigens. Serum specimens collected from 10 blood donors gave negative or low titers in PHA and indirect IFL tests ($\leq$10, one was 20-40) and no precipitin bands were formed.

Table 2. Immune Response in a Patient with Fusobacterium necrophorum Septicemia Measured by Passive Hemagglutination (PHA), Indirect Immunofluorescence (IFL), and Agar Gel Diffusion (AGD)

Serum Specimens Collected after Symptoms Appeared	Patient's Strain of F. necrophorum		
	HA	IFL	AGD
7 days	10[a]	10	0[b]
10 days	10	40	0
3 weeks	320	320	2
4 weeks	320	320	1
21 weeks	10	40	1

[a] Reciprocal titer.

[b] Number of precipitin bands.

In 1939, Laporte and Brocard (20) detected flocculating antibody to F. necrophorum in six patients with septicemia, but they did not detect antibody to this organism in normal individuals.

Our patient with B. thetaiotaomicron septicemia showed a tube agglutination titer of up to 1:80 and precipitin bands by AGD with the patient's strain of B. thetaiotaomicron. No precipitin bands by AGD and tube agglutination titers no higher than 1:20 were found when this patient's sera were tested with four strains of B. fragilis.

The five patients with B. fragilis septicemia also showed an immune response with homologous strains. The tube agglutination titers varied from 1:40 to 1:160 depending upon time of serum collection, and from 1 to 4 precipitin bands were formed by AGD. Again, the 10 blood donors that served as controls usually showed tube agglutination titers of ≤1:10; titers of the control sera never exceeded 1:20.

Immune Response in Eight Patients with Bacteroides Septicemia or Pyothorax

In 1975, we (19) published another human immune response study on eight patients: seven of these patients had septicemia and one patient had pyothorax. Six of the seven cases of septicemia were B. fragilis and the other was B. thetaiotaomicron. The serologic tests used to study the immune response included: tube agglutination, indirect IFL, and AGD. All patients' sera were positive, 1:40 to 1:160, by tube agglutination and indirect IFL. All patients' sera formed one or more precipitin bands with homologous strains by AGD. Two to four-fold increases in titer seen in the agglutination test were also seen in the indirect FA test, indicating that twofold changes, or higher, with these testing procedures represented true changes in antibody based on reproducibility.

Agglutinating and indirect IFL antibody titers in the normal human adults included in our study were usually 1:10 and never exceeded 1:10, whereas antibody titers measured by these two procedures in infected patients varied from 1:10 to 1:320. No precipitating antibodies were detected in these normal people, but precipitating antibody was demonstrated in all infected patients.

In our study there was an interesting association between antibiotic therapy and anaerobic infection in certain cases. Three patients with B. fragilis septicemia emerged during cephalothin therapy; two of these cases were associated with postoperative wound infections. The isolates of B. fragilis from each of these three cases showed in vitro resistance to cephalothin. Superinfection by the Bacteroides group after chemotherapy with such agents as neomycin and kanamycin has been previously noted by Finegold (9).

The four patients in our study with septicemia who received chloramphenicol survived the infection, whereas two of the remaining three patients who were treated with chemotherapeutic agents such as cephalothin, kanamycin, gentamicin, and/or ampicillin died of septicemia.

Septicemia occurred in five patients with chronic debilitating disease, including three with malignancy. There were only two cases of B. fragilis septicemia in the absence of chronic disease.

The immune response that we demonstrated in this study was detected in as little as five days and persisted for as long as 130 days. This shows the serological potential as a diagnostic aid for Bacteroides septicemia.

Rissing et al. (25) demonstrated precipitins to B. fragilis in 50% of 12 patients with bacteremia whereas we showed precipitins in 100% of our patients.

The immune response in patients infected with certain anaerobic bacteria, as well as in normal adults, has been investigated by certain other immunological techniques. For example, Quick et al. (24) demonstrated antibody titers of 1:4 to B. fragilis, F. nucleatum, and Fusobacterium mortiferum in normal subjects by the sensitive PHA procedure. Antibodies to the same three antigens were also detected in maternal or cord serum. Three patients infected with anaerobic Gram-negative bacilli showed elevated titers to antigens of B. fragilis and Fusobacterium.

CROSSED IMMUNOELECTROPHORESIS (CIE)

CIE with intermediate gel has been reported previously as a useful technique for the serodiagnosis of candidiasis (1,28), Pseudonas aeruginosa (11), actinomycosis (13) and Mycobacterium leprae infections (3). We have, therefore, evaluated CIE with intermediate gel as a diagnosis of B. fragilis septicemia. These findings are preliminary since only one case was investigated; however, the results seemed worthy of report. In 1975 at Emory University Hospital in Atlanta, Georgia, we had a Caucasian male who was admitted to the hospital with a diagnosis of tumor of the colon. He developed peritonitis and septicemia following removal of the colonic tumor. Blood cultures and a specimen from the abdominal wound yielded pure cultures of B. fragilis.

Bacterial Strains

The bacterial isolates used for the preparation of standard antigens and antisera were B. fragilis (337-75) isolated from a blood culture and B. fragilis (338-75) isolated from an abdominal wound.

These organisms were identified according to the methods of Holdeman, Cato, and Moore (12).

Serum Specimens

Serum specimens were collected from the patient two days after the onset of fever (acute serum), eight days after onset of fever, and 25 days after onset of fever. Merthiolate was added to the serum specimens in a final concentration of 1:5000. The sera were stored at -65 C until tested.

Preparation of Antisera

B. fragilis strains 337-75 and 338-75 were used as antigens for the preparation of antisera. Each strain was grown on brain heart infusion agar (BHIA), supplemented with 5% sheep blood, 0.5% yeast extract, 0.0005% hemin, and 0.00005% Vitamin K_1. The BHIA plates were incubated for 48 h at 37 C in an anaerobe chamber (Coy Manufacturing Co., Ann Arbor, Michigan) in an atmosphere of 80% N_2, 10% CO_2, and 10% H_2 (Matheson Gas Co., Atlanta, Ga.). Vaccines containing approximately 2 x 10^9 cells/ml were prepared from these cultures according to the method of Lambe (16). Albino New Zealand rabbits were bled prior to immunization and immunized following the schedule of Lambe (16). The rabbits were bled one week after the last injection. Merthiolate was added to the sera in a final concentration of 1:5000. The sera were stored at -65 C. The preimmunization rabbit sera, the immune rabbit sera, and the patient's sera were titered by the agglutination test following the protocol of Lambe (16).

Preparation of Globulin

Hyperimmune rabbit sera with equivalent agglutination titers were pooled. The globulin fraction of the pooled antisera was obtained by precipitation with an equal volume of 70% saturated ammonium sulfate according to the procedure of Hebert et al. (10). The protein content of the globulin preparation was determined by the method of Lowry et al. (21) and was adjusted to a final concentration of 20 mg/ml by dialysis against polyethylene glycol (molecular weight, 15,000-20,000, Matheson, Coleman, and Bell, Manufacturing Chemist, Norwood, Ohio).

Preparation of Cytoplasmic Antigens

Cytoplasmic antigens were prepared from 48 h cultures of *B.* fragilis strains 337-75 and 338-75 grown on supplemented BHIA at 37 C in the anaerobe chamber. The cells were harvested with sterile physiological saline (PSS), washed three times with PSS, and stored at -65 C until needed. The cytoplasmic antigens were prepared from the washed cells by sonication. After centrifugation at 1500 x g for 30 min at 4 C, the cell debris was discarded and the supernatant fluid containing the cytoplasmic antigens was centrifuged for 60 min at 105, 000 x g at 4 C in the Beckman L2-65B ultracentrifuge.

Cytoplasmic antigens for 337-75 and 338-75 were a suspension of sonicated cells grown at one time on the culture medium; these are called a single sonicate. A pool of six suspensions of sonicated cells grown on six different occasions are called a pooled sonicate; a pooled sonicate was studied for 338-75 only.

Crossed Immunoelectrophoresis Procedure

Crossed immunoelectrophoresis (CIE) was performed as described by Weeke (30). Tris (hydroxymethyl) aminomethane-barbital buffer, ionic strength 0.02, pH 8.6 was used. Electrophoresis was performed with either a Behring Diagnostic electrophoresis chamber and an LKB 3371 E DC power supply or an LKB 2117 multiphor electrophoresis chamber and a Buchler voltage and current regulated power supply. A 5 ul quantity of cytoplasmic antigen solution containing either 1.5 mg/ml, 3 mg/ml or 6 mg/ml was electrophoresed in the first dimension with 10 V/cm for 35 min. In the second dimension, electrophoresis was performed with 1-2 V/cm overnight. After electrophoresis in the second dimension, the slides were rinsed, dried, and stained according to the procedure of Weeke (30).

CIE Antigen-Antibody Reference Systems

Antigen-antibody reference systems for B. fragilis 337-75 and B. fragilis 338-75 were developed using cytoplasmic antigens prepared from a single sonicate of 337-75 or 338-75, and specific rabbit antiserum to either 337-75 or 338-75. A 338-75 reference system using a pooled sonicate was investigated also. The optimal antigen concentration for 337-75 was 3 mg/ml and the optimal globulin concentration was 5 ul/cm^2. This 337-75 reference system produced six precipitates, labeled rockets 1,2,3,4,5 and 6 plus what appeared as a single band of precipitates labeled area A (Fig. 1). The 338-75 reference system was developed with an optimal antigen concentration of 3 mg/ml and a globulin concentration of 5 ul/cm^2. This 338-75 reference system produced four precipitates, labeled rockets 2,3,4,5 plus area A (Fig. 2). The 338-75 reference system with the pooled sonicates of six batches of cells produced seven precipitates labeled rockets 2,3,4,5,6,7, and 8 plus area A (Fig. 3). The appearance of more rockets with the pool of six sonicates as compared to fewer rockets with a single sonicate agreed with the report of investigators of another reference system (14). These results are summarized in Table 3.

CIE with Patient's Serum in the Intermediate Gel

CIE with intermediate gel described by Axelsen (1,2) was used to detect antibodies to B. fragilis in the three serum specimens of the

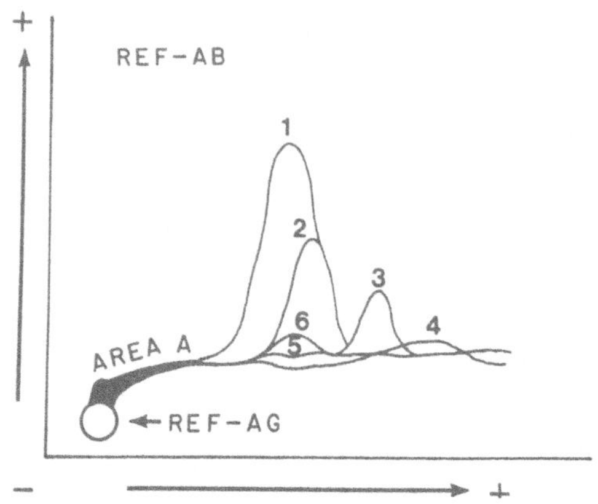

Fig. 1. Schematic drawing of crossed immunoelectrophoresis of the 337-75 reference system. The reference antigen (REF-AG), a single sonicate of 337-75, was electrophoresed in the horizontal direction. The reference antibody (REF-AB), rabbit anti-337-75, was added before electrophoresis in the vertical direction.

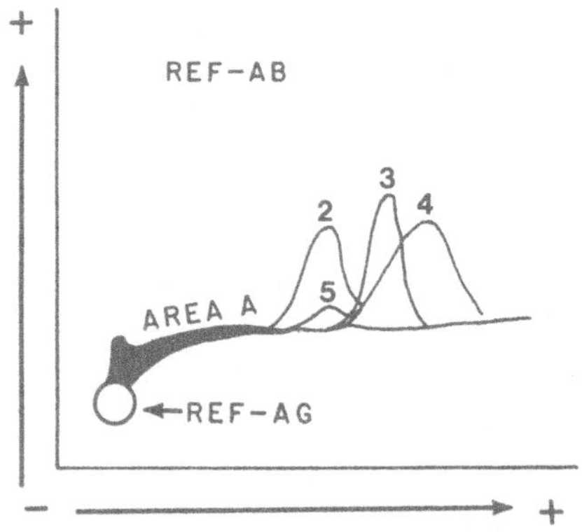

Fig. 2. Schematic drawing of crossed immunoelectrophoresis of the 338-75 reference system. The reference antigen (REF-AG), a single sonicate of 338-75, was electrophoresed in the horizontal direction. The reference antibody (REF-AB), rabbit anti-338-75, was added before electrophoresis in the vertical direction.

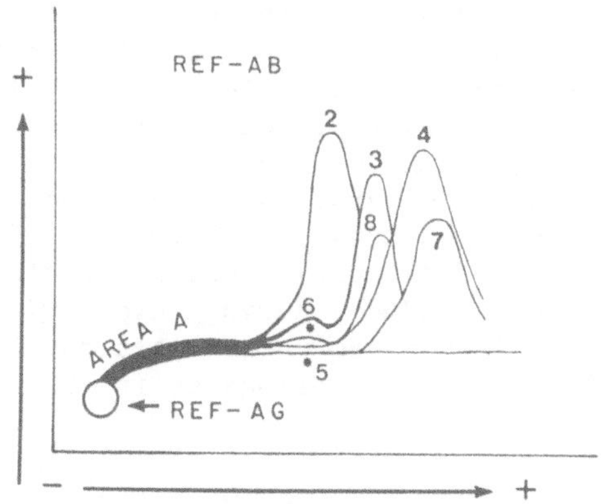

Fig. 3. Schematic drawing of crossed immunoelectrophoresis of the 338-75 reference system. The reference antigen (REF-AG), a pool of six sonicates of 338-75, was electrophoresed in the horizontal direction. The reference antibody (REF-AB), rabbit anti-338-75, was added before electrophoresis in the vertical direction.

patient. The intermediate gel contained 100 ul of the patient's serum. First and second dimensional electrophoreses were run as described for CIE. The 337-75 reference system which was run with a single sonicated antigen and an intermediate gel showed one precipitate, rocket 4, with the acute serum, three precipitates, rockets 2,

Table 3. Reference Systems of *B.* fragilis (337-75) and *B.* fragilis (338-75) with Homologous Rabbit Antiserum. Comparison of Single and Pooled Sonicates

Number of Antigens		
337-75 (Single Sonicate)	338-75 (Single Sonicate)	338-75 (6 Pooled Sonicates)
1		
2	2	2
3	3	3
4	4	4
5	5	5
6		6
		7
		8
(Area A)	(Area A)	(Area A)

4 and 5, with the eight day serum, and three precipitates, rockets 2, 4 and 5 with the 25 day serum (Table 4). The 338-75 reference system with a single sonicated antigen and an intermediate gel showed a total of five precipitates, rockets 2,4,6,9, and 10, in the patient's three serum samples (Table 5). An example of rockets formed in the intermediate gel containing patient's serum is illustrated in Fig. 4. Thus, the patient produced antibodies 2,4,5,6,9, and 10 to the two B. fragilis isolates over a 25 day period after infection. Antibodies 1,3,7, and 8 were not produced during this period. Antibodies 9 and 10 emerged from area A when the patient's serum was used, although antibodies 9 and 10 were not delineated in the reference systems.

Tandem CIE

The results obtained with CIE of the reference antigen-antibody systems and with CIE of the patient's sera in an intermediate gel suggested antigenic difference between B. fragilis strains 337-75 and 338-75. Therefore, tandem CIE described by Kroll (15) was used to compare the precipitates of these two cytoplasmic sonicates. The cytoplasmic antigens were placed in the wells and allowed to absorb into the agar. After absorption was complete the wells were filled with molten agarose. The first and second dimensional electrophoreses were run as described for CIE. There were two precipitates of identity and two precipitates of non-identity when these two cytoplasmic antigens were tested against anti-337-75 globulin. There were also two precipitates of identity and one precipitate of non-identity when these two antigens were tested against anti-338-75 globulin.

Table 4. B. fragilis 337-75 Reference System With Patient Serum in Intermediate Gel

Reference System 337-75 Antigen (Single Sonicate)	Patient Serum 2 day (acute)	8 day	25 day
1			
2		2	2
3			
4	4	4	4
5		5	5
6			
Area A			

Table 5. *B. fragilis* 338-75 Reference System With Patient Serum in Intermediate Gel

Reference System 338-75 Antigen (Single Sonicate)	Patient Serum 2 day (acute)	8 day	25 day
2		2	2
3			
4	4	4	4
5			
	6		
Area A	9		9
	10	10	10

CIE with Intermediate Gel with Rabbit Globulin

The results obtained in tandem CIE for the comparison of antigens was confirmed with CIE by intermediate gel for comparison of the antisera. Anti-337-75 globulin in the intermediate gel retained all the precipitates of the 338-75 reference system. However, with anti-338-75 globulin in the intermediate gel, precipitate number 1 of the 337-75 reference system was not retained in the intermediate gel.

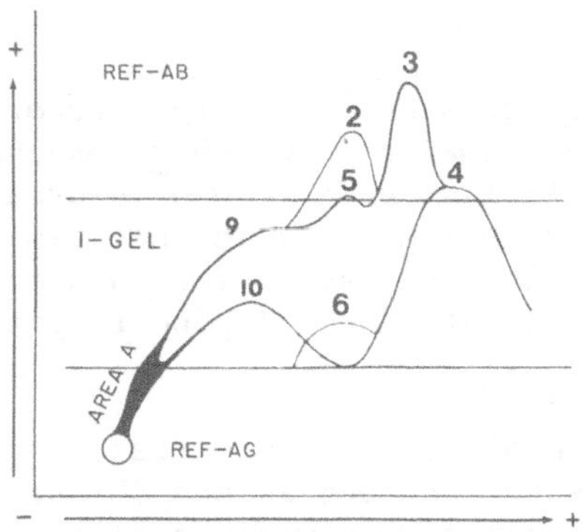

Fig. 4. Schematic drawing of crossed immunoelectrophoresis of the 338-75 reference system with the patient's acute serum in the intermediate gel. The reference antigen (REF-AG), a single sonicate of 338-75, was electrophoresed in the horizontal direction. The patient's acute serum was placed in the intermediate gel (I-GEL) and the reference antibody, rabbit anti-338-75, was placed in the area marked REF-AB.

Discussion of CIE

CIE with intermediate gel provided a sensitive method for detecting antibodies to *B. fragilis*. An antibody response was detected as early as two days after the onset of fever; this is the first report of detection of antibodies to *B. fragilis* within two days after onset of fever in a case of septicemia. CIE with intermediate gel may prove a rapid diagnosis since the best anaerobic culture methods currently used may require several days or longer to isolate and identify *B. fragilis*.

These preliminary CIE results indicate that it may be necessary to use either a polyvalent antigen or a polyvalent antiserum for the *B. fragilis* reference system. These polyvalent reagents should include all of the antigens of *B. fragilis* (17).

IMMUNE RESPONSE TO ANAEROBIC COCCI

Little information is available on the immune response to anaerobic coccal infection. The anaerobic cocci have been frequently implicated in a wide range of infections which we reported in 1974 (18). These infections ranged from simple, benign skin infections to more severe diseases such as deep cavity abscesses, osteomyelitis, and septicemia. In the last few years, hip replacement has become more common and anaerobic infection has been a complication. Too often these cultures yield no growth. In 1977, Evanski et al. (8) reported 387 operations which yielded nine infections, three of which were Peptococcus species. Nelson (23) reported 16 cases of deep sepsis after total hip replacement and described peptococci in three instances.

Taylor et al. (29) from London in 1979 reported two cases of infected total hip replacements in which *P. magnus* was isolated in pure culture from the implant when it was removed. It was estimated that more than 50,000 organisms were isolated in the broth after washing the prosthesis in each case. The indirect FA test and the ELISA method were used to study the immune response in these two cases.

Serum samples from 91 blood donors tested against the *P. magnus* isolates were negative by indirect FA and ELISA. Serum samples taken from both patients preoperatively were negative at all dilutions tested, but sera taken at intervals after operation showed strong fluorescence, suggesting that *P. magnus* was acquired at or after the time of the operation. These findings support the view that the antibody response to *P. magnus* was specific and directed against the organisms infecting the hip prosthesis.

Taylor et al. (29) also reported four further cases of infections in joint prosthesis from: P. acnes, P. magnus, P. asaccharolyticus, and Peptococcus not speciated. In each case they were isolated in pure culture. These findings demonstrate the value of storing patients' sera obtained before operation and during the period of postoperative care. Antibody levels made retrospectively support the validity of the bacteriological findings and also help to speculate as to the time the infection was acquired.

SUMMARY

An immune response to anaerobes has been shown in such diseases as septicemia, wound infection, and hip infection. Immunological procedures that have proven reliable in detecting antibody production in anaerobic infections include: passive hemagglutination, indirect fluorescent antibody, agglutination, agar gel diffusion, crossed immunoelectrophoresis, and ELISA.

LITERATURE CITED

1. Axelsen, N.H. 1973. Quantitative immunoelectrophoretic methods as tools for a polyvalent approach to standardization in the immunochemistry of Candida albicans. Infect. Immun. 7: 949-960.

2. Axelsen, N.H. 1973. Intermediate gel in crossed and in fused rocket immunoelectrophoresis. Scand. J. Immunol. 2 (Suppl. 1): 71-77.

3. Axelsen, N.H., M. Harboe, A. Closs, and T. Godal. 1974. BCG antibody profiles in tuberculoid and lepromatous leprosy. Infect. Immun. 9: 952-958.

4. Chow, A.W., and L.B. Guze. 1974. Bacteroidaceae bacteremia: clinical experience with 112 patients. Med. (Baltimore) 53: 93-126.

5. Danielsson, D., and D.W. Lambe, Jr. 1980. Immunology of anaerobic bacterial infections. In R.A. Good and J. Day (ed.), Immunology of Human Infection. Plenum Pub. Corp., New York.

6. Danielsson, D., D.W. Lambe, Jr., and S. Persson. 1972. The immune response in a patient to an infection with Bacteroides fragilis subsp. fragilis and Clostridium difficile. Acta. Pathol. Microbiol. Scand. (B) 80: 709-712.

7. Danielsson, D., D.W. Lambe, Jr., and S. Persson. 1974. Immune response to anaerobic infections, p. 173-191. In A. Balows, R.M. Dehaan, V.R. Dowell, and L.B. Guze (ed.), Anaerobic bacteria: Role in disease. Charles C. Thomas, Springfield.

8. Evanski, P.M., T.R. Waugh, C.A. Prietto, and C.F. Orofino. 1977. Anaerobic infection after total hip replacement. Report of three cases. Clin. Orthop. 126: 178-180.

9. Finegold, S.M. 1968. Infections due to anaerobes. Med. Times 96: 174-187.

10. Hebert, G.A., D.L. Pelham, and B. Pittman. 1973. Determination of the optimal ammonium sulfate concentration for the fractionation of rabbit, sheep, horse, and goat antisera. Appl. Microbiol. 25: 26-36.

11. Højby, N., and N.H. Axelsen. 1973. Identification and quantitation of precipitins against Pseudomonas aeruginosa in patients with cystic fibrosis by means of crossed immunoelectrophoresis with intermediate gel. Acta. Pathol. Microbiol. Scand. (B) 81: 298-308.

12. Holdeman, L.V., E.P. Cato, and W.E.C. Moore. 1977. Anaerobe Laboratory Manual, 4th ed. Virginia Polytechnic Institute and State University, Blacksburg.

13. Holmberg, K., C. Nord, and T. Wadström. 1975. Serological studies of Actinomyces israelii by crossed immunoelectrophoresis: Standard antigen-antibody system for A. israelii. Infect. Immun. 12: 387-397.

14. Holmberg, K., C. Nord, and T. Wadström. 1975. Serological studies of Actinomyces israelii by crossed immunoelectrophoresis: Taxonomic and diagnostic applications. Infect. Immun. 12: 398-403.

15. Krøll, J. 1973. Tandem-crossed immunoelectrophoresis. Scand. J. Immunol. 2 (Suppl. 1): 57-59.

16. Lambe, D.W., Jr. 1976. Determination of Bacteroides melaninogenicus serogroups by fluorescent antibody staining. Appl. Microbiol. 28: 561-567.

17. Lambe, D.W., Jr., and D.A. Moroz. 1976. Serogrouping of Bacteroides fragilis subsp. fragilis by the agglutination test. J. Clin. Microbiol. 3: 586-592.

18. Lambe, D.W., Jr., D.H. Vroon, and C.W. Rietz. 1974. Infections due to anaerobic cocci. In A. Balows, R.M. DeHaan, V.R. Dowell, and L.B. Guze (ed.), Anaerobic bacteria: Role in disease. Charles C. Thomas, Springfield.

19. Lambe, D.W., Jr., D. Danielsson, D.H. Vroon, and R.K. Carver. 1975. Immune response in eight patients infected with Bacteroides fragilis. J. Infect. Dis. 131: 499-508.

20. Laporte, A., and H. Brocard. 1939. La réaction de floculation du sérum en présence d'un extrait alcoolique microbien dans les infections a Bacillus funduliformis. C.R. Soc. Biol. (Paris). 131: 4-7.

21. Lowry, O.H., N.J. Rosebrough, A.L. Farr, and R.J. Randall. 1951. Protein measurement with the Folin phenol reagent. J. Biol. Chem. 193: 265-275.

22. Monteiro, E., J. Fossey, M. Shiner, B.S. Draser, and A.C. Allison. 1971. Antibacterial antibodies in rectal and colonic mucosa in ulcerative colitis. Lancet 1: 249-251.

23. Nelson, J.P. 1977. Deep infection following total hip arthroplasty. J. Bone Joint Surg. (AM) 59: 1042-1044.

24. Quick, J.D., H.S. Goldberg, and A.C. Sonnenwirth. 1972. Human antibody to Bacteroidaceae. Amer. J. Clin. Nutr. 25: 1351-1356.

25. Rissing, J.P., J.G. Crowder, J.W. Smith, and A. White. 1974. Detection of Bacteroides fragilis infection by precipitating antibody. J. Infect. Dis. 130: 70-73.

26. Schwan, A., and A.-C. Rydén. 1978. The clinical importance of anaerobic bacteria in wound infections after gastrointestinal surgery. Scand. J. Infect. Dis. 10: 119-125.

27. Schwan, A., and A.-C. Rydén. 1978. Antibody response in thirteen patients with Bacteroides fragilis infections. Scand. J. Infect. Dis. 10: 213-218.

28. Swendsen, P.J., and N.H. Axelsen. 1972. A modified antigen-antibody crossed electrophoresis characterizing the specificity and titre of human precipitins against Candida albicans. J. Immunol. Meth. 1: 169-176.

29. Taylor, A.G., W.J. Fincham, M.A. Golding, and J. Cook. 1979. Infection of total hip prostheses by Peptococcus magnus: an immunofluorescence and ELISA study of two cases. J. Clin. Pathol. 32: 61-65.

30. Weeke, B. 1973. Crossed immunoelectrophoresis. Scand. J. Immunol. 2 (Suppl. 1): 15-35.

31. Wilson, W.R., W.F. Martin, C.J. Wilkowske, and J.A. Washington. 1972. Anaerobic bacteremia. Mayo Clin. Proc. 47: 639-646.

IMMUNE RESPONSE TO ANAEROBIC WOUND INFECTIONS

Anna Schwan

Institute of Clinical Bacteriology
University of Uppsala
S-75122 Uppsala, Sweden

INTRODUCTION

The increased knowledge of anaerobic bacteria, their occurrence, cultivation and identification has raised the question of their pathologic significance. The engagement of immunological defense mechanisms in anaerobic infections is, therefore, of great interest. Many severe infections associated with Bacteroides fragilis have been described, and there are a number of reports concerning the antibody response to these bacteria.

Various techniques of demonstrating antibody response in anaerobic infection have been used.

Tube agglutination (TA) has been used in several reports (Table 1). Antibody response has been found to B. fragilis and Fusobacterium varium (1,2,3,9,15). TA is a simple method to detect antibodies to surface antigen. It is not very sensitive, and an important drawback is the tendency of some strains to agglutinate spontaneously. Antibodies to B. fragilis in sera from healthy persons have been found in very low titers of 1:10 or less.

It is not suitable to do a quantitative determination of antibodies with agar gel diffusion (AGD) tests. Instead a qualitative examination of antigens can be performed. The test has been performed using ultrasonic bacterial extracts both with heterologous and homologous strains (1,2,9,12). Rissing (12) found no precipitating antibodies against B. fragilis in sera from 20 healthy persons, nor did Lambe (9) in 10 control sera.

The more sensitive passive hemagglutination (PHA) test has also

Table 1. Methods Used for Demonstrating Antibodies to Anaerobic Bacteria

Method	Strains	Authors
Tube agglutination	Bacteroides fragilis	Danielsson et al., 1972
	B. fragilis, Fusobacterium varium	Danielsson et al., 1974
	B. fragilis, F. varium	Danielsson et al., 1974
	B. fragilis	Lambe et al., 1975
	B. fragilis	Schwan & Ryden, 1978
Agar gel diffusion	B. fragilis	Danielsson et al., 1972
	B. fragilis, Fusobacterium necrophorum	Danielsson et al., 1974
	B. fragilis	Lambe et al., 1975
Passive hem-agglutination	B. fragilis, F. varium	Danielsson et al., 1974
	B. fragilis, F. necrophorum	Danielsson et al., 1974
	B. fragilis	Schwan & Ryden, 1978
Indirect immuno-fluorescence	B. fragilis, Clostridium difficile	Danielsson et al., 1972
	B. fragilis, F. varium, Clostridium perfringens	Danielsson et al., 1974
	B. fragilis, F. necrophorum, C. difficile	Danielsson et al., 1974
	B. fragilis	Lambe et al., 1975
	B. fragilis, C. perfringens, Gram-positive cocci	Schwan & Ryden, 1978
	Peptococcus magnus	Taylor et al., 1979
Enzyme linked immunosorbent assay	P. magnus	Taylor et al., 1979

been used for detecting antibody response in infections with B. fragilis and Fusobacterium (2,3,15). Antibodies to heat-stable polysaccharides and lipopolysaccharides are detected by this test. Using PHA antibodies to B. fragilis in sera from healthy individuals have been found in titers of 1:40 or less.

With indirect immunofluorescence (IFL) the immune response of the different immunglobulin classes can be determined easily by using antihuman IgG, IgA and IgM. The immunofluorescent (IFL) test measures antibodies to various types of surface antigens, both heat-stable and heat-labile. Immunofluorescence has been used in several studies, all examining antibody response to the patient's own strains (1,2,3,9, 14,15,16). Serum antibodies to B. fragilis, fusobacteria, clostridia, and Gram-positive cocci have been demonstrated with IFL. Danielsson and co-workers (2) have described a patient in whom antibody response to an isolated strain of B. fragilis was demonstrated both with IFL, AGD and TA, whereas antibodies to Clostridium difficile were demonstrated only by IFL. Antibodies to B. fragilis in healthy individuals have been found in titers of 1:20 or less using antihuman IgG.

Taylor and co-workers (16) described antibody response to Peptococcus magnus in two patients with infections after total hip replacement. The antibody response was followed with indirect immunofluorescence and the ELISA-technique. The antigen used for ELISA was suspended, ground, lyophilized bacteria. Thus, this test and the AGD measure antibodies not only to surface antigens, as the other three methods used, but also to intracellular antigens.

The studies mentioned thus far have dealt with the antibody response to the patient's strain. By demonstrating antibodies to heterologous B. fragilis strains the clinical significance of an isolated B. fragilis could be estimated, or a clinical suspicion of an anaerobic infection - not bacteriologically verified - could be strengthened. Various immunological methods have been used for this purpose.

Agar gel diffusion (Table 2) was used by Rissing and co-workers (12), who demonstrated precipitating antibodies to B. fragilis in 50% of 12 patients with B. fragilis bacteremia and 44% of nine patients with wound infections using heterologous strains of B. fragilis and Bacteroides thetaiotaomicron as antigen. Sera from patients with lung abscesses from whom no cultures were obtained were positive in five of eight cases.

Okubadejo and others (11) used counterimmunoelectrophoresis (CIEP) with antigen from two different B. fragilis strains. They found IgG antibody response in paired sera from 66% of 149 patients with B. fragilis infections; 98% of 109 controls were negative. As stated by the authors a positive CIEP indicates a current infection,

Table 2. Methods Used for Diagnosing Bacteroides Infections by Demonstrating Antibodies to Heterologous Bacteroides Strains

Method	Antigen	Authors
Agar gel diffusion	B. fragilis B. thetaiotaomicron	Rissing et al., 1974
Counterimmuno-electrophoresis	B. fragilis	Okubadejo et al., 1978
Complement fixation test	B. fragilis	Ross and Gilmore, 1978
Radioactive antigen-binding assay	B. fragilis	Kasper et al., 1978

while a negative is not conclusive.

Ross and Gilmore (13) demonstrated antibody titer changes to B. fragilis in five patients with postoperative abdominal infections by a complement fixation test. No immune response was found in 20 control sera.

Kasper et al. (8) demonstrated antibody titer changes to B. fragilis in nine women with pelvic inflammatory disease (PID) from which B. fragilis was isolated. They used a radioactive antigen binding assay with capsular polysaccharide of a B. fragilis type strain as antigen. Thirty-seven women with PID from which other organisms were isolated or who had no signs of PID had no such antibody titer changes.

In the anaerobe laboratory at the Institute of Clinical Bacteriology in Uppsala we have examined wound cultures after abdominal surgery wishing to demonstrate (i) the number of anaerobic bacteria present, and (ii) the immune response, if any, to some of the isolated anaerobes.

As antibodies to various anaerobes can be found not only in patients' but also in control sera, it is essential to examine sera from healthy individuals. Without knowledge of normal serum titers it is difficult to estimate the clinical value of a patient's serum antibody titer in a single serum specimen.

We examined sera from healthy blood donors with IFL using anti-human IgG, looking for antibodies to one strain each of B. fragilis, Bacteroides vulgatus, Fusobacterium nucleatum, Clostridium ramosum, Clostridium sporogenes, Clostridium perfringens, Peptococcus prevotii, P. magnus, Peptococcus asaccharolyticus and Peptostreptococcus anaerobius; all of these strains were isolated from clinical specimens.

MATERIALS AND METHODS

Patients

Fifty-four patients treated at the Department of Surgery, University Hospital, Uppsala, were included in the study. The patients were randomly selected from those showing signs of wound infection after abdominal surgery. Three patients with abdominal abscesses unrelated to surgery were also included.

Sampling and Transport

The specimens were collected with a sterile cotton swab and placed in modified Stuart's medium (5). Fluid material was aspirated with a sterile syringe and injected into a sterile gassed tube (97% CO_2, 3% H_2) or into anaerobic blood culture bottles. All specimens were immediately transported to the laboratory for cultivation.

Culture and Identification

Media used for isolation of aerobes included blood agar with and without Gentian violet, hematin and phenol-red-mannitol agar. All plates were incubated at 37 C; the hematin agar and Gentian violet agar plates were incubated in an atmosphere containing 5% CO_2. Standard biochemical procedures were followed for identification of the aerobic bacteria. Anaerobes were isolated on Brain Heart Infusion Agar base (Difco Laboratories, Detroit, Mich., USA) with the addition of 0.5% yeast extract (Difco Laboratories), 5% sheep blood, menadione 0.5 ug/ml (Sigma Chem., St. Louis, Mo., USA) and hemin 5 ug/ml (Sigma Chem.). The plates were used within 2 h of preparation or stored under strict anaerobic conditions until used. Inoculated plates were incubated at 37 C in anaerobic jars using the Gas Pak system (BBL, Maryland, USA). The plates were examined for growth after 48 and 96 h. The methods described by Holdeman and Moore (7) were used for identifying anaerobic bacteria.

Definition of Wound Infection and Beginning of Infection

A wound was said to be infected when it contained pus visible to the naked eye (17). The day of operation was considered the beginning of the infection. When the patients were operated because of an abdominal abscess, the beginning of infection was more difficult to decide. We chose a day when the patient first showed signs of pain and fever.

Serum Specimens from Patients

Serum samples from the patients were collected as soon as possible after the isolation of the anaerobic strains and at various intervals depending on the availability of the patients. Serum samples were frozen in small portions and stored at -70 C until used.

Serum Specimens from Blood Donors

Serum samples were collected from 56 healthy blood donors, 37 men and 19 women. Mean age of the male blood donors was 36 years (range 20-59) and of the female blood donors was 35 years (range 21-55). The sera were inactivated for 30 min at 56 C and kept frozen at -70 C until used. Indirect IFL tests using antihuman IgG were made against the anaerobic strains other than _B._ fragilis. The _B._ fragilis patients' sera were examined with indirect IFL using antihuman IgG, IgA and IgM as well as with PHA and TA.

Preparation of Antigens

The strains were cultivated for 48 h on the same agar plates used for primary isolation (14). The bacteria were harvested in sterile phosphate-buffered saline (PBS). For TA tests whole bacterial cells were treated with 3% formalin for 1 h and washed 3 times in sterile PBS. The bacterial suspension was diluted to approximately 10^9 cells/ml.

Untreated, whole bacterial cells washed 3 times in PBS at a concentration of approximately 10^8 cells/ml were used as antigen for the indirect IFL.

The supernatant of bacterial cells, suspended in PBS to about 25-30 mg wet weight/ml and boiled for 2 h was used as antigen in passive HA tests.

Indirect IFL

A 0.01 ml sample of the bacterial suspension was smeared on a glass slide and dried in air. The bacteria were covered with 0.01 ml of the serum specimen diluted 1:10 through 1:1280 in two-fold increments in PBS containing 4% bovine serum albumin (BSA). The slides were incubated in a moist chamber at 37 C for 30 min, washed with PBS for 10 min and dried in air. The smears were then covered with 0.01 ml of fluorescein isothiocyanate (FITC)-labeled antihuman IgG, IgA and IgM (DAKO-immunoglobulins a/s, Copenhagen, Denmark), respectively, incubated and washed as above. The slides were mounted under a cover glass with phosphate-buffered glycerin. The slides were read under a Leitz Orthoplan fluorescence microscope equipped with incident light, an Osram ABO 200 mercury lamp and a KP 490 as primary filter and a TK 510/K515 as the secondary filter. A magnification of 450 x was used.

The criteria used for recording the specific fluorescent staining of the bacteria were as follows: 3+, intensely fluorescent margins, well-marked edges; 2+, faintly fluorescent margins, edges usually well-marked; 1+, barely distinguishable fluorescent margins with diffuse edges. 3+ and 2+ were regarded as positive reactions; 1+ and no visible bacteria was regarded a negative reaction. A four-fold or greater change of titer was considered significant.

Passive HA

Sheep red blood cells (SRBC) were washed three times in PBS and used as carriers of the bacterial antigens. One part of a 2% suspension of SRBC in PBS was incubated with one part of the supernatant of the boiled bacteria at 37 C for 60 min. After centrifugation the sensitized SRBC were washed three times in PBS and suspended to a density of 1% in PBS, containing normal rabbit serum (NRS) 1:200, previously absorbed with SRBC.

The tests were performed in V-shaped microplates. Serum specimens were diluted two-fold with PBS + NRS 1:200, starting at a dilution of 1:10. To 0.025 ml of diluted serum 0.025 ml sensitized SRBC was added. The microplates were incubated at 37 C and read after 1 h. A further reading was done after incubation at 4 C overnight. Serum with unsensitized SRBC and sensitized SRBC in PBS were always included as controls. Serum specimens were diluted two-fold in PBS, starting at a dilution of 1:10; 0.5 ml of the serum dilutions was added to an equal volume of the appropriate antigen. The tubes were incubated at 37 C and read after 24 h. Antigen controls in PBS were always included. The highest serum dilution giving visible agglutination was considered the agglutination titer.

Antibody titers in control serum, pooled from five healthy lab workers, were examined for all strains. A four-fold or greater titer change was considered significant (3).

RESULTS AND DISCUSSION

Patients' Immune Response

The immune response of 13 patients with B. fragilis infections was followed (Table 3). The majority of the patients had wound infections after surgery on the large bowel, the gall-bladder or appendix. Two patients had abscesses not related to surgery. Ten of the Bacteroides strains were B. fragilis, three were B. thetaiotaomicron. Bacteroides grew in pure culture from three patients; additional anaerobes were found in seven of the cases.

Significant immune response was found with IFL in 12 of 13 cases (Table 4). The highest titers were observed for IgG; a titer of 1:640 or more was found in 8 of 13 patients. A four-fold or greater decrease of titer was seen in all cases except one, where the first serum sample was collected 74 days after the beginning of infection when it is possible that the peak of the infection had already passed.

Eight patients showed a four-fold change in IgA antibody titer, but never reached the values shown for IgG.

Most of the patients had no change in IgM antibody titer; only four cases where the IgG and IgA titers were very high showed significant decrease. The absence of IgM response indicates previous contact with the antigen.

Control serum tested against all strains showed a titer of 1:20 or less against all three classes of immunoglobulins.

Table 3. Thirteen Patients with B. fragilis Wound Infections

Infection	Number of Patients
Abscess, not related to surgery	2
Postoperative infections	
Laparotomy	1
Operation on gallbladder	3 (2)[a]
Appendectomy	2
Operation on large bowel	5 (1)[a]

[a] Figures in brackets indicate pure cultures.

Table 4. Significant Titer Changes in 13 Patients with B. fragilis Infections

Serological Test		Number of Cases
Indirect immunofluorescence		
	IgG	12
	IgA	8
	IgM	4
Passive hemagglutination		11
Tube agglutination (nine cases)		6

By PHA increased antibody titers were detected in all cases (Table 4). In most of them (11 of 13) a significant change was observed. They were lower than the corresponding IgG titers, using the indirect IFL technique, in all cases but one. Control serum showed titers of 1:20 or less.

TA tests gave significant titer change in fewer patients (six of nine) than the other two methods used (Table 4). They were mostly found in cases where the titers demonstrated with indirect IFL and PHA were very high. They did, however, exhibit the same pattern as with PHA. The titers never exceeded 1:160 in the TA tests. Control serum showed a titer of 1:10 or less against all strains.

From 10 patients whose wound cultures grew anaerobic cocci significant titer change was found in three cases.

When cocci were isolated in mixed cultures with other anaerobes, the titers were, if possible, measured against all strains (Table 5). Thus, B. fragilis and anaerobic cocci were found together in five cases. In three of these titers were significantly changed against the Bacteroides strains but remained unchanged against the cocci. In the fourth case both titers were significantly reduced, whereas in the fifth case no titer changes were found.

From two patients whose wound cultures yielded C. perfringens no significant titer change was found (Table 5).

The immune reaction of the different immunoglobulins was studied only with the IFL technique. In all cases antibodies of the IgG and IgA classes seemed to be involved, the IgA to a smaller degree.

Table 5. Immune Response to Some Anaerobic Strains Isolated from Wound Infections

Strain	Total Number of Isolates	Titer Change	
		Significant	Not Significant
Gram-positive cocci	10[a]	3	7
Clostridium spp.	1		1
C. perfringens	2		2

[a] 1 pure culture; 5 together with B. fragilis; 4 together with aerobes.

The presence of IgM antibodies was not studied before and after mercaptoethanol reduction when PHA was performed. Danielsson et al. (2) showed that the IgM antibody titer did not change significantly after reduction. They concluded that IgG and possibly IgA are the participating antibodies in PHA.

According to our findings the rise in antibody titer seems to come within one week. Okubadejo and co-workers (11), using CIEP, found antibodies seven to ten days after the onset of infection. Lambe (9) found antibodies, in one case, after five days. Samples with very short intervals would be needed to determine the exact time. It is important to note that the beginning of the infection in these studies is not exactly known. The number of days before the antibody response is detectable is estimated from a calculated date for the onset of infection, or from the date when the Bacteroides strain was isolated.

According to Lambe (9) antibodies in some patients persisted for over four months. Okubadejo (11) gives the figure of three to six weeks. We have found increased antibody titers in some cases for as long as five months, even though healing was not delayed.

Case Reports

For four patients in the study a more detailed description of the immune response is given.

The first patient, AE, (Fig. 1) was an elderly man with a pelvic abscess which developed after rectal excision was performed for cancer of the rectum. The infection healed quickly after surgical

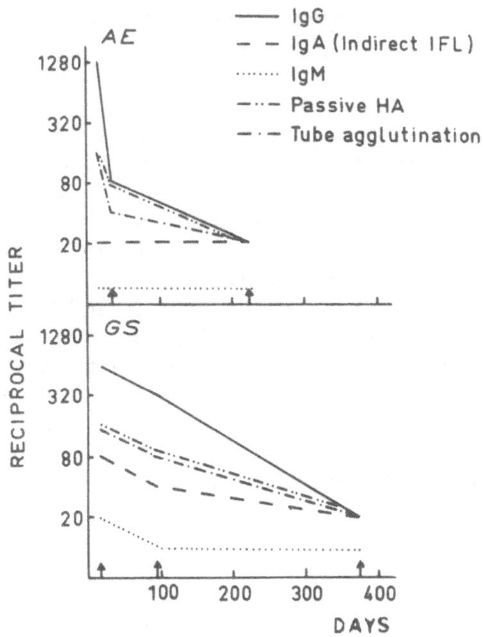

Fig. 1. Antibody response to B. fragilis in two patients with wound infections of short duration.

drainage. The first serum sample had a very high IgG titer that decreased fast initially and was normal again after seven to eight months. No involvement of IgA or IgM was observed. The curves for PHA and TA show the same pattern as for IgG measured by indirect IFL.

GS (Fig. 1) was a 63-year-old female with a wound infection after cholecystectomy. The infection healed promptly after incision. The serum samples show an almost linear decrease of IgG and IgA titer; no involvement of IgM was observed. Two and a half months after the infection the IgG titer was still high. The antibody response measured by PHA and TA followed the IgG titer. No further serum sample was obtained until one year later when the antibody level was normal.

Patients AE and GS both had infections that healed after incision and without antibiotic treatment. The duration of the infection was short. In both cases the elevated titer started to decrease during the early convalescent period. The very steep slope of the

IgG curve in case AE is not compatible with the half-life of IgG and must be explained by the variation of the method.

FE (Fig. 2), an 87-year-old female, had a retroperitoneal abscess after perforation of a sigmoidal diverticulum, and DK (Fig. 2), a 61-year-old female with hemiplegia, had a wound abscess after appendectomy. In both cases the antibody response persisted for a long time and dropped slowly as compared to cases AE and GS. The IgG level had not normalized one year after the beginning of the infection. The antibody titers studied by PHA and TA decreased faster than the IgG titer which persisted during the beginning of the infection. In both cases the IgG titers were high initially.

The long and complicated infections of FE and DK are well illustrated in the titer curves. The IgG titers are high initially and persist for a considerable period in both cases. Even one year after

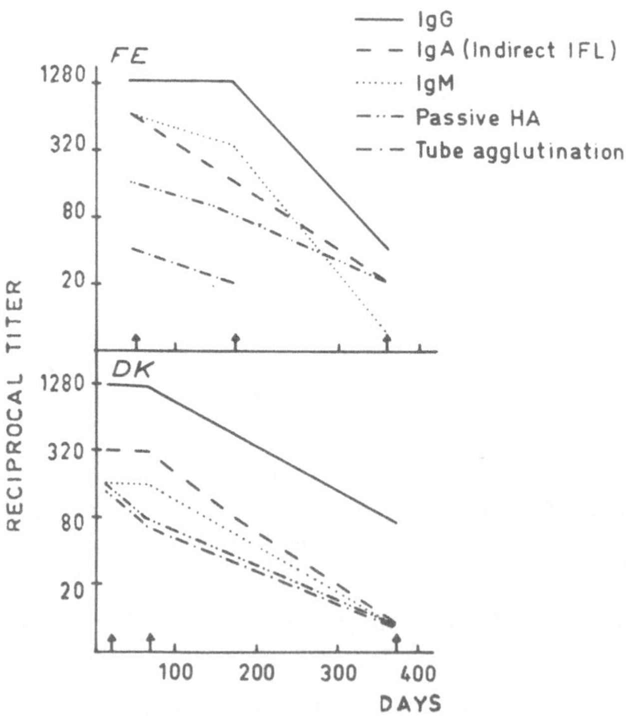

Fig. 2. Antibody response to B. fragilis in two patients with long-standing wound infections.

the beginning of the infection the titers have not normalized. In case FE the long-standing IgM response indicates a persisting antigen stimulation.

Antibodies in Normal Serum

Antibodies to B. fragilis in normal serum never exceeded a titer of 1:20.

A few persons had titers of 1:40 against B. vulgatus (Fig. 3). This difference is possibly because B. vulgatus is more common than B. fragilis in the bowel flora. Obviously the immune system is activated very little by the Bacteroides species in normal persons.

The increased antibody titers against the B. fragilis strains isolated from the infected patients provide evidence that these strains were responsible for the infections. This conclusion is, however, based on convalescent sera since no acute sera were obtained.

Antibodies against F. nucleatum were found in all serum specimens; titers of 1:40-1:160 were most common (Fig. 3).

The sera were tested against three strains of clostridia, namely Clostridium ramosum, C. sporogenes and C. perfringens.

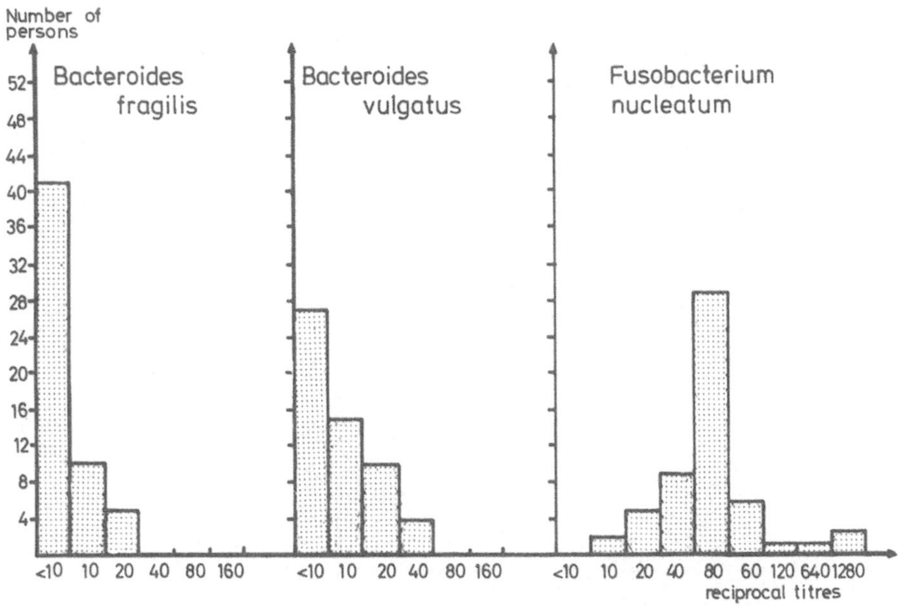

Fig. 3. Antibody titers in sera from 56 healthy blood donors.

For C. perfringens all sera had titers of 1:320 or more (Fig. 4); for C. sporogenes a majority of the titers were also very high. Against C. ramosum, on the other hand, very low antibody titers were found in normal serum. Danielsson (4) and others have also noted very high antibody titers against C. perfringens in both patient's and control serum. We cannot explain these different titers against the clostridia, but they are certainly very interesting, as the role of C. perfringens in connective tissue disorders has been discussed by some authors. Månsson and Olhagen (10) found antibodies to C. perfringens alpha-toxin in sera from patients with rheumatoid arthritis. They did not, however, find elevated antibody titers in control sera. For different strains of anaerobic cocci the results were varying.

Antibodies against P. anaerobius and P. asaccharolyticus were found in most sera, often in very high titers (Fig. 5). Few, or low titer, antibodies were found against P. prevotii and P. magnus. Taylor and others (16) have examined sera from 91 blood donors for antibodies to P. magnus and report similar results using indirect IFL and the ELISA-technique. The pathologic significance of an isolated strain of cocci is difficult to estimate because of these varying control titers. Probably the role of anaerobic Gram-positive cocci in abdominal wound infection is less important than that of B. fragilis. In experimental infection a synergism between B. fragilis and Gram-positive cocci has been demonstrated (6).

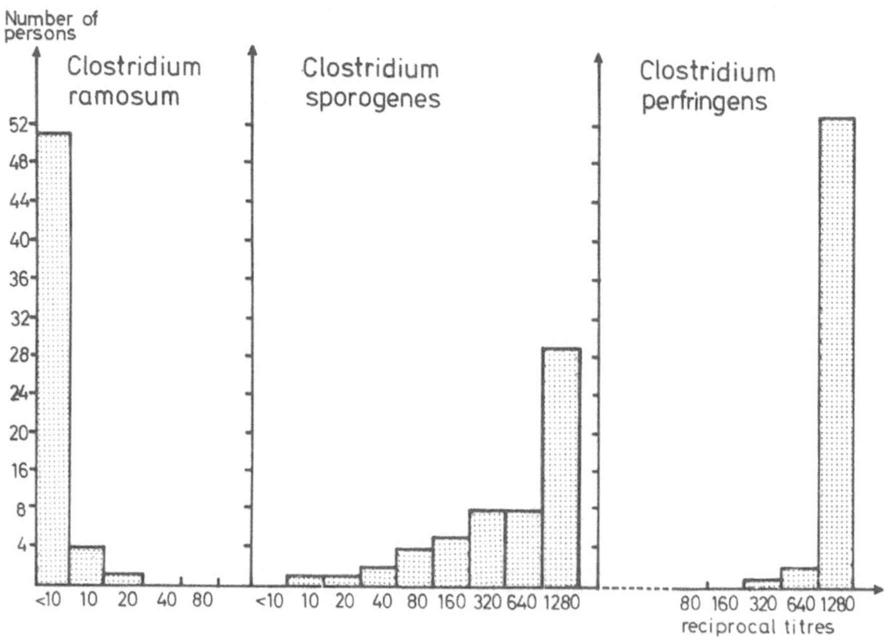

Fig. 4. Antibody titers in sera from 56 healthy blood donors.

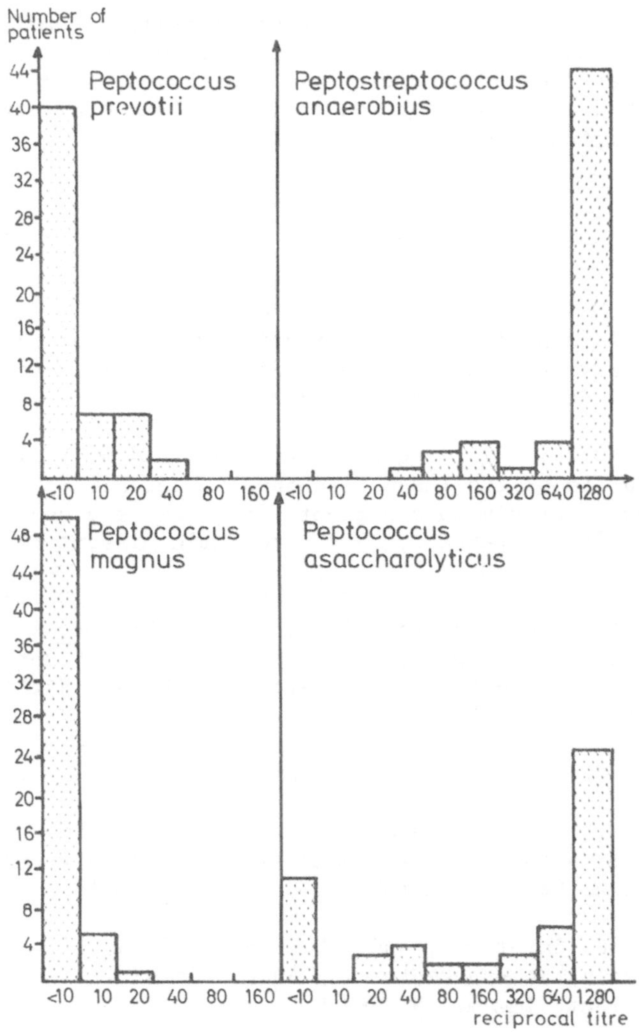

Fig. 5. Antibody titers in sera from 56 healthy blood donors.

SUMMARY

B. fragilis is an important pathogen in wound infection. Serum antibodies are detectable about one week after the onset of the infection and can persist for several months. IgG and IgA are mainly involved in the immune response. Titers against *B.* fragilis in control sera are low.

The pathogenicity of the anaerobic Gram-positive cocci and the clostridia is difficult to prove, as control titers are sometimes very high. C. perfringens is definitely a pathogen in cases of gas gangrene, but this organism might be a commensal in other types of abdominal wound infections.

LITERATURE CITED

1. Danielsson, D., D.W. Lambe, and S. Persson. 1972. The immune response in a patient to an infection with Bacteroides fragilis ss. fragilis and Clostridium difficile. Acta Pathol. Microbiol. Scand. (B) 80: 709-712.

2. Danielsson, D., J. Kjellander, S. Persson, and S. Wallensten. Investigation of the immune response to aerobic and anaerobic intestinal bacteria in a patient with Crohn's disease. Uppsala. In S. Persson, 1974. Academic Dissertation.

3. Danielsson, D., D.W. Lambe, and S. Persson. 1974. Immune response to anaerobic infections, p. 173-191. In A. Balows, R.M. Dehaan, V.R. Dowell, and L.B. Guze (ed.), Anaerobic bacteria: Role in disease. Charles C. Thomas, Springfield, Ill.

4. Danielsson, D.: Personal communication

5. Gastrin, B., L. -O. Kallings, and A. Marcetic. 1968. The survival time for different bacteria in various transport media. Acta Pathol. Microbiol. Scand. 74: 371.

6. Hill, G.B., S. Osterhout, and P.C. Pratt. 1974. Liver abscess production by non-spore-forming anaerobic bacteria in a mouse model. Infect. Immun. 9: 599-603.

7. Holdeman, L.V., E.P. Cato, and W.E.C. Moore. (ed.) 1977. Anaerobe Laboratory Manual, 4th ed. Virginia Polytechnic Institute and State University, Blacksburg.

8. Kasper, D.L., D.A. Eschenbach, M.E. Hayes, and K.K. Holmes. 1978. Quantitative determination of serum antibody response to the capsular polysaccharide of Bacteroides fragilis ssp. in women with pelvic inflammatory disease. J. Infect. Dis. 138: 74-80.

9. Lambe, D.W., D. Danielsson, D.H. Vroon, and R.K. Carver. 1975. Immune response in eight patients infected with Bacteroides fragilis. J. Infect. Dis. 131: 499-508.

10. Månsson, J., and B. Olhagen. 1966. Intestinal Clostridium perfringens in rheumatoid arthritis and other connective tissue disorders. Acta Rheum. Scand. 12: 167-174.

11. Okubadejo, O.A., N.F. Lightfoot, and W.G. Hewitt. 1978. Diagnosis of Bacteroides fragilis infection with counter-immunoelectrophoresis. J. Clin. Pathol. 31: 1078-1082.

12. Rissing, J.P., J.G. Crowder, J.W. Smith, and A. White. 1974. Detection of Bacteroides fragilis infection by precipitin antibody. J. Inf. Dis. 130: 70-73.

13. Ross, C.A.C., and R.F. Gilmore. 1978. Serological diagnosis of Bacteroides fragilis infections by a complement fixation test. J. Clin. Pathol. 31: 1083-1084.

14. Schwan, A., and A.-C. Rydén. 1978. The clinical importance of anaerobic bacteria in wound infections after gastrointestinal surgery. Scand. J. Infect. Dis. 10: 119-125.

15. Schwan, A., and A.-C. Rydén. 1978. Antibody response in thirteen patients with Bacteroides fragilis infections. Scand. J. Infect. Dis. 10: 213-218.

16. Taylor, A.G., W.J. Fincham, M.A. Golding, and J. Cook. 1979. Infection of total hip prostheses by Peptococcus magnus: an immunofluorescence and ELISA study of two cases. J. Clin. Pathol. 32: 61-65.

17. Williams, R.E.O., R. Blowers, L.P. Garrod, and R.A. Shooter. 1966. Hospital infection. Causes and prevention. 2nd ed., p. 181. Lloyd-Luke, London.

IMMUNE RESPONSES OF HAMSTERS AND HUMANS WITH ANTIBIOTIC-ASSOCIATED COLITIS

Joseph Silva, Rodney Lusk, Robert Fekety, Kenneth Wilson, Donald Batts, David Mason, and Daniel Spratt

University of Michigan Medical Center
Department of Internal Medicine
Division of Infectious Diseases
Ann Arbor, Michigan 48109

INTRODUCTION

The Golden Syrian hamster has served as a model for antibiotic-associated colitis of humans and has been instrumental in discovering its pathogenesis (4,18). Toxigenic Clostridium difficile have been implicated as the major cause of antibiotic-associated colitis (AAC) in both hamsters and humans (5,10,20). While clindamycin first focused attention on this lesion, many other antibiotics have been implicated subsequently following either parenteral or oral administrations. AAC also varies greatly in its clinical presentation in humans and in its geographic distribution (17,23).

In recent years, drugs such as rifampin, diphenylhydantoin, levamisole, and niridazole have been associated with altered states of cellular immunity, by causing either immunosuppression or hypersensitivity. Similarly, since 1970 data has accumulated which stresses the importance of cellular immunity in enigmatic gastrointestinal illnesses such as Crohn's disease (7) and ulcerative colitis (16). Because of these data, we studied the importance of immune responses of humans and hamsters to C. difficile and its toxin.

METHODS

Patient Identification

The immune status of 44 patients with antibiotic-associated diarrhea seen at either the University of Michigan or its affiliated hospitals was studied. In addition, stool or blood of AAC patients sent to us were examined. These studies were completed between March, 1975, and January, 1979. Diarrhea was defined as five or more loose bowel movements on a single day. When possible, patients had sigmoidoscopy, colonoscopy and colonic biopsies to diagnose pseudomembranous colitis (PMC).

Lymphocyte Transformations in Patients

Studies of lymphocyte transformation with human blood were performed in triplicate as previously described (22). In brief, microcultures were established with 100,000 lymphocytes per well. Transformation was assayed quantitatively by measuring ^{3}H-thymidine incorporation. The stimulants employed were phytohemagglutinin-P (PHA, Difco, Detroit, Mich.; 75 ug/ml), Concanavalin A (Con A) (Calbiochem), clindamycin phosphate (8 and 80 ug/ml) and ampicillin trihydrate (8 and 80 ug/ml) (Upjohn Company, Kalamazoo, Mich.); streptokinase-streptodornase (SK-SD) and candidal antigen. Results are expressed as stimulation indices (SI) which is defined as the ratio of scintillation counts per ten min of mitogen-stimulated lymphocytes to counts obtained during incubation without mitogens.

Lymphocyte Transformations in Hamsters

Different lots of one to two-month-old Golden Syrian hamsters bred by Charles River Breeding Colonies (Lakeview, N.J. and Wilmington, Mass.) were used. Ten groups, each composed of 15 hamsters, were injected with sterile saline, or with sublethal doses of clindamycin phosphate (Upjohn Company) or ampicillin trihydrate (Bristol Laboratories), with or without complete Freund's adjuvant (CFA) (Grand Island Biological, New York), as shown in Table 1. All substances were administered by subcutaneous injection between the scapulae. All initial injections were followed in 14 days by booster injections with the same materials. After seven more days, four hamsters from each group were sacrificed by cervical separation following light anesthesia with ether.

Spleens were removed aseptically and placed in individual plastic Petri dishes containing RPMI-1640 (Grand Island Biological, Grand Island, N.Y.), disrupted by teasing with fine-tipped forceps and pipetting to break cell clumps. The cells were then placed in large Falcon tubes and allowed to settle briefly. The cell suspension was drawn off and the cells were washed once with phosphate buffer saline (pH 7.4). Lymphocytes were resuspended in a mixture of RPMI-1640 tissue culture media containing 10% heat-inactivated fetal calf serum with no antibiotics and counted in a hemocytometer.

Lymphocyte cultures were established in quadruplicate in microtiter plates. One hundred thousand lymphocytes/microtiter well were

Table 1. Immunization Regimens Given to Hamsters

Control Groups			
1.	Saline	0.3cc	
2.	CFA[a]	0.3cc	
Antibiotic Groups			
		mg/kg	
3.	Clindamycin	0.25	
4.	Clindamycin	0.025	
5.	Ampicillin	0.25	
6.	Ampicillin	0.025	
Antibiotic and CFA Groups			
		mg/kg	
7.	Clindamycin	0.25	+ 0.3cc CFA
8.	Clindamycin	0.025	+ 0.3cc CFA
9.	Ampicillin	0.25	+ 0.3cc CFA
10.	Ampicillin	0.025	+ 0.3cc CFA

[a] Complete Freund's adjuvant.

cultured with the following stimulants: clindamycin phosphate (8 and 80 ug/ml), ampicillin (8 and 80 ug/ml), Con A (6.25, 1.56 and 0.38 ug/ml) (Sigma Chemical, St. Louis, MO), and Con A in the previous concentrations with clindamycin phosphate (8 and 80 ug/ml).

All cultures were incubated at 37 C in a 5% CO_2 humidified atmosphere. At 66 h of incubation, one uCi of ^{3}H-thymidine (specific activity 20 Ci/m mole, New England Nuclear, Boston, MA) was added to each well. Six hours later those cultures were harvested onto glass fiber filter paper with an Otto-Hiller multiple sample precipitator. The filter papers were washed several times with 0.85% NaCl, 5% trichloroacetic acid, absolute methanol and then dried. The dried samples were immersed in toluene scintillator (Liquoflor 42 ml/l toluene, New England Nuclear) and the radioactivity measured with a Beckman liquid scintillation counter. The average counts of the quadruplicate filter papers were calculated and expressed as scintillation counts recorded per min (cpm). At 114 h this procedure was repeated with cultures containing only antigens.

Skin Tests

Skin testing for immediate sensitivity in humans to clindamycin was determined by intradermally injecting clindamycin phosphate (8 and 80 ug/ml). A positive test result was read if wheal and flare were observed within 20 min. Appropriate control solutions (saline and codeine) were also employed. Candida (1:100), SK-SD (40/20 U), dermatophytin, and tuberculoprotein (intermediate strength) were also applied in 0.1 ml volumes by the Mantoux technique to determine delayed hypersensitivity and were read 48 and 72 h after placement.

Antibody Studies

Direct immunofluorescent examination of colon biopsy specimens were performed in the Clinical Immunology Laboratory at the University of Michigan by Dr. Michael Deegan. Fluorescein isothiocyanate was conjugated to commercially obtained antisera against human IgG, IgA, IgM, C3, C4, and fibrinogen.

HLA determinations were performed by the microdroplet cytotoxicity test as described by Terasaki et al. (24). ABO typing was performed by standard agglutination techniques.

Tests for complement- and noncomplement-dependent serum antibodies to clindamycin were performed by Mr. John Judd of the Simpson Institute at the University of Michigan as follows. Human group erythrocytes were pretreated with clindamycin phosphate and saline. Serum specimens from the patients in our study group and control subjects were added to these cells with and without additional guinea pig complement. Cells were observed for agglutination or lysis at room temperature and at 37 C and were studied by the indirect antiglobulin test.

Carcinoembryonic antigen was measured by a modified assay (12) using a radioimmune assay kit which is commercially available (Hoffmann-La Roche, Inc.).

Testing for Clostridial Toxin

A microculture technique was employed which measures the cytotoxicity of fecal filtrates obtained from hamsters or humans when incubated for 24 h with Walker carcinoma cells and human foreskin fibroblasts (HFF) (21). This assay was also used to study toxins produced by clostridia previously isolated from human cases with AAC when grown in brain heart infusion broth. Neutralization of all toxic specimens in this assay was then attempted with horse antisera produced to toxin(s) of Clostridium sordellii, and on some specimens with rabbit antisera produced to toxin(s) of C. difficile. Neutralizations were performed by an in vitro assay in which the appropriate clostridial antitoxin was added to the test sample for 30 min at 37 C, intermittently mixed, and then added (100 ul) to a 200 ul microtiter well. After 24 h, neutralization was considered positive if a reduction of 50% or more occurred in the cytotoxicity of the highest dilution of filtrate used.

Production of Somatic Antibodies to C. difficile

Seven rabbits were immunized with intravenous doses of C. difficile strain 49A grown in broth or on agar. Organisms were washed twice with phosphate buffered saline and injected into marginal ear veins. Injections started with 10^6 organisms and were doubled daily until 10^8-10^9 organisms were administered. This highest dose was repeated every five days for six injections. Animals were bled for antibody analysis one week after the last injection. Agglutination tests were performed at room temperature using a tube dilution technique in which samples were centrifuged for 10 min at 5000 x g.

Partial Purification of C. difficile Toxin for Immunoprecipitation Tests and Production of Antibodies in Rabbits

Toxin of C. difficile was partially purified as described by Harvie et al. (14). C. difficile was incubated anaerobically for 24 h in pre-reduced, buffered brain heart infusion (BHI) broth. Organisms were separated from the BHI broth by centrifugation and filtration. The supernatant was mixed continously with $(NH_4)_2SO_4$ (50% vol/vol) overnight at 4 C. This solution was then centrifuged and the supernatant was discarded. The pellet was resuspended in phosphate buffered saline, pH 7.6 (PBS). The suspension was dialyzed against PBS for seven exchanges (vol/vol, 1:100) over one week. The dialysate was sterilized by membrane filtration and the volume adjusted to produce >50% toxicity at 10^{-4}/ml in the microtoxicity test with HFF and Walker carcinoma cells.

Production of Antitoxins to C. difficile Toxin

Thirteen rabbits were immunized by one of 13 regimens (Table 2). The general scheme involved daily immunizations for four days followed by an alternative route on the fifth day. Various combinations of subcutaneous, intravenous, and oral routes were employed. The amount of toxin administered daily was that contained in a 10^{-2}/ml dilution of filtrate produced from a broth culture of C. difficile and partially purified as indicated above. Aliquots of this toxic filtrate were also treated by heating (56 C x 30 min) or by mixing with 60 U of C. sordellii antitoxin prior to injection. Other portions of toxin (10^{-2}/ml) were also mixed with 0.4 ml CFA (Difco).

Detection of Antibodies to C. difficile

Counterimmunoelectrophoresis was performed according to the method of Axelsen et al. (3) as modified by Batts et al. (unpublished). In brief, conditions employed included 0.8% agarose in

Table 2. Results of Rabbit Immunizations with Partially-Purified _C_. difficile

Toxin Treatment: Heating (56 C x 30 min)	Toxin Treatment: Chemical	Days Administered and Route: 1→4	Days Administered and Route: 5th	Antibody Assays: Precipi-tating	Antibody Assays: Neutral-izing
Unheated	-	Oral	SQ[a]	-	-
	CFA	Oral	IP[b]	3 lines	-
	CFA	Oral	Oral	-	-
	CFA	SQ	IP	3 lines	-
Heated	-	Oral	SQ	-	-
	CFA	Oral	IP	3 lines	-
	-	Oral	IP	1 line	-
	CFA	SQ	IP	1 line	-
Unheated	_C_. sordellii antitoxin	SQ	IV[c]	1 line	+/-
Heated	-	SQ	IV	1 line	-
Unheated	-	SQ	IV	2 lines	-
Unheated	Endotoxin IV	IV	IV	1 line	-
Unheated	Cold incubation	SQ	IP	1 line	-

[a] Subcutaneous.

[b] Intraperitoneal.

[c] Intravenous.

cacodylic acid (IS = 0.0125%, pH 6.2, Sigma), 7 mm distances between wells, prior electrophoresis of antibody for 30 min, loading of the antigen (toxin sample), and re-electrophoresis (30 min, 10 MA of constant current), and appropriate gel washes and staining with amido black.

The sera were studied for agglutination and neutralizing antibodies, and also for precipitating antibodies to clostridial toxins which were produced in vitro in anaerobic culture (19).

RESULTS

Lymphocyte Transformations of Humans with PMC

Stimulation indices of 33 normal controls who had not received clindamycin or other antibiotics in the previous two months are compared to results obtained on 18 patients with biopsy-proven PMC and 11 patients with antibiotic-associated diarrhea without biopsy-proven PMC. Fifteen patients with antibiotic diarrhea who had no visualization procedures or biopsies performed either because of medical contraindications or because they were not under our direct control were also assessed (Table 3). Thirty of the 33 normal controls showed stimulation indices to PHA-P which were within the normal range of 50-200. Three other controls were slightly decreased below our normal range for this control group. All control subjects had lymphocytes with SI's which were <1 in the presence of clindamycin or ampicillin (at both 8 or 80 ug/ml concentrations).

Table 3. Lymphocyte Transformation Studies in Humans

Number of Subjects Studied	Antibiotic Associated Diarrhea	Status of Colon	Stimulation Indices with Antigens: PHA	Clindamycin (8 ug/ml)	Ampicillin (8 ug/ml)
Controls					
33	No	Normal	50-200	<1	<1
Patients				Range for Patients	
18	Yes	PMC[a]	NL-4 ↓-14[b]	NL-12 ↑-2	NL-13 ↑-1
11	Yes	No PMC	NL-2 ↓-9[b]	NL-11	NL-11
15	Yes	Not Visualized	NL-4 ↓-11[b]	NL-15	NL-15

[a] Pseudomembranous colitis.

[b] $p < 0.005$ when compared with PHA results of normal controls.

Eighteen patients had biopsy-proven pseudomembranous enterocolitis. PHA responses were normal in only four patients, being decreased in 14. While lymphocytes of 12 patients with biopsy-proven AAC had no responses to clindamycin or ampicillin, one and two patients had increased stimulation indices to ampicillin and clindamycin respectively. Of 11 patients with diarrhea but no pseudomembranous enterocolitis demonstrated by sigmoidoscopy, nine had diminutions in lymphocyte transformations to PHA. None of these 11 patients had abnormal responses to either clindamycin or ampicillin. There were 15 other patients with diarrhea who could not undergo visualization studies of their colons. While seven of these 15 had either C. difficile and/or toxin present in their stool and clinically fit the pattern of pseudomembranous enterocolitis, only four of these 15 patients had normal transformational responses to phytohemagglutinin. However, none of them demonstrated abnormal increases in their SI's to clindamycin or ampicillin. Also (in data not shown in Table 3) lymphocytes from 14/17 and 12/14 patients with PMC had no reactions to SK-SD or candidal antigens respectively. Only two and three patients showed normal lymphocyte transformations to these antigens respectively.

Lymphocyte Transformations of Hamsters

Table 4 shows the results of lymphocyte transformations obtained with splenic mononuclear cells from hamsters challenged with one of two doses of either clindamycin or ampicillin, with or without CFA. No dramatic increases occurred in lymphocyte transformations to clindamycin or ampicillin "antigens" whether or not these antibiotics were delivered with CFA. These sublethal doses of antibiotics caused no clinical disease in the recipients and their splenic lymphocytes showed normal transformational response to PPD.

Table 5 shows the lymphocyte transformations of splenic lymphocytes of hamsters given ampicillin or clindamycin. The data are expressed in scintillation counts per minute x 10^3 for either cultures containing no antigens or varying concentrations of Con A. The maximal responses of their lymphocytes to Con A in the group challenged only with saline was 32.1 to 24.3 x 10^3 when tested at Con A concentrations of 6.25 ug/ml and 1.56 ug/ml. Ampicillin appeared to have no effect on lymphocyte transformation. In contrast, a depression occurred in stimulation indices in animals challenged with clindamycin. While the numbers of animals studied were small, these data suggest an association between altered lymphocyte transformations and receipt of clindamycin. One important aspect is that these data imply that no antibiotic hypersensitivity was induced in these hamsters following antibiotic challenge.

Distribution of HLA and Blood Group Antigens in Patients

Table 6 shows the distribution of HLA antigens either at the

Table 4. Mean Values of Stimulation Indices of Splenic Lymphocytes from Hamsters Challenged With Clindamycin or Ampicillin

Antigen Tested in vitro	Stimulation Indices following Challenge with Clindamycin				Antigen Tested in vitro	Stimulation Indices following Challenge with Ampicillin			
	Clinda 0.25 mg	Clinda 0.25 mg + CFA[a]	Clinda 0.025 mg	Clinda 0.025 mg + CFA		Ampi 0.25 mg	Ampi 0.25 mg + CFA	Ampi 0.025 mg	Ampi 0.025 mg + CFA
None	4.3[b]	1.9	10.4	13.5	None	2.0	1.4	2.3	2.4
Clindamycin 8 ug/ml	5.5	1.8	3.4	2.2	Ampicillin 8 ug/ml	10.4	1.3	2.6	1.1
Clindamycin 80 ug/ml	4.4	0.9	2.9	2.0	Ampicillin 80 ug/ml	9.9	2.6	1.7	1.7
PPD	2.7	1.5	3.9	2.9	PPD	2.4	1.6	3.0	1.7

[a] Complete Freund's adjuvant.

[b] Numbers expressed as the group mean of scintillation indices recorded when splenic lymphocytes were incubated with the indicated antigen (4 animals/group).

Table 5. Splenic Lymphocytes of Lymphocyte Transformations of Hamsters Challenged with Ampicillin and Clindamycin Without CFA ($\pm$cpm[a] x 10^3)

Mitogen Tested	Antibiotic Administered (mg/kg) Ampi 0.25	Ampi 0.025	Clind 0.25	Clind 0.025	Saline
None	0.1[b]	1.4	0.4	0.7	0.8
Con A (ug/ml)					
6.25	36.6	28.7	3.7[b]	1.3[b]	32.1
1.56	19.2	28.4	11.3	1.6[b]	24.3
0.38	1.5	1.5	7.1	1.0	3.0

[a] Values represent means of scintillation counts of groups each containing four animals.

[b] $p < 0.025$ from test values obtained with lymphocytes obtained from hamsters given ampicillin at concentrations of Con A indicated.

Table 6. HLA Antigen Distribution

Group	Patient Number	1st Sublocus Antigen	2nd Sublocus Antigen	ABO/Rh
	1	3, 10	50	A-
PMC	2	2, 9	15, 17	O-
biopsy	3	2, 29	14, 18	O+
proven	4	-	14, 17	O+
	5	2	7, 12	O
	6	9	18, 27	A+
	7	1, 2	8, 13	B+
	8	1, 28	12, 17	A+
	9	19	7, 50	AB+
NO	10	2	15, 27	A-
PMC	11	10	12, 50	A+
visualized	12	1, 3	17, 50	O+
	13	2, 9	-	O+
	14	3	50	A-

first or second sublocus as determined in 14 patients. Blood group typing is also indicated. Twenty-five patients had received clindamycin and had developed diarrhea. Six patients had proven PMC and eight patients with diarrhea were negative for PMC on sigmoidoscopy. There were no significant HLA antigen associations in the eight patients without PMC. Two of six patients with PMC had HLA type 14 at the second sublocus. The expected frequency for this antigen was 0.35, which indicates a slight increase in this haplotype. There were no abnormal frequencies for any of the ABO or other blood group antigens examined.

Results of Skin Tests in Humans

Skin tests to 8 or 80 ug/0.1 ml saline or clindamycin were performed in six patients with biopsy-proven PMC, and in seven patients with antibiotic-induced diarrhea who did not have their colons visualized. None of these patients demonstrated an immediate reaction (wheal and flare) to clindamycin. Only one patient demonstrated positive delayed responses to commonly employed skin test antigens (Candida, PPD, SK-SD, dermatophytin) when studied 48 to 72 h. These data indicate that our patients were deficient in cell-mediated immunity of the delayed type.

Studies of Abnormal Serum Antibodies

Table 7 shows the results of studying our patients with antibiotic-associated diarrhea, 11 of which were biopsy-proven. No abnormal antibodies of the agglutinating type were found when human erythrocytes were pretreated with clindamycin and patients' sera were added to this system either with or without the addition of complement. These data seem to indicate that there were no abnormal hemagglutinating antibodies to the inducing antibiotics found in their

Table 7. Abnormal Antibodies in Antibiotic-Associated Diarrhea and Colitis

Group	Number of Patients	Rheumatoid Factor	ANA	Ab to RBC's + Clindamycin
Colon visualized				
PMC	11	0	0	0
No PMC	14	3	1	0
Colon not visualized	17	2	1	0

serum. We did not perform these studies following the addition of C. difficile toxin to human erythrocytes. In preliminary studies we also found that C. difficile toxin was not hemolytic to human, porcine, sheep, horse, hamster, or dog erythrocytes. However in the microcytotoxicity test, the toxin when present at a titer of 10^{-2} / ml causes human erythrocytes to hemagglutinate.

The presence of rheumatoid factor and antinuclear antibodies in sera from a few patients was not unusual for this elderly population. Furthermore five patients with rheumatoid factor had rheumatoid arthritis or other collagen-vascular diseases.

Immunofluorescent Studies

Three patients had colon biopsy specimens examined by indirect immunofluorescent techniques. In two of three patients the biopsies showed pseudomembranous enterocolitis while one had a normal biopsy. Colon biopsies of all three patients showed moderate numbers of IgA cells and occasional IgM bearing-plasma cells in the submucosa. Immunofluoresence with IgG, C3 and C4 conjugates (human) were all negative. The results in these three specimens seem to indicate no role for immune-complex deposition in these few patients studied.

Determination of Carcinoembryonic Antigen (CEA)

CEA determinations were performed on sera of 17 patients with antibiotic-associated diarrhea and 15 control subjects. The mean and range of CEA determinations for patients with biopsy-proven PMC clearly indicate that CEA increases during active colitis (Table 8). Patients who had only diarrhea and not PMC on biopsy similarly had an increase in CEA (7.8 ng/ml). However this group mean value and range were lower than that seen in the patients in the biopsy-proven group. In five other patients whose colons were not visualized or biopsied, the lowest mean CEA value (4.3 ng/ml) was found.

Status of Antibodies to C. difficile Toxin in Patients with AAC

Twenty-four patients have successfully recovered from antibiotic-associated colitis. Toxin was found in the stools of these patients in fecal filtrate dilutions ranging from 10^{-1} to 10^{-4}. All stools toxic in the microculture assay were neutralized by C. sordellii antitoxin. Samples of convalescent sera from all 24 patients (obtained two to six weeks after resolution of their diarrhea) were studied for their capability to neutralize partially-purified C. difficile toxin which was produced in BHI broth cultures. No patient's serum reduced the cytotoxicity of these cultural filtrates containing C. difficile toxin even at highest dilution of toxicity. Two of these 24 patients had relapses following vancomycin therapy and even following recovery, no neutralizing antibodies were found in these patients' serum.

Table 8. Carcinoembryonic Antigen in Antibiotic-Associated Diarrhea

Group	Number	Mean CEA (ng/ml)	Range (ng/ml)
Normal controls	15	3.2	0.5 - 4.5
Antibiotic-associated diarrhea			
PMC proven	8	20.7	11.8 - 28.8
No PMC proven	4	7.8	4.3 - 10.6
Colon not visualized	5	4.3	2.1 - 7.2

Two other patients of these 24 patients had C. difficile toxin found in their serum which was obtained when they were acutely ill. The toxin titer in their blood was 10^{-1} and it was neutralized by C. sordellii antitoxin and by heating their serum (56 C x 30 min). Sera from these two patients never subsequently showed any neutralizing antibodies when studied in convalescence.

Sera from 16 of these 24 patients were studied for their capability to agglutinate dilutions of 18 h broth cultures of C. difficile. No patient's serum was found to agglutinate these organisms when studied following manipulation of a variety of incubational and other physical conditions.

Rabbit Immunizations with C. difficile and its Toxin

All seven rabbits immunized with whole C. difficile organisms showed agglutination antibodies with titers ranging from 1:64 to 1:4,096. Sera from the seven rabbits also agglutinated C. sordellii in dilutional titers essentially as high as for C. difficile. As a control test organism, Clostridium innocuum isolates were not agglutinated.

Precipitating antibodies were also ellicited in rabbits immunized with C. difficile toxin which was partially purified by ammonium sulfate precipitation. Rabbits were challenged (Table 2) with either subcutaneous toxin (either heated or unheated, with or without CFA or with the antigen-antibody complex given subcutaneously, or with orally administered C. difficile toxin (heated or unheated, with or without CFA). Most of these methods produced at least one precipitating antibody and others, two or even three lines. There were discrete precipitating lines particularly in the wells which employed C. difficile toxin which was administered by the subcutaneous and/or oral routes. Three of six rabbits given C. difficile toxin intraperitoneally (IP) produced three lines of precipitating antibody. No differences were seen in the precipitating lines whether the antitoxin containing fraction was heated or unheated prior to immunization. None of these antisera neutralized C. difficile toxin in microtiter cytotoxicity tests.

Similarly, in passive radial immunodiffusion assays which were performed in 1% agarose, lines of identity were seen with antisera produced by intravenous administrations of either whole C. difficile organisms or its purified toxin (partially purified C. difficile was contained in the center well). These data suggest that the C. difficile toxin may be protoplasmic as the organisms used in intravenous challenges were extensively washed in buffered saline prior to administration.

The only animal found to possess a limited neutralization effect in its sera for C. difficile toxin was the one challenged with the combination of C. difficile toxin and C. sordellii antitoxin (which were incubated prior to intravenous delivery). Undiluted serum from this animal at eight weeks post-immunization on two occasions produced a 50% reduction in cytotoxicity of a 10^{-2} dilution of crude of C. difficile toxin when tested in the tissue culture assay. These results are encouraging regarding the production of an effective neutralizing antibody.

DISCUSSION

The role of C. difficile in the pathogenesis of antibiotic-associated colitis (AAC) appears well established. This organism was implicated by several groups working independently (4,5,10,18, 20). Inducing antibiotics have included the cephalosporins, tetracyclines, erythromycin, penicillins, aminoglycosides and lincomycins (8,15). The unifying mechanism is the elaboration of a highly lethal toxin which appears to interact very rapidly with cell mucosal surfaces (1). These mucosal cells then rapidly vacuolate and the villous tips degenerate (as occurs in vitro with fibroblast monolayers). The underlying lamina propria is then freely exposed to other organisms and substances within the fecal stream.

Two of our patients had C. difficile type toxin in their blood. This toxin may account for the occasional clinical presentation of "toxemia" in some patients and maybe their encephalopathy. However, we were unable to demonstrate neutralizing, precipitating or agglutinating antibodies in the serum of patients who have recovered upon successful treatment of their AAC. Whether there are other natural immune responses to C. difficile and its toxin is unknown.

No unique host susceptibility has been defined by lymphocyte haplotyping although we found a slight predisposition or co-association with haplotype 14 at the second sublocus in three of our patients with biopsy-proven AAC. Similarly, antibiotics did not induce haptenic antibodies which were complement- and/or noncomplement-dependent as assayed in an erythrocyte system. No increased frequency of abnormal antibodies was found such as rheumatoid factor or antinuclear antibody in patients with antibiotic-associated diarrhea. One interesting aspect of our search for auto-antibodies and antigens was that there were increases in CEA in patients with antibiotic-associated diarrhea and colitis. This is not surprising as serum CEA elevations have been found in other intestinal inflammatory diseases and malignancies. Whether this antigen will prove to be an effective way to sequentially follow patients with AAC following therapy remains to be studied.

The epidemiology of this disease is yet undefined. C. difficile has been isolated from the vaginal vault in 10% to 15% of women sampled in one study (13) and in lesser numbers in fecal samples of normal humans (9). The lack of a selective medium for C. difficile has hampered the discovery of its transmission routes. However, George and Finegold have employed a selective medium which contains cefoxitin and cycloserine (11). We have had some experience with this medium and it appears promising. The employment of this medium may well reveal that there are marked geographical variances in isolation of C. difficile, thus explaining the sporadic reports of AAC. Alternatively, there may be explanations for this occurrence based on varying immunity within our patient population.

Our studies of the immunity in patients with either AAC proven by biopsy or sigmoidoscopy may offer an alternative explanation. The majority of our patients demonstrated defective cell-mediated immunity. We found specific hypersensitive reactions to either clindamycin or ampicillin in only two patients. Quite clearly the large majority of our patients were defective on skin testing to a variety of antigens which indicate their relatively anergic state. Also their lymphocyte transformations in vitro were defective to both nonspecific mitogens (Con A, PHA) and to specific antigens (Candida and SK-SD). Hamsters immunized with sublethal doses of ampicillin or clindamycin with or without CFA demonstrated no hypersensitivity to these antibiotics in lymphocyte cultures. In fact, it appeared that animals challenged with clindamycin had an inhibition of lymphocyte transformations. These data seem to indicate that a hypersensitivity state to the inducing antibiotic is an unlikely explanation for AAC in humans or hamsters.

It may be that antibodies to C. difficile exist prior to infection with C. difficile or are synthesized during infection to defend against C. difficile and its toxin. In our attempts to detect these antibodies against C. difficile or its toxin, several interesting observations were made. First, while it was relatively easy to generate precipitating antibodies to antigens of *C*. difficle, these antibodies were not of a neutralizing type. Multiple routes and combinations of immunization regimens were employed. Precipitating antibodies were frequently generated to partially-purified preparations of the toxin (with or without Freund's adjuvant) either by subcutaneous, intraperitoneal and/or oral administrations in various combinations. Lines of identity were also found in passive immunodiffusion experiments using antisera from animals given either washed whole organisms or the partially-purified toxin of *C*. difficile. These data indicate that *C*. difficile toxin contains ample amounts of protoplasmic toxin. It is also interesting that heated partially purified toxin administered by oral or subcutaneous routes produced similar precipitating antibodies. Previously, heat lability has been one hallmark of this toxin. Heating destroys the toxin's lethal effect following intraperitoneal injection into hamsters, the vascular permeability effects in rabbit skin, and the cytotoxicity for fibroblastic monolayers. This physicochemical property may point the way to the future of using nontoxic vaccines in human populations. Allo et al. (2) have recently demonstrated that hamsters can be passively protected by administrations of *C*. sordellii antitoxin against challenges of antibiotic known to induce lethal colitis or intracecal injections of *C*. difficile toxin. While orally-administered vancomycin in hamsters and humans appears effective in treating AAC (5,6, 8,15), a toxoid approach may be an effective way for eliminating this disease in selective patients.

CONCLUSIONS

These observations indicate patients with AAC have marked impairment in cell-mediated immunity of the delayed type as studied by skin tests to commonly occurring antigens and in vitro lymphocyte cultures. No acute hypersensitivity to clindamycin or ampicillin was found on skin testing or lymphocyte testing with these two antibiotics except in two patients. Patients with AAC showed no uniform HLA haplotyping predisposition or increased incidence of autoantibodies. These patients did have increased incidence of serum CEA during the acute phases of AAC. Sera of two patients with acute AAC produced *C*. difficile-like toxic effects in tissue culture. No patient with AAC was found to have serum antibodies (agglutinating, neutralizing or precipitating) when studied two to six weeks following resolution of this disease.

Immunization of hamsters with sublethal concentrations of ampicillin or clindamycin failed to produce hypersensitivity of splenic lymphocytes to either antibiotic, although clindamycin recipients demonstrated hyporesponsiveness of their lymphocytes to common mitogens.

Partially-purified toxin of C. difficile produced serum precipitating antibodies in rabbits following administration in a variety of routes such as subcutaneous, intraperitoneal, intravenous, and even orally. It did not matter if the toxin was rendered nonlethal by heating prior to administration in terms of antibody responses. No neutralizing antibodies were generated. These data suggest that although the toxin can be manipulated by heating to produce an innocuous toxoid, hamsters do not produce neutralizing antibodies following challenge with this material. Approaches are underway to further characterize C. difficile toxin and ways to generate neutralizing antibodies with other toxoids.

ACKNOWLEDGMENTS

Sponsored in part by the Upjohn Company of Kalamazoo, Michigan and the National Institutes of Health.

LITERATURE CITED

1. Abrams, G.D., M. Allo, G. Rifkin, R. Fekety, and J. Silva. 1978. Mucosal damage due to Clostridium difficile toxin: Similarity to clindamycin-associated typhlitis. The 18th Interscience Conference on Antimicrobial Agents and Chemotherapy. Atlanta, Ga., October.

2. Allo, M., J. Silva, R. Fekety, G. Rifkin, and H. Waskin. 1979. Prevention of clindamycin-induced colitis in hamsters by Clostridium sordellii antitoxin. Gastroent. 76: 351.

3. Axelsen, N.H., J. Kroll, and B. Weeke. 1973. A manual of quantitative immunoelectrophoresis, methods and applications. Scand. J. Immunol. 2 (Suppl. 1) Universitetsforlaget, Oslo.

4. Bartlett, J.G., A.B. Onderdonk, R.L. Cisneros, and D.L. Kasper. 1977. Clindamycin-associated colitis due to a toxin-producing species of Clostridium in hamsters. J. Infect. Dis. 136: 70.

5. Bartlett, J.G., T.W. Chang, M. Gurwith, S.L. Gorbach, and A.B. Onderdonk. 1978. Antibiotic-associated pseudomembranous colitis due to toxin-producing clostridia. New Engl. J. Med. 298: 531.

6. Browne, R.A., R. Fekety, J. Silva, D.I. Boyd, C.O. Work, and G.D. Abrams. 1977. The protective effect of vancomycin on clindamycin-induced colitis in hamsters. Johns Hopkins Med. J. 141: 183.

7. Dykes, P.W. 1972. Immunology of Crohn's disease. Gastroent. 1: 349.

8. Fekety, R. 1979. Prevention and treatment of antibiotic-associated colitis. Microbiology. pp. 276-279.

9. George, W.L., V.L. Sutter, and S.M. Finegold. 1978. Toxigenicity and antimicrobial susceptibility of Clostridium difficile, a cause of antimicrobial agent-associated colitis. Curr. Microbiol. 1: 55.

10. George, W.L., V.L. Sutter, E.J.C. Goldstein, S.L. Ludwig, and S.M. Finegold. 1978. Aetiology of antimicrobial-agent-associated colitis. Lancet 1: 802.

11. George, W.L., V.L. Sutter, D. Citron, and S.M. Finegold. 1979. Selective and differential medium for isolation of Clostridium difficile. J. Clin. Microbiol. 9: 214.

12. Gerfo, P.L., J. Krupey, and H.J. Hansen. 1971. Demonstration of an antigen common to several varieties of neoplasia. Assay using zirconyl phosphate gel. New Engl. J. Med. 285: 138.

13. Hafiz, S., M.G. McEntergart, R.S. Morton, and S.A. Waitkins. 1975. Clostridium difficile in the urogenital tract of males and females. Lancet 1: 420.

14. Harvie, N., S. Ellis, D. Mason, M. Allo, G. Rifkin, J. Silva, and R. Fekety. 1978. Isolation and purification of a Clostridium difficile toxin that causes colitis in the Syrian hamster. The 18th Interscience Conference on Antimicrobial Agents and Chemotherapy. Atlanta, Ga., October.

15. Keighley, M.R.B, D.W. Burdon, Y. Arabi, J. Alexander-Williams, H. Thompson, D. Youngs, M. Johnson, S. Bentley, R.H. George, and G.A.G. Mogg. 1978. Randomised controlled trial of vancomycin for pseudomembranous colitis and postoperative diarrhea. Br. Med. J. 2: 1667.

16. Kraft, S.C., and J.B. Kirsner. 1971. Immunological apparatus of the gut and inflammatory bowel disease. Gastroent. 60: 922.

17. Lusk, R.H., F.R. Fekety, J. Silva, T. Bodendorfer, B.J. Devine, H. Kawanishi, L. Korff, D. Nakauchi, S. Rogers, and S.B. Siskin. 1977. Gastrointestinal side effects of clindamycin and ampicillin therapy. J. Infect. Dis. 135 (Suppl.): S111.

18. Lusk, R.H., R. Fekety, J. Silva, R.A. Browne, D.H. Ringler, and G.D. Abrams. 1978. Clindamycin-induced enterocolitis in hamsters. J. Infect. Dis. 137: 464.

19. Mancini, G., A.O. Carbonara, and J.F. Heremans. 1965. Immunochemical quantitation of antigens by single radial immunodiffusion. Immunochemistry 2: 235.

20. Rifkin, G.D., R. Fekety, J. Silva, and R.B. Sack. 1977. Antibiotic-induced colitis: implication of a toxin neutralized by Clostridium sordellii antitoxin. Lancet 2: 1103.

21. Rifkin, G.D., R. Fekety, and J. Silva. 1978. Neutralization by Clostridium sordellii antitoxin of toxins implicated in clindamycin-induced cecitis in the hamster. Gastroent. 75: 422.

22. Simon, M.R., J. Silva, D. Freier, J. Bruner, and R. Williams. 1977. Tuberculin-specific transfer factor in dogs. Infect. Immun. 18: 73.

23. Tedesco, F.J. 1976. Clindamycin-associated colitis. Am. J. Dig. Dis. 21: 26.

24. Terasaki, P.I., M. Van Diepow, C.I. Davidson, and M.R. Mickey. 1969. Serotyping for homotransplantation XXIV heart transplantation. Amer. J. Cardiol. 24: 500.

SYSTEMIC IMMUNE RESPONSES TO ORAL ANAEROBIC ORGANISMS

Robert J. Genco, Jørgen Slots, Christian Mouton, and
P. Murray

Department of Oral Biology and Periodontal Disease
Clinical Research Center
State University of New York at Buffalo
School of Dentistry
Buffalo, New York

INTRODUCTION

Periodontal diseases such as gingivitis and periodontitis are common infections of man after the fourth decade of life. Gingivitis also effects children and young adults, however, periodontitis, which results in loss of alveolar bone, is much less common in children than in adults. Most forms of periodontal disease represent long standing infections by anaerobic organisms. They are most likely mixed infections and hence, precise information about the infecting organisms is difficult to ascertain. As with most chronic bacterial infections, there is a delicate balance between host defense mechanisms and virulence factors expressed by the bacteria. Although direct effects of the organisms likely account for some of the pathology, the course, severity and eventual outcome of periodontal disease is thought to be determined to a large extent by host responses to the infecting organisms.

The common form of adult periodontitis has been studied in detail and overall features of the disease have been conveniently divided into the following four stages (38): (i) the initial lesion; (ii) the early lesion; (iii) the established lesion; and (iv) the advanced lesion. The initial lesion exhibits features resembling an acute vasculitis with a large number of neutrophils found migrating through the vessels at the junctional epithelium into the gingival crevice. The early lesion is characterized by the presence of a dense infiltrate of small and medium sized lymphocytes immediately subjacent to the gingival sulcus. Most of the lymphocytes found are

B cells although a small percentage are T cells. Pathologic alterations in fibroblasts and loss of connective tissue substance adjacent to subgingival epithelium are found at this stage. The disease subsequently progresses to the established lesion at which time plasma cells predominate in the connective tissue, however, extensive bone destruction has not yet occurred. Some of the features of acute inflammation continue to persist. The advanced lesions are exceedingly complex and resemble in most respects those in other long term chronic inflammatory diseases. In the advanced lesions are many of the features of the established lesion with plasma cells predominating, some acute inflammatory cells present and collagen destruction. The advanced lesion, however, is distinguished from the established lesion by the presence of alveolar bone resorption; at this point the disease is called periodontitis. The microbial flora which accumulates at the gingival margin and in the periodontal pocket serves as the source of inciting agents for periodontal tissue destruction.

The essential role of microorganisms in the etiology of periodontal disease is suggested by human and animal studies. Studies of human periodontal disease show that there are large accumulations of bacteria associated with periodontal tissues. In established periodontitis lesions in adults, Bacteroides asaccharolyticus, Bacteroides melaninogenicus subsp. intermedius, Fusobacterium nucleatum and Actinomyces species are prominent members of the subgingival flora. Representative strains of oral Actinomyces viscosus and Actinomyces naeslundii have been shown to cause periodontal bone loss in conventional hamsters (12) and in germ free rats (13). Animal evidence to support the role of B. asaccharolyticus comes mainly from monkey studies (See this issue, Slots, et al.) in which the numbers of B. asaccharolyticus increase with the severity of disease and when the numbers of subgingival B. asaccharolyticus are reduced, bone regeneration occurs.

A less common form of periodontitis is found in teenagers and young adults and is termed juvenile periodontitis. Often juvenile periodontitis lesions are localized to the first molars and incisors and this disease is called "periodontosis" or localized juvenile periodontitis, abbreviated as LJP. The periodontal or subgingival microflora in LJP shows a predominance of Actinobacillus actinomycetemcomitans and Capnocytophaga species (25,26,33). It appears that there is specificity of the microflora differentiating LJP from the adult form of periodontitis. It is likely that other organisms will be found in other forms of periodontal disease. For example, Loesche et al. (20) found in children with Down's syndrome, which is often complicated by periodontal disease, that the subgingival flora had large numbers of clostridial species.

There were many early reports of a systemic immune response to oral organisms in periodontal disease (6,22). This is not surprising, since periodontal infections result from an accumulation of large numbers of organisms in subgingival sites in contact with the gingiva. Not only is the bacterial mass large and potential antigenic challenge great, but the area of infected gingival tissues surrounding the teeth may reach 40-50 cm^2 and much of the gingival epithelium exposed to organisms is ulcerated and likely allows easy access to immunocompetent cells. In addition, it is well documented that transient bacteremias occur even during procedures like toothbrushing and chewing of food. Organisms that are found in the bloodstream under these circumstances are often those which are recoverable from the subgingival area and hence, likely come from this area. Organisms which gain repeated access to the bloodstream would be expected to induce an immune response.

CELL-MEDIATED IMMUNITY TO ORAL ORGANISMS

Considerable evidence has accumulated which shows that a significant cell-mediated immune response to periodontal organisms occurs in patients with gingivitis and periodontitis. For example, Ivanyi and Lehner (11) and Horton et al. (10) have shown that patients with gingivitis and periodontitis exhibit a lymphoproliferative response to dental plaque and plaque organisms. In addition, Lehner (19) has shown that patients with adult periodontitis and gingivitis respond to periodontal organisms such as F. nucleatum, Bacteroides melaninogenicus and Veillonella. More recently, Patters et al. (29) have shown specificity in the cellular immune response in adult periodontitis. Sixty-two per cent of subjects with adult periodontitis show a lymphoproliferative response to B. asaccharolyticus whereas none of the normals or edentulous patients and only 14% of those with gingivitis showed this lymphoproliferative response. In addition, they showed a marked increase in responsiveness of patients to A. viscosus in subjects with gingivitis and periodontitis, 92% and 77% respectively, of these patients in these two categories have a lymphoproliferative response to A. viscosus, whereas only 20% of normal subjects gave such a response. Since both of these organisms induced little or no response in cord blood and normal subjects showed reduced or minimal response to these organisms, the interpretation of these results is that the lymphoproliferative response is likely specific to antigens in the bacterial preparations used to stimulate the lymphocytes in vitro.

STUDIES OF SERUM ANTIBODIES IN PERIODONTAL DISEASE

Studies of serum antibodies in periodontal disease in the past have been hampered mainly by lack of appropriate oral organisms with which to study the disease-related antibody responses. Recently, two organisms, B. asaccharolyticus and A. actinomycetemcomitans have been identified as prominent organisms in adult periodontitis and localized juvenile periodontitis respectively. Studies of human antibodies to these two organisms has provided evidence of a specific immune response associated with periodontal infection. Studies to be discussed here have been carried out in our laboratories with these two organisms. The serologic groupings of the organisms were assessed with rabbit sera prior to investigating human serum reactions. The human serum reactions were assessed by two-dimensional gel diffusion precipitin analysis to assess antigens to which the humans reacted. The human immune responses were also assessed by ELISA which detects low as well as high level responses and allows identification of the isotype of the antibody.

ANTIBODIES TO BACTERIA IN ADULT PERIODONTITIS

Antibody production to periodontal organisms in adult periodontitis is a prominent response seen to periodontal disease. Topical application of antigens to the gingiva induces a serum antibody response and accumulations of plasma cells containing specific antibody (30,32).

Antibodies to oral organisms have been demonstrated in the serum of patients with periodontal disease. For example, antibodies reactive with A. naeslundii and Actinomyces israelii (8,27), Leptotrichia buccalis (7,9,21,22), Fusobacterium species (15), Treponema microdentium (36), Veillonella alcalescens (6) and Bacterionema matruchotii (8) have been demonstrated in periodontal patients. Some of the studies show direct correlation between antibody titer and severity of disease (6,27), while the others report no clear relationship.

The antigenic analysis of the B. asaccharolyticus and B. melaninogenicus subspecies has provided an interesting and clear cut definition of serologic groupings in this heterogeneous group of organisms. It was found that rabbit antisera directed to oral B. asaccharolyticus strains failed to react with the non-oral strains of B. asaccharolyticus (23,31). Lambe (16) and Lambe and Jerris (17) reported earlier that antisera to the non-oral B. asaccharolyticus did not react with organisms of the B. melaninogenicus subsp. intermedius or B. melaninogenicus subsp. melaninogenicus groups of organisms and antisera to the latter two failed to react with the non-oral B. asaccharolyticus establishing serotypes among the recognized subspecies of B. melaninogenicus.

The definition of a clear cut serologic group consisting of B. asaccharolyticus strains derived from the oral cavity prompted a further investigation of these organisms, and since there were no detectable common antigens between the oral and non-oral strains of B. asaccharolyticus, it was felt that they may be indeed different species. Biochemical analysis and end product analysis revealed that there were few biochemical differences, however, both groups of organisms were asaccharolytic so they are biochemically inactive with respect to carbohydrate fermentation and these tests would not be expected to be helpful in differentiation. More definitive information with respect to these two groups or organisms comes from collaborative studies with Dr. Alan Coykendall in which the GC ratios and DNA homologies clearly showed that oral B. asaccharolyticus may be a different species from the non-oral B. asaccharolyticus. Accordingly, Bacteroides gingivalis has been proposed as the new name for oral B. asaccharolyticus, however, we will refer to these organisms as B. asaccharolyticus of oral source since the proposal for a change in name is under consideration.

Armed with this information we sought to study antibodies directed to oral B. asaccharolyticus using precipitin in gel and ELISA. By gel diffusion, it was found that 40% of adult periodontitis sera had precipitating antibodies to B. asaccharolyticus whereas a smaller but significant percentage of those with gingivitis and normals had antibodies to this organism detectable by precipitin analysis. Better differentiation of antibody levels of patient and control groups was obtained using ELISA. The background antibody levels were determined from a series of sera derived from individuals with no periodontal disease. The samples included umbilical cord sera, as well as sera from infants, young children, adolescents and healthy adults. Antibodies directed to solubilized antigens from oral B. asaccharolyticus by ELISA were titered and the immunoglobulin class determined (24). Umbilical cord sera contained only IgG antibodies and no detectable IgA or IgM attesting to the specificity of ELISA. The infants' sera contained little IgG, IgA or IgM antibody, however, as the age of the group tested increased, isotype specific patterns were detected. IgM antibody levels were first detected and plateaued at adult levels from six months to six years of age. IgG antibody levels reached adult levels only in the adults and IgA levels were constantly increasing, and in this cross-sectional analysis reached the highest levels in the adults. Screening of patients and age matched control sera by ELISA using antigens of oral B. melaninogenicus subsp. intermedius and B. asaccharolyticus showed higher titers to B. asaccharolyticus in the adult periodontitis group but no differences in titers to the B. melaninogenicus subsp. intermedius antigens.

The IgG antibody levels to oral B. asaccharolyticus of patients with adult periodontitis and localized juvenile periodontitis are compared to those of normal subjects. As can be seen in Table 1, the IgG levels of antibody are significantly elevated in patients with adult periodontitis, however, they are at normal levels in patients with localized juvenile periodontitis and lower than normal levels in edentulous subjects. In contrast, IgM antibodies are elevated in the localized juvenile periodontitis patients and at or near control levels in the adult periodontitis patients. IgA antibodies to B. asaccharolyticus were the same in both adult and localized juvenile periodontitis patients and not different from the control levels.

These studies show that there are elevated IgG antibody levels

Table 1. Level[a] of Serum IgG Antibodies Reacting to Oral Bacteroides asaccharolyticus-extracted Antigens in Groups of Patients with Various Periodontal Conditions

Group[b]		Mean EU-G ± SD
Adult periodontitis	n = 34	257.5 ± 468.4[b]
Acute necrotizing ulcerative gingivitis	n = 12	46.0 ± 46.7
Localized juvenile periodontitis	n = 41	60.5 ± 88.8
Post-localized juvenile periodontitis	n = 9	86.8 ± 52.6
Normal adults	n = 56	55.7 ± 64.6

[a] Expressed as ELISA Units (EU) relative to a positive serum reference pool.
[b] Significant difference from Normal Adults (P <.05), Mann-Whitney test.

in patients with adult periodontitis and they correlate with findings of Slots (34) and Tanner et al. (37) of high levels of B. asaccharolyticus found in the lesions of patients with adult periodontitis. The specificity of the immune response to B. asaccharolyticus was assessed by studying the cross-reactions with oral B. melaninogenicus subsp. intermedius and by absorption. Cells of B. asaccharolyticus removed the antibodies detectable by ELISA to B. asaccharolyticus-soluble antigens whereas absorption with B. melaninogenicus subsp. intermedius or A. actinomycetemcomitans failed to absorb this antibody activity.

Antigens involved in the immune response to B. asaccharolyticus and the differential isotype response to B. asaccharolyticus is being studied further to determine if antibodies can provide evidence of disease severity, or act as indicators of impending disease. Further analysis is being made to determine if the antibody levels change with therapy and if they can be used to monitor therapy.

HUMAN SERUM ANTIBODIES TO A. ACTINOMYCETEMCOMITANS

The antibody response to A. actinomycetemcomitans was assessed by screening human sera by gel diffusion tests and it is apparent that humans reacted with distinct patterns to the four reference strains used. Some human sera formed precipitin bands with components of strain Y4 as well as with ATCC strains 29522 and 29524 reacting with at least one and sometimes more than one common antigen shared by these strains. Other human sera reacted strongly with ATCC strain 29523 and failed to react with the other three strains.

Rabbit sera directed to these four strains confirmed that there are at least two serotypes represented among these four strains. We designate these as serotype a, which is represented by the reference strain ATCC 29523, and the other serotype b, which is represented by the other three strains Y-4, ATCC 29522 and ATCC 29524. Reference human and rabbit sera react with at least one antigen specific to these strains, one common to the serotype a and the other common to serotype b. These antigens are heat stable, retaining their antigenicity after boiling at 100 C for 30 min. Patient and control sera were screened by gel diffusion with soluble sonic extracts of all four strains so that immune responses to one or the other serotype would not be missed. In Table 2 the results of the screening of the human sera with representatives of the two serotypes of A. actinomycetemcomitans are given. It can be seen that about 70% of the subjects in the LJP group reacted by forming bands of precipitate with one or the other serotype whereas only 10-20% of subjects with other forms of periodontal disease such as ANUG, post-LJP, GJP or adult periodontitis reacted. Very few subjects who exhibited normal periodontal tissues reacted; these included the normal controls, the non-diseased siblings of the LJP subjects, or edentulous subjects. The precipitin screening studies show that the LJP patients have a statistically significantly higher prevalence of individuals with precipitating antibodies to A. actinomycetemcomitans than other periodontal disease groups or normal individuals.

The disease LJP follows a familial tendency and the antibodies to one or another serotype were also found to follow this familial tendency in five families studied. The results of a typical family studied are shown in Fig. 1. In this gel diffusion pattern the three diseased siblings reacted with one major antigen of A. actinomycetemcomitans strain Y4 whereas the mother and the two nondiseased siblings failed to react. A similar pattern was found for the other families, that is, all the members of the family were diseased or reacted to the Actinobacillus or reacted with either one or the other serotype among the reference strains (Table 3).

The culturing of the A. actinomycetemcomitans was made feasible by the development of a selective medium which allows detection and enumeration of as little as 0.001% of the total flora as A. actinomycetemcomitans (35). Using this medium, samples from a group of periodontally normal individuals, and a group of untreated LJP patients were cultured for A. actinomycetemcomitans. Six to seven gingival or subgingival sites were cultured as well as samples taken from the cheek, tongue and saliva of each subject. Normal subjects (seven out of eight) had no detectable A. actinomycetemcomitans in their subgingival flora and one subject had an average of 0.008% of the subgingival flora composed of A. actinomycetemcomitans. None of the normal subjects had detectable Actinobacillus in their saliva, buccal mucosa or tongue with the exception of the subject who had a small percentage in his subgingival flora. In contrast, all patients with LJP had

Table 2. Serum Antibodies to Actinobacillus actinomycetemcomitans in Periodontal and Control Subjects

Group	n	$\bar{X}$ Age (range)	% of Individuals with Serum Precipitins to: Y4	ATCC 29523	Y4 and/or[b] ATCC 29523
Periodontal patients[a]					
Localized juvenile periodontitis (LJP)	52	20 (13-30)	56%	42%	69%
Generalized juvenile periodontitis (GJP)	12	21 (14-29)	8%	16%	25%
Post-juvenile periodontitis (Post-JP)	9	39 (31-56)	11%	11%	22%
Acute necrotizing ulcerative gingivitis (ANUG)	11	24 (17-32)	9%	9%	17%
Adult periodontitis	48	38 (27-62)	10%	6%	15%
Edentulous	9	55 (49-65)	11%	11%	11%
Control subjects					
Asymptomatic siblings in families with LJP	12	15 (9-23)	0%	8%	8%
Normals	29	29 (20-56)	6%	3%	10%

[a] LJP refers to patients with localized (molar-incisor) form of juvenile periodontitis; GJP, to the generalized form of juvenile periodontitis; post-JP, to those adults (>30 yrs.) with evidence of having had juvenile periodontitis; ANUG, to acute necrotizing ulcerative gingivitis.

[b] Significance of differences in % individuals with serum precipitins to Y4 and/or ATCC 29523 between groups using the Yates' Corrected Chi-square Analysis.

LJP vs. GJP, post-JP and ANUG	$p < 0.025$
LJP vs. adult periodontitis	$p < 0.001$
LJP vs. edentulous	n.s.
LJP vs. asymptomatic siblings	$p < 0.05$
LJP vs. normals	$p < 0.01$

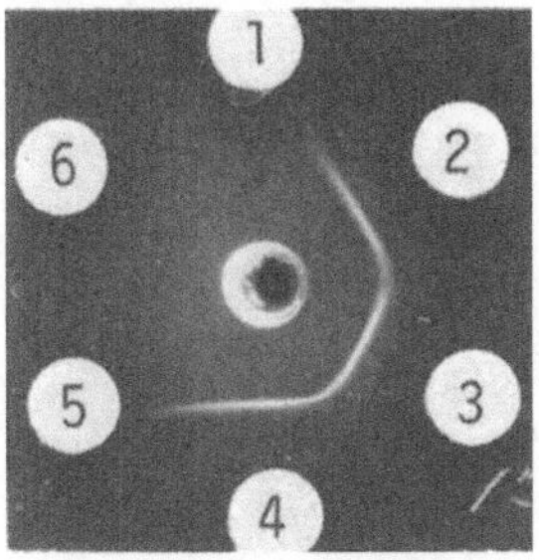

Fig. 1. Gel diffusion test of serum from a family with localized juvenile periodontitis with Actinobacillus actinomycetemcomitans. Central well contains a sonic extract of A. actinomycetemcomitans strain Y4 at 10 mg protein per ml, and the peripheral wells contain serum from members of one family. Well 1, mother, normal periodontium; wells 2,3,and 4 contain sera from siblings affected by LJP; and wells 5 and 6 contain sera from siblings with normal periodontal tissues.

detectable and sometimes high percentages (1-15%) of the total flora of many subgingival areas comprised of A. actinomycetemcomitans. Most of the LJP patients tested for this organism in other oral sites also showed a small but significant percentage of the flora comprised of Actinobacillus. A comparison of the antibody response of the normal and LJP subjects correlated directly with the microbiological findings using the gel diffusion precipitin test. Using ELISA the IgG antibodies to A. actinomycetemcomitans were assessed and little or no antibody of this class was detected in the normal group. In contrast, the LJP group had precipitating antibodies and high levels of IgG and sometimes IgM and IgA antibodies; the latter were detectable by ELISA. In general, there was good correlation between the precipitin test and ELISA in assessment of serum antibody to A. actinomycetemcomitans using sonic extracts of the organism as antigen source. Both assays showed antibody in most LJP patients who had cultivable A. actinomycetemcomitans in their oral flora. Neither assay showed significant antibody in normals.

In summary, the bacteriological and serum antibody studies with A. actinomycetemcomitans show clearly that patients with LJP have a marked serum response mainly of IgG antibodies to Actinobacillus which show serotype specificity. These antibodies correlate with the finding of large numbers of the organisms in the subgingival sites of periodontal infection and likely result from this periodontal infection. In pilot studies with a group of patients with GJP it was found that few or none have IgG antibodies to A. actinomycetemcomitans suggesting that either they do not have the organism, or that they are infected with the organism and have failed to form antibodies to the organism. It is tempting to speculate that low levels of antibodies

Table 3. Serum Precipitins to Type A[a] or Type B Actinobacillus actinomycetemcomitans in Families with LJP

Family	Individual (Age)	Relationship[b]	Diagnosis[c]	Serum Precipitins to *A.* actinomycetemcomitans Type A (29523)	Type B (Y4/29522/29524)
Kol	M (40)	m	LJP	–	+
	D (19)	s	Normal	–	–
	D (17)	d	Normal	–	–
	V (14)	d	LJP	–	+
Buc	M (55)	m	Normal	–	–
	L (19)	d	LJP	–	+
	V (17)	d	LJP	–	+
	G (15)	d	LJP	–	+
	W (12)	s	Normal	–	–
	J (9)	d	Normal	–	–
Mer	K (19)	d	LJP	–	+
	V (17)	d	LJP	–	+
	T (15)	d	LJP	–	+
Spr	R (24)	s	LJP	+	–
	R (22)	s	Normal	–	–
	F (19)	d	Normal	–	–
	R (16)	s	Normal	–	–
	M (13)	d	Normal	–	–
	E (10)	d	Normal	–	–
Cas	M (23)	s	Normal	+	–
	C (20)	s	LJP	+	–
	C (19)	d	Normal	–	–

[a] Reactions with a or b antigens which are serotype specific are noted here. The Type A reference strain is ATCC 29523 and for Type B reference strains Y4, ATCC 29522 and 29524 are used. Reactions with Actinobacillus common antigens occurred in some sera, but they are not tabulated here.

[b] m stands for mother, s for son and d for daughter.

[c] Diagnosis is based upon radiographic evidence of alveolar bone loss.

fail to prevent the disease from becoming localized (as it does in the more common LJP) and the disease then becomes generalized. The localized form is known to go into remission in the late teens or early 20's and again, it is tempting to speculate that the reason it goes into remission is because antibodies are formed.

PATHOGENIC POTENTIAL OF A. ACTINOMYCETEMCOMITANS AND NEUTROPHIL STUDIES

Taichman et al. showed that A. actinomycetemcomitans produces a leukocidin which shows marked toxic activity to human neutrophils with lesser activity on human monocytes (39). Tsai et al. (39) showed that the same set of sera described here from LJP patients and controls have the ability to neutralize this leukocidin. Eighty-nine per cent of the patients with LJP have antibody which neutralizes the leukocidin as compared to around 20-30% of normals and adult periodontitis patients.

THE STUDY OF NEUTROPHIL FUNCTION IN PERIODONTAL DISEASE

Several laboratories, including ours, have been studying the functional capabilities of neutrophils in various forms of periodontal disease. In 1977 Cianciola et al. (3) described a peripheral neutrophil chemotactic defect in 9/9 patients with LJP. Clark et al. (4), Lavine et al. (18), and Van Dyke et al. (40) confirmed a depressed cell-associated neutrophil chemotactic response in patients with LJP. Chemotactic studies of 55 patients with LJP have been reported in these papaers and 81% show neutrophil chemotactic defects. On the other hand, few patients with adult periodontitis show depressed neutrophil chemotactic responses. The function of peripheral neutrophils was assessed in diseased and non-diseased siblings in 14 families in which two or more siblings suffered from juvenile periodontitis. Cianciola et al. (3) report that depressed neutrophil chemotactic responses to several standard chemotactic agents were found not only in the diseased siblings, but also in 9/13 non-diseased siblings. These findings suggest that the depressed neutrophil chemotactic response occurs in the absence of overt periodontal disease and it is likely not secondary to the disease. It is tempting to speculate that the depressed chemotactic response preceeds development of overt LJP, and may even predispose to development of the disease. Longitudinal studies comparing non-diseased siblings with normal neutrophil function, to those with depressed chemotaxis, will be essential in assessing the role of any of the neutrophil dyscrasia observed in the non-diseased siblings. The studies of neutrophil chemotaxis in LJP patients and their families, and the clinical experiments of nature in patients with primary or secondary immunodeficiencies affecting neutrophils, point to a role for this cell in periodontal diseases. It has been known for a number of years that patients with compromised neutrophil function such as those with agranulocytosis (1,14), cyclic neutropenia (5), and the Chediak-

Higashi syndrome (38) often have very severe destructive periodontal disease. These clinical observations, as well as the demonstration of depressed neutrophil chemotaxis in juvenile periodontitis point to the neutrophil as a major protective cell acting against the periodontal microflora.

UNIQUE NEUTROPHIL-ACTINOBACILLUS ANTIBODY INTERACTIONS INVOLVED IN JUVENILE FORMS OF PERIODONTAL DISEASE

Based upon the studies of neutrophils, and of antibodies to the microflora in localized forms of juvenile periodontitis, the following hypothesis is set forth to explain the clinical features of the disease: (i) The depressed neutrophil chemotactic response preceeds overt periodontal infection in certain families. (ii) A subgingival overgrowth of organisms such as A. actinomycetemcomitans occurs which inhibits neutrophil function at the local site by production of a leukocidin. This further depresses the potential for the neutrophil protective function, and predisposes to further overgrowth by this and probably other organisms such as Capnocytophaga. (iii) Alveolar bone loss, connective tissue loss and other features of LJP occur. (iv) At some point an immune response to the A. actinomycetemcomitans antigens including the leukocidin, and heat stable serotype antigens occurs, with serum antibody production. The antibodies inhibit the leukocidal activity of the organism, and other antibodies may also be bactericidal and opsonic leading to restoration of the protective capabilities of the local neutrophil. This and possibly other protective factors lead to resolution of the infection and the disease goes into remission. In the event that antibodies do not form, the disease progresses to the generalized form.

Several features of this hypothesis of the unique host bacterial interactions in LJP need to be proven; however, they are approachable experimentally. Some of the questions that remain are the following: (i) What is the cause of the depressed neutrophil in chemotaxis found in patients with juvenile periodontitis? Is it genetic or environmental (caused by subclinical infection with bacteria or viruses) or both? (ii) What is the nature of the depressed neutrophil chemotactic response seen in juvenile periodontitis? Is it a homogeneous defect, does it vary with the patient? What is the biochemical basis of the reduced locomotory response? (iii) How do the infecting anaerobes such as A. actinomycetemcomitans and Capnocytophaga species, as well as others found in lesions of LJP patients, lead to tissue destruction? (iv) What is the basis of the strong antibody response seen to A. actinomycetemcomitans in LJP? What is the precise role of these antibodies in the disease process?

IMMUNOLOGIC PROFILE OF PERIODONTAL PATIENTS

A summary of immune responses and phagocytic cell functional aberrations is provided in Table 4. From the studies of immune re-

Table 4. Immunologic Profile of Periodontal Patients

Response or Function	Patient Group: Gingivitis	Adult Periodontitis	Localized Juvenile Periodontitis
Serum antibodies	Present to many oral organisms at low levels Elevated to Actinomyces	Elevated IgG antibodies to *A.* viscosus Elevated IgG antibodies to *B.* asaccharolyticus	Elevated IgG serum, precipitins and antitoxin activity to *A.* actinomycetemcomitans
Neutrophil chemotaxis	Normal	Normal; elevated in some	Depressed in 70-80% Occasional patients with depressed monocyte chemotaxis
Cellular immunity	*A.* viscosus >90% positive *B.* asaccharolyticus 15% positive Dental plaque positive	*A.* viscosus 80% positive *B.* asaccharolyticus 60% positive Dental plaque strong positive	Strong response to *A.* viscosus, *B.* asaccharolyticus, Capnocytophaga

actions in periodontal diseases of the past decade, clear differences between diseased patients' immune reactivity and that of normal controls is apparent suggesting that periodontal infections are associated with significant systemic immune reactions. Furthermore, it is becoming increasingly clear that various clinically distinct forms of periodontal disease can be characterized by distinct immunologic profiles. In gingivitis, low levels of serum antibodies to many organisms are seen and elevated antibody levels to Actinomyces species, a predominant subgingival organism in this condition, is apparent. The lymphoproliferative response to A. viscosus is elevated while the response to B. asaccharolyticus, an organism not common in gingivitis, is low. In contrast, patients with the adult form of periodontitis have elevated serum antibodies as well as lymphoproliferative responses to B. asaccharolyticus, an organism often isolated in large numbers from the periodontal lesions of these patients. In gingivitis and adult periodontitis, which are related conditions differing in severity and affecting most of the population, neutrophil chemotactic function is often normal. In contrast, subjects with juvenile periodontitis, either the localized or the generalized form, often have depressed neutrophil chemotactic responses which may account for their unusual susceptibility to periodontal disease.

Patients with the localized form of juvenile periodontitis have elevated antibody levels to A. actinomycetemcomitans, an organism which is prominent in their lesions.

The precise role of the antibodies in the etiopathology of periodontal disease is unclear in gingivitis and the related adult form of periodontitis. It is tempting to speculate, however, that the depressed neutrophil function in juvenile periodontitis accounts at least in part for the unusual susceptibility of these patients to periodontal infection, and that subsequent production of antibodies to the infecting organisms such as A. actinomycetemcomitans leads to remission of the disease, a feature which may account for its localization.

LITERATURE CITED

1. Bauer, W.H. 1946. The supporting tissues of the tooth in acute secondary agranulocytosis (arsphenamin neutropenia). J. Dent. Res. 25: 501.

2. Behni, T., C.C. Tsai, W. McArthur, N.S. Taichman, and R.J. Genco. 1979. Inhibition of Y4 leukotoxic activity by sera from juvenile periodontitis patients. J. Dent. Res. 58A: Abstr. 116.

3. Cianciola, L.J. 1979. Neutrophil chemotaxis in non-diseased siblings. J. Dent. Res. 58A: Abstract.

4. Clark, R.A., R.C. Page, and G. Wilde. 1977. The defective neutrophil chemotaxis in juvenile periodontitis. Infect. Immun. 18: 694.

5. Cohen, D.W., and A.L. Morris. 1961. A periodontal manifestation of cyclic neutropenia. J. Periodont. 32: 159.

6. Evans, R.T., S. Spaeth, and S.E. Mergenhagen. 1966. Bactериocidal antibody in mammalian serum to obligatory anaerobic gram negative bacteria. J. Immun. 97: 112.

7. Genco, R.J., P.A. Mashimo, G. Krygier, and S.A. Ellison. 1974. Antibody-mediated effects on the periodontium. J. Periodont. 45: 330.

8. Gilmour, M.N., and R.J. Nisengard. 1974. Interaction between serum titer to filamentous bacteria and their relationship to human periodontal disease. Arch. Oral Biol. 19: 959.

9. Hawley, C.E., and W.A. Falker, Jr. 1975. Antigens of Leptotrichia buccalis II. Their reaction, complement fixing IgM in human serum. J. Periodont. Res. 10: 216.

10. Horton, J.E., J.J. Oppenheim, and S.E. Mergenhagen. 1974. The role for cell-mediated immunity in the pathogenesis of periodontal disease. J. Periodont. 45: 351.

11. Ivanyi, L., and T. Lehner. 1970. Stimulation of lymphocyte transformation by bacterial antigens in patients with periodontal disease. Arch. Oral Biol. 15: 1089.

12. Jordan, H.V., and P.H. Keyes. 1964. Aerobic gram positive filamentous bacteria as etiologic agents of experimental periodontal disease in hamsters. Arch. Oral Biol. 9: 401.

13. Jordan, H.V., R.J. Fitzgerald, and H.R. Stanley. 1965. Plaque formation and periodontal pathology in gnotobiotic rats infected with an oral actinomycete. Am. J. Pathol. 47: 1157.

14. Kostman, R. 1975. Infantile genetic agranulocytosis. Acta. Paedtr. Scand. 64: 362.

15. Kristoffersen, T., and T. Hofstad. 1970. Antibodies in humans to an isolated antigen from oral fusobacteria. J. Periodont. Res. 5: 110.

16. Lambe, D.W. 1974. Determination of Bacteroides melaninogenicus serogroups by fluorescent antibody staining. Appl. Micro. 28: 561.

17. Lambe, D.W., and R.J. Jerris. 1976. Description of a polyvalent conjugate and a new serogroup of Bacteroides melaninogenicus by fluorescent antibody staining. J. Clin. Micro. 3: 506.

18. Lavine, W.S., E.G. Maderazo, J. Stolman, P.A. Ward, R.B. Cogan, I. Greenblatt, and P.B. Robertson. 1979. Impaired neutrophil chemotaxis in patients with juvenile and rapidly progressing periodontitis. J. Periodont. Res. 14: 10.

19. Lehner, T. 1972. Cell-mediated immune responses in oral diseases; a review. J. Oral Pathol. 1: 39.

20. Loesche, W.J., R.N. Hockett, and S.A. Syed. 1972. The predominant cultivable flora of tooth surface plaque removed from institutionalized subjects. Arch. Oral Biol. 17: 1311.

21. Mashimo, P.A., R.J. Genco, and S.A. Ellison. 1976. Antibodies reactive with Leptotrichia buccalis in human serum from infancy to adulthood. Arch. Oral Biol. 21: 277.

22. Mergenhagen, S.E., W.C. DeAraujo, and H.E. Vara. 1965. Antibody to Leptotrichia buccalis in human serum. Arch. Oral Biol. 10: 29.

23. Mouton, C., J. Slots, and R.J. Genco. 1979. Serology of Bacteroides melaninogenicus (BM) by the indirect fluorescent antibody technique (IFAT). J. Dent. Res. (Special Issue) 58A: Abstr. 56.

24. Mouton, C., J. Slots, and R.J. Genco. 1979. Serum antibodies to oral Bacteroides melaninogenicus ss. intermedius (BMI) in humans. Am. Soc. Micro. Abstr. EH8.

25. Newman, M.G., S.S. Socransky, E.D. Savitt, D.A. Propas, and P. Crawford. 1976. Studies on the microbiology of periodontosis. J. Periodont. 7: 373.

26. Newman, M.G., and S.S. Socransky. 1977. Predominant cultivable microbiota in periodontosis. J. Periodont. Res. 12: 102.

27. Nisengard, R.J., and E.H. Beutner. 1970. Immunologic studies of periodontal disease. V. IgG type antibodies and skin test responses to Actinomyces and mixed oral flora. J. Periodont. 41: 149.

28. Page, R.C., and H.E. Schroeder. 1976. Pathogenesis of inflammatory periodontal disease. Lab. Invest. 83: 235.

29. Patters, M.R., R.J. Genco, M.J. Reed, and P.A. Mashimo. 1976. Blastogenic response of human lymphocytes to oral bacterial antigens. Comparison of individuals with periodontal disease to normal and edentulous subjects. Infect. Immun. 14: 1213.

30. Ranney, R.R. 1970. Specific antibody in gingiva and submandibular nodes of monkeys with allergic periodontitis. J. Periodont. Res. 5: 1.

31. Reed, M.J., J. Slots, C. Mouton, and R.J. Genco. 1980. Antigenic studies of oral and non-oral black pigmented Bacteroides strains. Infect. Immun. (Submitted).

32. Rizzo, A.A., and C.T. Mitchell. 1966. Chronic allergic inflammation induced by repeated deposition of antigen in rabbit gingival pockets. Periodont. 4: 5.

33. Slots, J. 1976. The predominant cultivable organisms of juvenile periodontitis. Scand. J. Dent. Res. 84: 1.

34. Slots, J. 1977. The predominant cultivable microflora of advanced periodontitis. Scand. J. Dent. Res. 85: 1114.

35. Slots, J., H.S. Reynolds, and R.J. Genco. 1980. Actinobacillus actinomycetemcomitans in periodontal disease in man. I. A cross-sectional microbiological investigation. Infect. Immun. (Submitted).

36. Steinberg, A.D., and S.N. Gershoff. 1968. Quantitative differences in spirochetal antibody observed in periodontal disease. J. Periodont. 39: 286.

37. Tanner, A.C.R., C. Haffer, G.T. Bratthall, R.A. Visconti, and S.S. Socransky. 1979. A study of bacteria associated with advancing periodontitis in man. J. Clin. Periodont. 6: 278.

38. Temple, T.R., H.R. Kimball, S. Kakehashi, and C.R. Amen. 1972. Host factors in periodontal disease: Periodontal manifestations of Chediak-Higashi syndrome. J. Periodont. Res. 7: 26.

39. Tsai, C.C., W. McArthur, T. Behni, B.F. Hammond, and N.S. Taichman. 1979. Extraction and partial characterization of a leukotoxin from a plaque derived gram negative microorganisms. Infect. Immun. 25: 427.

40. Van Dyke, T.E., H. Horoszewicz, L.J. Cianciola, and R.J. Genco. 1980. Neutrophil chemotaxis dysfunction in human periodontitis. Infect. Immun. 27: 124.

CLINICAL SUMMARY OF CONFERENCE

Joseph Silva, Jr.

Department of Internal Medicine
Division of Infectious Diseases
University of Michigan Medical Center
Ann Arbor, Michigan 48109

A summary of this conference is quite a challenge. Clinicians look at basic microbiological data differently than microbiologists because we are obviously confronted with different problems. I learned a great deal in preparing my comments. I've taken the liberty to separate the presentations according to how I viewed the various topics. I think the best place to start is at the patient's bedside with the clinician.

Dr. Lambe addressed the key essentials if a microbiological laboratory is to adequately support the clinician. And, all the things I heard in the last three days indicate that many in attendance are working towards this goal. The essentials are: to isolate the important organisms from a bacteriologically congested specimen, to identify the organisms accurately, and to give antibiotic susceptibility data that is reliable to the clinician. The clinician is the one that is often going to "drop the ball". "Sample procurement" appears as an easy task for laboratory workers, but for most clinicians it's burdensome. The task is to bypass the background flora. The sample should be collected deep, obviously by a syringe technique, or sterile catheter, if fluid is present; but if none is present, a two swab technique is the technique of choice. The place we frequently fail is transporting the specimen from the bedside, operating room, or clinic to the laboratory. Somehow, we have to improve techniques of transporting samples to a central laboratory. I wish one of you would take up this challenge and invent some type of dye that can be placed in a carrying medium, so that once the system is open, a color fuse is triggered in 20 minutes so that the specimen will turn a very nice red or blue color to recognize that the specified time is exceeded. Towards this goal, Dr. Chan presented a new cultural system that I found intriguing. I believe some of us should employ it who do not wish to incur the expense of a glove box or other systems.

Dr. Holdeman's comments were very interesting. I don't know why physicians agonize about naming new species; I find it very interesting. The academicians need to remain a step or two ahead of the practicing physician. And I think many physicians welcome the new names. It brings some excitement and vigor to their practice. Dr. Holdeman's discussion, particularly of the new speciations, was very exciting. We need to move out of this bacteriological dark age and move into a position so that we can readily classify an organism. Once the properties are known, clinicians can often provide more meaningful specimens. These newly named organisms will obtain a personality so they have a clinical Gestalt for the clinician just as they relate to the pneumococcus, or staphylococci, etc. So I urge you to keep moving in this direction.

It's also interesting to me that some of the newer named genera and species, such as Capnocytophaga, Bacteroides disiens, and Bacteroides bivius would never have been discussed in papers by Drs. Williams or Hill if they weren't appropriately given a name. And I gave up counting how many times I heard Bacteroides asaccharolyticus. This is a good example how a new name has now given credence to periodontal disease studies.

I'm not going to discuss much of the antibiotic data presented by Mr. Laslie and Dr. Lambe. More defined mechanics for developing a standardized disk method for antibiotic susceptibility testing of anaerobes are desperately needed. I enjoyed their harlequin colored slides. They were beautiful and I think more antibiotic data should be presented in that fashion.

Dr. Sanders came over from New Orleans and, in a "machine-gun" fashion, presented much antibiotic susceptibility data. I think we should look closely at his data in comparison to patterns which exist in our hospitals. He studied approximately 800 isolates of anaerobes. I'm worried about some of the trends that I detect in this antibiotic susceptibility data. His MIC's of B. fragilis for carbenicillin are very high; others have not noted this degree of resistance. I think it also demonstrates how the cephalosporins, particularly cephalothin and cephamandole inhibit many of the anaerobes in vitro. This point should be stressed to our surgical colleagues since they sometimes fly in a bacteriological void and just believe that the cephalosporins are only adequate for aerobic Gram-negative rods. I think one important point of Dr. Sanders' data was the resistance of Fusobacterium, Eubacterium, and Propionibacterium to metronidazole. He also stressed that drainage and antibiotic therapy aimed at specific organisms are important, and I certainly agree with these concepts. Furthermore in the discussion period he made a startling observation that of 17 patients with lung abscess who were treated with metronidazole a favorable response rate of only 30% was seen. This, I believe, is less than most other clinicians see. He should probably look at the mechanism of how metronidazole penetrates the lung and gets into the sputum. Are there inhibitors of the bactericidal activity of metronidazole in the lung fluids or in the sputum? Clearly, in other clinical situations such as treatment of brain abscess and for prophylactic use before colonic surgery, metronidazole has been of value against anaerobes.

Dr. DelBene gave a nice presentation on the beta-lactamases of B. fragilis and also of other anaerobes. I was startled by some of the frequencies of plasmid carriage he noted, for example, 93% of B. fragilis isolates carried plasmids. Obviously, not every plasmid is transporting antibiotic resistance. He also said that over half the isolates of Bacteroides melaninogenicus, and 30% of clostridia carry plasmids. It is obvious that antibiotics were around prior to man identifying them. Organisms have developed so that they can produce enzymes which protect the organisms from an antibiotic produced by another microbial group. I don't believe the anaerobes are different from other groups of organisms in which emergence of antibiotic resistance is apparent. Therefore, more knowledge about the lactamases that are found in these organisms is very important. Some of the newer agents such as clavulinic acid can inhibit some enzymes. For these reasons some of the semi-synthetic penicillins like cloxacillin, or the new cephalomycin, cefoxitin, may be useful.

Dr. DelBene also gave an excellent review of the clinical relevance of beta-lactamase producing strains found in the literature. He addressed some of the abdominal models such as described by Louie et al., and Thadepalli's clinical study from Cook County Hospital where they had over 100 cases of penetrating abdominal wounds. These data suggest that beta-lactamases must be considered in current therapy.

I thought Dr. Moore gave an excellent talk about fecal flora and future trends concerning grants. I think it can be accepted that we probably know more about the lunar surface than we know about the anaerobic flora of a substance that all of us produce daily, but most of us intellectually ignore. The studies of anaerobic fecal flora of stool samples that he presented were difficult to accomplish. The one thing that I am going to urge my clinicians to think about is the large and variable number of organisms found in stool samples. Dr. Moore mentioned that the number of organisms per gram wet weight of feces is 5×10^{10}. This density prompted him to comment that no one should ever feel alone in this world. It is commonly stated in standard textbooks and the pharmaceutical literature that Bacteroides fragilis is the most common anaerobe in the stool. And yet, in a few fecal samples his group studied, Bacteroides fragilis was 29th in the list of commonly-occurring organisms. In fact, Bacteroides vulgatus was the most commonly-occurring organism in the two different study groups. The marked increase that occurs in flora numbers when passing from the ileum to the cecum was also important to note. Lastly, he mentioned the various alterations that occur in the flora with stress and I'm a firm believer in this concept. We likely do not have any bacterial or fungal population in our body that is the same day to day. He just showed a few examples of how numbers of these organisms can vary. Probably when the bottom line comes in on these data, it's going to be like looking at the Holland Tunnel in New York City with a varying traffic going in and out.

Dr. Gale Hill presented some excellent data concerning the anaerobic flora in the female genital tract. A lot of competition occurs in this ecological niche. I think she's quite right, we have to move from the days of just thinking that lactobacilli and streptococci are the major flora and that simple pH changes determine the floral content. She showed in her cultural data that there are many different anaerobes within the genital tract, often eight to nine different anaerobic genera in each cultural sample. Clearly this site is a dynamic system. We currently have only a small inkling of the complexity; some data indicating a decrease in aerobes before menstruation, I think, highlight these changes. In this setting B. fragilis, although not a prominent organism in the vaginal tract, clearly is a very important pathogen.

Dr. Nichols presented an excellent discussion concerning anaerobic infections in the surgical patient. I think he brought up two very important points for us. The first is that the stomach may not be the efficient digester of bacteria as many may believe. Gastric contents contain many anaerobes. We should probably keep reassessing the normal content of anaerobes in these cavities of various patient populations. We may define subgroups that need one type of antibiotic prophylaxis versus others that don't need any. He stressed several times that parasurgical infections are caused by two to five different anaerobic genera per patient. His studies on antibiotic prophylaxis are very interesting. He showed the data from an old study in which neomycin and erythromycin were given at one and two o'clock in the afternoon and 11 o'clock at night preceding colonic surgery. With this regimen, both aerobic and anaerobic flora of the stool were reduced by 3 to 4 logarithms. This treatment is now referred to as the Condon-Nichols regimen. It is prescribed pre-operatively in many hospitals throughout the United States before colonic surgery.

Dr. Nichols also showed data from a recently published study which he termed VA Study Part II. The three prophylactic regimens given pre-operatively included cephalothin alone, versus (2) oral neomycin and erythromycin, with or (3) without, intravenous cephalothin. Here again he showed that the key in reducing para-operative infection was to achieve levels of antibiotics in the lumen of the gut which reduced bacterial numbers. A 6% rate of post-operative infection was found with neomycin and erythromycin (with or without cephalothin) versus 39% when cephalothin was given alone. I think these recent data will be widely quoted. As an aside, many in this audience have provided data for Dr. Nichols and his colleagues to capitalize on, as he indicated in his talk, he is an anaerobic prostelyte. You couldn't have a better proponent of anaerobic bacteriology, and he'll spread the word to his surgical colleagues.

In the same theme, Dr. Onderdonk discussed an experimental model for abscess formation. These elegant studies showed that there is synergism between aerobes and anaerobes. The cooperation between these organisms must be a fantastic event, not only in causing disease, but also in abetting anaerobes in whatever they were intended to normally do on our body surfaces. I think his use of antibiotic probes like clindamycin and gentamicin have demonstrated the biphasic aspects to these infections. The interesting thing to me is his collaboration with Dr. Kasper in terms of working out the mechanism. What is unique about Bacteroides fragilis in causing these infections? I don't know if Bacteroides fragilis has a capsule. From their data one recognizes that whatever is on the outer surface, capsule or not, has a very important role in terms of making this species of Bacteroides very virulent. Dr. Onderdonk's recent data, concerning metronidazole in this model is exciting. He found that this drug reduced the numbers of E. coli and Bacteroides fragilis within the artificially induced intra-abdominal abscess. More work is needed to explore the antibiotic effect of metronidazole for Gram-negative aerobic bacilli.

An area to be discussed by Dr. Danielsson is that of the serological responses reported in anaerobic disease and periodontal disease. However, I do have several brief comments on a few of these papers. The first comment concerns the excellent discussion by Dr. Lauwers concerning Campylobacter enteritis. I believe that every large laboratory should be looking for Campylobacter jejuni which is a common cause of diarrhea. Clinically it acts like many of the so-called viral diarrheas; the clue is that the patient has notable fever and more abdominal cramps. Bile staining of stools begins the sequence and then bloody diarrhea intervenes. Unfortunately, many of these children develop disseminated disease with endocarditis, peritonitis, and reactive arthritis. We have to alert our clinicians to the existence of this new type of disease. It's a treatable cause of diarrhea and responds nicely to erythromycin, tetracycline, chloramphenicol, etc. Often when clinicians deal with patients who have bacillary sepsis, the agents frequently employed are penicillin, cephalothin, or ampicillin. Campylobacter is very often resistant to these antibiotics. The history is important in anticipating this diagnosis. Recently the CDC has described an outbreak of Campylobacter in abattoir workers. Historical points to consider are: do they live on a farm; do they have a sick dog; do they work around a meat-oriented industry, such as a slaughter house?

The data presented by Dr. Danielsson concerning the role of anaerobes in Crohn's disease was provocative. This disease is searching for a pathogen. My own bias is there has to be an organism lying either at the gut surface or in the stool that is provoking granulomatous formations. He discussed the various etiopathogenic mechanisms that are potential candidates to cause this disease. I found his data concerning the effects of azothioprine and 6-mercaptopurine on various anaerobes very interesting. He found that Peptostreptococcus and Fusobacterium varium and Fusobacterium necrophorum are sensitive to very high concentrations of these drugs. We have recently looked at the bactericidal activity of methotrexate on several genera of anaerobes, and found that they don't have carrier proteins to transport these very "weak" antibiotics across their membranes and therefore do not have much, if any, antibiotic properties. Dr. Danielsson's bacteriological effects may depend on new mechanisms which effect metabolic activities besides those of antibacteriosis. We should begin studying some of our cancer patients in terms of their mechanisms of diarrhea. As he showed in some beautiful fluorescent slides, immunoglobulin production at the mucosal surface is very active in Crohn's disease. His data concerning metronidazole may also point the way in eventually working out the mechanism of this disease. While he did not have much control on the fecal flora of his controls, this antibiotic reduced the fecal flora by several logarithms in his patients with Crohn's disease.

The periodontal papers were exciting. I never knew there was so much work in both immunity and anaerobic microflora associated with this disease. The build-up of plaques and the number of organisms that Dr. Williams demonstrated to occur over 24 hours in an experimental animal was astounding. And the transmission electron micrograph showing organisms contained in a dental plaque was truly amazing. The models of dentogingival disease that Drs. Slots and Genco showed should eventually provide the answer. The improvement in cataloging anaerobic organisms such as Capnocytophaga is an important advance. Dr. Genco also showed that periodontal disease can lead to alterations in immunological responses of circulating leukocytes. No longer should we view gingivodental disease as only a superficial illness.

Serology of anaerobic infections is the way that microbiology has to move into the future. We have to move away from identifying these organisms by their footprints of metabolic activity. But rather we need to identify them with other techniques that we've heard today ranging from passive hemagglutination, the direct fluorescent antibody technique to gel diffusions, employing electric current or not, antigen binding, or ELISA techniques. The onset of antibody responses in patients with anaerobic infections occurred within three to five days in studies presented by Dr. Danielsson, Dr. Lambe, and Dr. Rissing.

In summary, I found this to be a very exciting conference. I learned a great deal throughout the day and from discussions with course participants. I know that many attending this conference have similar feelings. And we thank you, the audience, for your good questions.

MICROBIOLOGICAL SUMMARY OF CONFERENCE

Dan Danielsson

Department of Clinical Microbiology and Immunology
Central County Hospital
S-701 85 Orebro, Sweden

I didn't realize what I had agreed to when I promised to make the microbiological summary, but when I saw the program, I was also very tempted because it had a content that really attracted me. During the last three days, we have been sitting for approximately 20 h listening to various aspects of anaerobes and anaerobic infection. I recall a story about a young boy whose father was a microbiologist, and this father used to work a bit on Sundays. One Sunday morning he took his young boy with him. While the father was doing some work in the lab, he let his young boy look at some slides in the microscope, and the boy saw some tiny blue rods. He asked his father what type of bacteria this was, and he said, they are diphtheroids. The boy was pleased with this and he looked at another slide and saw some other kinds of blue rods, and he again asked his father what bacteria they were. The father looked in the microscope and said they are diphtheroids. And the boy looked at a third slide and again he saw some blue rods that looked a little bit different. And so he had to ask his father, and he said well, they are anaerobic diphtheroids. "But Daddy," said the boy, "are diphtheroids allowed to look like whatever they want to?" I thought this simple story might well form the basis for a microbiological summary of this conference.

It's very important for us active in a field like anaerobic bacteriology which is still rapidly growing to come together and get a few things straightened out. And I really think that this conference has managed especially by bringing all the microbiologists together with the clinicians and dentists. That has been a very good blend. Dwight Lambe has commented now and then about continuing education, and I must admit, it has been continuing education for me for three days.

On the first morning of this conference, Dr. Holdeman took us on a most interesting trip in her lecture of newer anaerobic species. And she brought up a most important question, what is a species? She gave several examples on how the species have changed their names during the years. Dr. Holdeman stressed how important it is that we give the organisms the right medium to grow on so we can recognize them. It sounds logical and simple but we all know how difficult it can be many times. But we must take this as the platform from which we operate. Speciation is very important and we need to recognize what we see. And we not only need, we must recognize the individual organisms; and then Dwight Lambe stressed this also today. And this was also in Dr. Lambe's introductory lecture on cultivation of clinical specimens. And he beautifully illustrated the difference in growth on commercial media and freshly prepared media, and the importance of using pre-reduced media for biochemical studies. This is one of the prerequisites for successful growth of anaerobes. We all know this, and we must try to live up to it. Also clinical specimens must be properly collected. Dr. Silva has very nicely commented on that.

Dr. Nichols stressed how anxious the surgeon is to get the quick answer. And Dr. Lambe pointed out that we must not forget to Gram stain the clinical specimen.

We have heard during this conference several presentations on rapid methods. Dr. Phillips described how a preliminary diagnosis could be done of anaerobic infections by analysis of specimens with gas chromatography. And Kasper's rapid identification of specific antibodies against what we now have been calling the capsular polysaccharide. The capsular polysaccharide of B. fragilis has a great impact on rapid diagnosis. Dr. Rissing described the ELISA technique and how it also can be put into a practical situation.

Antibiotic susceptibility testing of anaerobes has its own inherent problems. We all know that we in clinical microbiology are responsible for routine testing, and we know the practical problems. We really need standardized methods for this. Mr. Laslie's and Dr. Lambe's report on the standardized disk technique was very interesting. I'm most grateful for the handout on the method they gave us. It will make it much easier for us to go home and compare the techniques we currently are using. In some laboratories it's considered that it's not very important to do sensitivity testing against anaerobes, but the reports here during this conference clearly point out that it is important. We are now facing, for example, clinically significant infections with B. fragilis strains which can be resistant to antibiotics which we rely upon. A resistance is coming against clindamycin, chloramphenicol, and metranidazole. It doesn't astonish me at all that they develop resistance.

Dr. Silva has commented on Dr. DelBene's most interesting report on the clinical significance of beta-lactamases. Something else that beta-lactamases are responsible for is resistance of B. fragilis against beta-lactam antibiotics. There is disagreement about the interaction of beta-lactam producers in mixed infections, and certainly they play a role especially in the compromised host.

This conference has had a series of excellent lectures by Drs. Williams, Slots, and Hill on normal flora of oral cavity, the gastrointestinal tract, and the genital tract. The genital anaerobic flora is unknown, which bothers clinicians. Many genital infections are not caused by the standard aerobic pathogens.

I regret that the impressive work carried out at the VPI Anaerobe Laboratory on the gastrointestinal flora has ceased because of lack of financial support. We now are at the stage when we try to treat patients with chronic diseases. It has been said to me that HLA typing would not have been possible if the surgeons had not started to make transplantations of kidneys. We know what an impact of new biological understanding HLA typing has provided. I understand it scares people when they take part of the very impressive data Ed Moore presented. But looking at the effects of therapy and trying to correlate this, for example, to the change of fecal flora, you must understand that we very often feel like amateurs compared to what they can accomplish at VPI. Important findings on juvenile periodontitis and localized or generalized gingivitis were presented. I really appreciated Dr. Slots' presentation on the monkey model, not because he had Swedish made equipment to measure bone loss in the monkeys, but he clearly illustrated that in this monkey model, B. asaccharolyticus is etiologically important and that was also beautifully illustrated by Dr. Williams that B. asaccharolyticus is important in periodontal disease. These data are similar to chronic inflammatory disease of the gastrointestinal tract.

Nearly two days of this conference has been dealing with immune response in infections with anaerobes and serology. And the design of this program was laboratory aspects, pathogenicity, human immune response, and serology, and this conference has given us what it promised. Dr. Silva gave an excellent presentation about pseudomembranous colitis.

Dr. Genco presented impressive work on the immune response of patients with periodontal diseases. It is clear from his presentation that immune responses both cellular and humoral accompany periodontal infections. In adult periodontitis, immunity to Bacteroides asaccharolyticus develops, and in juvenile periodontitis a marked antibody response to Actinobacillus actinomycetemcomitans is seen. The role of these antibodies remains to be elucidated. Dr. Genco suggested a protective role is likely since antibody-neutrophil interactions appear to provide major protective responses against the pathogenic oral flora in periodontal disease. Serology and immunology are techniques that have specificity built in them that are advantageous to us. And that's also why this program has been designed because Dr. Lambe had the feeling that these topics should be covered. Dr. Rissing gave an excellent presentation of the ELISA method.

Dr. Lambe gave an update on the serology of Bacteroidaceae. We must chemically define those antigens which are important, antigens which take part in the immune response, antigens which are important for serological diagnosis, etc.

Kasper's work of antigens of encapsulated strains of Bacteroides was interesting.

Dr. Onderdonk described the capsular polysaccharide. Now, we have animal models where we can let this organism adapt again, so it has its capsular polysaccharide. Two different colony types appear when you culture from these animals. And we have the same situation in gonococci. They can appear in different kinds of coats, so to speak, and they are still the same genotype, but they have other characteristics from an antigenic point of view.

Dr. Schwan presented data on the immune response and on the detection of antibodies with immune fluorescent techniques. High antibody titers appear against certain species of clostridia, but practically no antibody titers at all against other clostridia. What does it mean? What does it contribute to immunity, or what does it contribute to disease?

The two last talks on serology today were by Dr. Williams and Dr. Cummins. It's impressive work. P. acnes is so important in immune stimulation; this organism will certainly have great clinical implications in the future.

SUBJECT INDEX

GPSR Compliance

The European Union's (EU) General Product Safety Regulation (GPSR) is a set of rules that requires consumer products to be safe and our obligations to ensure this.

If you have any concerns about our products, you can contact us on ProductSafety@springernature.com

In case Publisher is established outside the EU, the EU authorized representative is:

Springer Nature Customer Service Center GmbH
Europaplatz 3
69115 Heidelberg, Germany

Batch number: 10683525

Printed by Printforce, the Netherlands